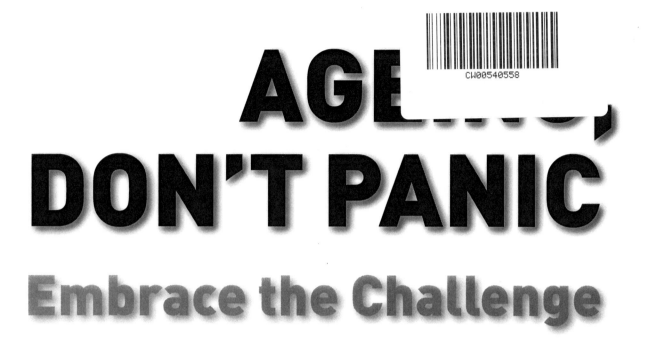

AGEING, DON'T PANIC

Embrace the Challenge

JOHN LUMLEY

Emeritus Professor of Vascular Surgery

Westminster Publishing Ltd
PO Box 50253, London EC2P 2WZ, United Kingdom
T & F : 0207 588 1098 - Email: sales@westminsterpublishing.org

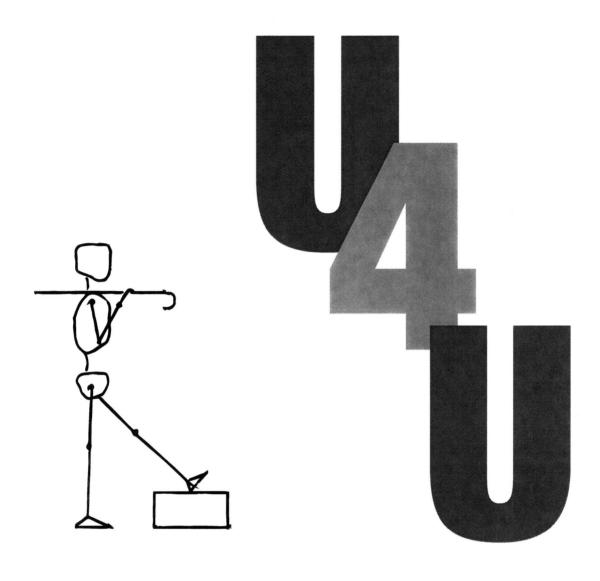

The demographic shift to an aging UK population is placing increasing demands on the NHS. The U4U Project is intended to stimulate elders to take control of their own destiny, and to look after themselves and each other. The aim is to challenge Government, Local Councils and Educational Institutions to facilitate this shift in responsibility. The text provides educational material for the project: please contact the editor to discuss further curricular development.

Teaches elders about themselves - so they can look after themselves and others

First published 2014

ISBN: 978-1-9998030-0-1

A catalogue record for this book is available from the British Library
Cover Design: Amina Dudhia
Typeset by Scribe Design, Margate, Kent
Produced by Westminster Publishing
Printed and Bound in EU

Contents

Contents

Preface

The UK is one of the most sophisticated societies in the world, and champions a National Health Service that for over half a century has been an institution to be proud of. However, rising costs of health care have challenged successive governments in the pursuit of excellence for the service. This has been further exacerbated by the cost of caring for an ageing population, and public expectation that public services are responsible for their health and wellbeing, and should be held to account for any failing.

Looking after your own health is a life long mission, but fortunately most of us do not have to spend much time worrying about it in our early years. It usually takes a life changing event, such as illness or retirement, to direct our attention to such matters.

This text challenges you to consider the changes that take place with ageing, and take personal responsibility for these events; addressing them when you are still in a position to plan and influence the quality of your later life. The U4U project facilitates this journey: it is an educational programme that considers ageing, addressing both its problems and their solutions

Topics extend from retirement to end-of-life issues, examining the body changes that occur with ageing, including frailty, disability and non-age-dependent disease (comorbidity). Additional topics include practical advice on housing, finance, electronic media, scams, safety, security, social care, care homes and advocacy.

It explores life changes and discusses ways of managing them. It is suggested that you dip into this material long before you personally require it and, by so doing, start giving the help to others that you would wish to receive yourself at a later date.

The aim of the U4U Project is to teach elders about themselves, so they can look after themselves and others. It:

- Increases your understanding of ageing
- Enables you to identify the problems of ageing
- Teaches you how to manage these problems
- Advises when to seek professional help
- Provides useful contacts

- Includes a glossary of medical terms
- Encourages you to help others

When facilities are inadequate – do something about it!

 # Chapter Authors

Sasha Sikdar
General Practitioner
Loneliness

James Berwin
Specialist Registrar, Trauma and
Orthopaedic Surgery
Falls Prevention

Nicola Bewes
Podiatrist
Putting your best foot, and leg, forward!

John Binding
Head of Services, Safeguarding Adults,
London Borough of Hackney
Safeguarding Adults

Carol Boswarthack
Head of Barbican and Community
Libraries, City of London
Love your Library

William Cooper
Art Educationalist, City of London
Enjoying Art

Carol Forde-Johnston
Lecturer Practitioner in Oxford University
Hospitals NHS Foundation Trust and
Oxford Brooks University
Wound Care; Post Hospital Nursing Care

Tony Graham
Accountant
Financial Advice for Elders

Edmund Green
Architect, Welsh School of Architecture
Homes for the Third Age

Sean Gregory
Director of Creative Learning, Barbican
Guildhall Creative Learning, London
Connecting with Music

Usha Grieve
Compassion in Dying
Planning for Your End of Life

Arthur Hawes
Archdeacon Emeritus of Lincoln
Spirituality, Health and Wellbeing

Pam Hibbs
Choosing a Care Home

Stella Howard
Trinity Laban Conservatoire of Music and
Dance
Dance

Chris Huckle
Musician and Librarian
Music in Public Libraries

Chapter Authors

Gwilym Tudor Jones
Researcher to MP on the Health Select Committee
Addressing the Mental and Physical Needs of the Individual

Davina Lilly
Leader on Homelessness and Rough Sleeping in the City of London
Homelessness in the City of London

Sumaira Malik
Green Light Pharmacy
The Role of the Pharmacist in the Care of the Elderly

Jennifer Noel
Compassion in Dying
Planning for Your End of Life

Tim Oliver
Consultant Medical Oncologist
Cancer

Graham Peiser
A long term Resident
A Village Community Centre

Yvonne Pettingell
Senior Nurse, The Katherine House Hospice, Banbury
Palliative Care

Steve Playle
City of London Trading Standards Manager
Scams

Andrew Rogerson
Proactive Care of Older People Undergoing Surgery (POPS) Team, Department of Ageing and Health, Guys and St Thomas' NHS Foundation Trust
Having an Operation

Ilona Sarulakis
Head of Adult Social Care for the London Borough of Hackney
Safeguarding Adults

Richard Sherry
Clinical Psychologist
Geriatric Psychological Issues in Mental Health

Peter Tihany
Social Worker
Community Care; Caring

Martin Vernon
National Clinical Director for Older People NHS England
The Importance of Frailty, Living Well and Population Ageing

Kate Wakeling
Trinity Laban Conservatoire of Music and Dance
Dance

Kris Warren
Consultant in the Care of the Elderly
Dementia

David Wilcox
Writing at www.socialreporter.com
Computers

# Organisation of the text

The first section of the text considers the general problems of ageing and loneliness, the second health matters, the third the major changes that accompany retirement, the fourth addresses active ways to embrace ageing, and the final section discusses dependency.

Most topics are addressed from the reader's viewpoint, advising how you should respond to different situations; this format has been relaxed where an author is giving background information, or expressing personal experience. In some instances members of a Local Authority or a Charity have been asked to give an example of how specific problems are addressed or to define the law in a difficult area. Useful websites and other reading material are added to the relevant chapters, and in a glossary.

The Third Age

The UK population is living longer, but ageing does not come alone, you need to prepare for the changes you may encounter, taking on the responsibility of Self Regulation. The chapter on Social Isolation outlines the vulnerability and the potential loneliness that can occur in old age. Social Services, many Charities and multiple volunteers are available to provide support, but you must be willing to consider how they can help you when needed.

Health

You may be fortunate enough to have lived free of health problems, but these will present in later life, as we all die of something. However, minor and many major illnesses, including cancers and heart attacks, can be prevented or alleviated when recognised at an early stage.

The clinical problems of old age are grouped under the body system they primarily affect. Problems are identified by the symptoms they produce and, in some cases abnormal signs (e.g. a lump or tender area). A doctor diagnoses problems, and assesses their severity, by studying these symptoms and signs, and may then request appropriate investigations. The section begins with a chapter on health assessment, where the reader is taken through the medical approach to a patient's problems. Each chapter examines symptoms and signs that you may encounter in yourself or in others, and helps you decide whether they can be managed personally, or whether you should seek the advice of a pharmacist or a doctor. Detailed practical advice is given on areas that can be dealt with and the associated responsibilities considered. The section also considers how to prepare for a hospital admission and your return to the community.

Addressing Change

Retirement is likely to present the greatest change in you lifestyle in later life. This can be accompanied by a change in your financial resources and possibly moving house. If the latter, it may also involve changes in your circle of friends and the proximity to your family. This reappraisal of your lifestyle must include attention to the activities that include your health and wellbeing, as considered in the adjacent sections.

Activity

In earlier life, family commitments and full-time employment have meant you have not had to think about how to fill your time. As your family disperses and retirement looms you have to consider your time management and how to stay healthy. Managing old age extends beyond health matters, and this section considers how elders may fill their time. It emphasises the importance of being occupied, and how this can be achieved through outdoor pursuits and exploring the arts, as well as with exercise and the use of computers. The section includes a chapter on scams, and the avoidance that must be undertaken by the whole of society. This section advises on how you can link into community life with its wealth of resources.

Dependency

The final section is directed at a dependent individual, and their needs as they become less able to look after themselves. Although every effort should be made to retain your independence, there comes a time when you need to share some of this responsibility. The chapters consider the various measures that are in place to enable elders to stay in their own home, the care facilities that are available, how the system protects vulnerable adults and their entitlements; together with end of life issues, including advanced care planning, advocacy, probate, spirituality, palliative care and bereavement.

A chapter on homelessness may seem out of place in this text, but like patients with mental health problems, these individuals deserve specific care and are important in our social responsibility.

The Glossary provides definitions of medical and biological terms. A number of topics, such as frailty, loneliness, activity and entitlements, receive attention in more than one chapter. This emphasises the importance of these topics, and considers them from different perspectives.

A comprehensive index has been compiled for readers of the printed copy. This will facilitate reading a specific topic without missing information hidden in unsuspected places – ageing is a composite subject and a whole mind and body experience! It was not thought necessary to further enlarge the index with generic terms, such as GP, other professionals services and wellbeing, but beware there may be *multiple entries* on your chosen topic on any referenced page.

The aim of this text is to teach you about manageing yourself, and by so doing, enable you to look after both yourself and your peers. You are not alone, as Local Authorities, Community Groups, Charities and many individuals spend extensive time working in this area – while National Government has to address the political as well a the social implications of an ageing population. Although adding years to your life may be desirable, of equal importance is to add quality to your life, ensuring you enjoy and appreciate old age with its rich assortment of pleasures.

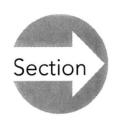

Section I

THE THIRD AGE

Chapter 1

Ageing

Ageing is a modern concept: the biblical reference is to three score years and ten, whereas in sixteenth century Britain, citizens died between forty and fifty years of age. By the beginning of the twentieth century this figure had increased by ten years, but the aged were considered socially disengaged, dependent and helpless members of society. The gradual increase in life expectancy during the course of the century was accompanied by a much-improved status for the elderly, positive reenforcement replacing the previous negative approach: **physiological** taking precedence over **chronological age**.

The number of octogenarians has doubled approximately every eleven years since 1945, and half of the babies born today are likely to reach 100 years of age.

Although the average **life expectancy** is increasing, the oldest person in the world has remained in the region of 130 for more than four centuries, and it is possible that modern medical and social care, while enabling you to live longer, are just shortening the ageing phase of life, rather than extending your overall lifespan.

At the present time **longevity** is leading to an increasing percentage of the aged in the UK population, and requiring increased medical and social needs. Family support is reducing, due to fewer children, women in full-time employment and employment being sited away from parental homes – resulting in a disparity of available care.

The **baby boom** of 1946–1964 that followed the Second World War has resulted in a current population of 5m over the age of 65. The over 85 cohort is increasing by 150,000/year (this figure was 660,000 in 1985; 1.5m in 2010; and estimated as 3.6m in 2035); by 2025, more than half the UK population will be over 50; and one in twelve over 80 by 2039. The elderly bulge has resulted in 6% of the population taking 43% of NHS resources and 65% of the hospital budget.

Thus the largest cohort of the population that could supplement the needs of social care is the aged themselves. Although the current statutory retirement age is being changed, there is still a substantial pool of retired skilled individuals, from all disciplines, with the potential of developing new social skills (page 237). The pool provides a voluntary body fully capable of running a **U4U Programme**.

The duration of any involvement and contributions is unknown – it could be short-term and eventually individuals may need the very support they are providing. Medical needs remain a separate specialist requirement, but an efficient age-support service can identify these needs earlier and more effectively.

Social services and a large number of charitable bodies and volunteers provide help for the aged, but companionship is usually short–term and many have to sell their homes and use their lifetime investments to afford long-term support: a new approach to this problem is urgently required.

Body changes

Theories on the factors influencing ageing abound, there are over 300, they include evolutionary adaptation, genetic predisposition, the toxic effects of the environmental, foodstuffs, bacteria and other factors that can change your genetic profile, and the current focus on telomere lengths in your chromosomes: shortened telomeres reduce the potential for replication, whereas their retention in cancer cells promotes replication of uncontrolled abnormal tissue.

Regardless of these various theories, in your latter years, you should be in control of and responsible for your own destiny, be able to retain credibility and dignity, and achieve a sense of fulfillment: this should be linked to a quality existence and peace of mind. You should be looking forward with pleasure to these later years, BUT old age does not come alone, it presents new challenges, some of which are unexpected, and new knowledge and skills may be needed to deal with them. Although it is common to regard old age as being 10–15 years older than you are, always add a note of realism on what it takes to maintain your health at its optimal level.

Ageing is accompanied by **frailty**, with progressive loss of strength and endurance; **disability**, when parts, such as your joints and lungs, undergo deterioration; and **comorbidity**, i.e. other diseases that are common, but not specific to ageing.

The most fearful problems to you, as an individual, probably relate to deterioration of your **mind** and **mobility**, while other problems that are particularly difficult to address are **loneliness** and **boredom**.

Old age is not a disease, or a terminal event, but the longer you live the more likely you are to die: the ageing body does undergo some **irreversible changes**. In the UK, it is estimated that 33% of the population between the ages of 50 and 60 are physically impaired, and this figure rises to 42% over the age of 65.

At the age of 30 your **heart** has ten times its needed capacity, and this falls by up to 1% every year thereafter. Similar reserves in the **lungs** and **kidneys** are also reduced, while the **genitourinary**

system is problematic in both sexes, the prostate enlarging in the male and the pelvic floor descending after pregnancy in the female. Your **gut** motility reduces, as does its power to absorb foodstuffs.

Your **height** reduces by a centimetre every decade and a kyphosis (hunch back) appears between 40 and 50. Your **gait** shortens and your feet begin to drag. Your bone strength reduces and muscle bulk falls: your trunk **girth** expands with fat deposition, as your thigh girth diminishes. **Weakness**, loss of balance, reduced **hearing**, poor **vision** and medication lead to 1 in 3 individuals over 65, and half of those over 80, having a memorable fall each year.

Your body water falls from 60 to 50%. Your **skin** looses its elastin and collagen content, causing it to be less flexible, and become thin and wrinkled. Your hair growth diminishes, particularly over the scalp, and hair becomes white due to loss of melanin. Your nails become brittle and ridged: one in three individuals over 65 cannot cut their own toenails. Changes in your **immune system** increase your vulnerability to infection and cancer. Neuroendocrine control reduces, affecting many body functions.

Intellectual changes are subtle: problem solving, memory, spontaneous thought, language and expression reduce, while creativity and imagination are retained. Personality is usually retained, but can be affected by stress, emotional factors and uncertainty.

Although individuals may prefer to consider themselves as a young mind in an old body, in the UK, there is a reported incidence of 16% **cognitive impairment** over the age of 65. Globally, it is suggested that 28% of the estimated 36 million demented individuals are undiagnosed: applying these figures to the UK equate to 283,000 of 400,000 (41%). The problem is accentuated by visual and hearing loss.

These multiple factors can be accelerated by many **risk factors**, particularly those considered in the cardiovascular disease and dietary chapters – hypertension, obesity, smoking and alcohol. Environmental factors include industrial toxins; foods contaminated with insecticides; and animal meat containing hormones and antibiotics. Genetic factor influence both susceptibility to disease, such as atheroma, and your natural resistance to the challenges of illness, accidents and toxins.

It is important to recognise these features, prepare for all these challenges, address fears, and to plan for potential change; you only have one go. It is reasonable to ignore the 10% of sudden deaths that you cannot influence, and address those you can.

Many people look on such events as inevitable, and prefer not to think about them in advance, considering that relatives or a state system will look after them, or they can afford the likely expense of carers. Nevertheless, there are preemptive measure that can help you ease ageing problems, and recognise comorbidity; by so doing you can improve your quality of life, and extend your independence.

These include personal, social, community, and environmental factors. Start with the risk factors – consider a balanced diet (page 70), regular exercise (page 245), alcohol in moderation and giving up smoking. You have probably not previously thought about safety at home, this is considered on page 298.

If you are loosing your independence, **address problems** of personal accommodation; archiving; personal hygiene; emergency contacts; wills; living wills; probate; funerals; end-of-life care; advocacy; and the power of attorney (page 345).

Chapter **2**

Self regulation in later life

Self regulation – a process that is greeted with much skepticism in Professional and Commercial circles, yet one that is expected of us when dealing with our personal affairs. From childhood onwards we are encouraged to develop personal responsibility and this is complicit with mature adulthood: but does this remain so to the end of our days, or are there moments when vulnerability appears and self regulation falters?

Throughout life you address changing circumstances, such as educational needs, employment, finances, friends, partners, family, accommodation and leisure activities. You are less likely to have considered the problems of ageing, unless this has been linked to supporting an ageing relative. Nevertheless, as you approach retirement, these problems deserve attention, turning them into manageable challenges.

In some societies the aged retain their seniority, maintaining a revered and venerable position within a family, while in others, being no longer a major earner can be accompanied by loss of position and respect, this in turn leading to a feeling of inadequacy and depression.

However, every age has its own pleasures, and surveys suggest that two thirds of the population enjoy old age, while a half of these consider it as the happiest period of their life. Capturing these joys requires self determination and application. Initial considerations are reemployment, and applying existing or new skills in the voluntary or commercial sectors. You are likely to acquire a different circle of friends and have to develop a new approach to time management.

It is a time to consider the things you said you wanted to try but had not previously had time for, such as educational pursuits, signing up for a degree or diploma in the arts or sciences, and acquiring new practical skills, such as in art, crafts and music. Consider opportunities to travel, adding adventure and fun (travel brochures themselves provide enjoyable reading). Do not neglect the need for regular exercise; enjoy your food, but be sure that new eating and drinking habits keep you at your optimal weight.

Although you are never too old to learn, set realistic achievable targets that enable you to reach your full potential. This includes examining your finances and balancing them with your needs.

As inheritance tax is around 40%, some consider the cost of everything you buy in later life can be looked on as a 40% reduction! You should write a will and obtain advise on legacies and trusts. You may be property-rich, but cash-short, and you need to consider if the size and position of your property equates to your long term needs. Will you need a car, and how are your driving skills likely to progress.

Aim to grow old with dignity and grace, retaining enthusiasm and independence, and living what you consider a quality lifestyle. Remain in control of your destiny: address matters of health and welfare, and maintain your personal appearance. Retirement enables you to relax your dress code for much of your time in your home, but make sure it is appropriate for other situations, including grooming your hands, nails and hair, and wearing suitable clothing and shoes. Similarly maintain the standards of your home environment to a level that you are proud of. Do not just sit back, eat, and be over-doctored, overprotected and over-patronised, abrogating all responsibility: such measures are certain to shorten your life span, and do little for the respect you deserve.

Advanced directives lay down how you wish your health to be managed, and appoint advocates on financial matters. Write your own obituary: a subject on which you are the expert, and can include all the bits you particularly want. You can plan and pay funeral expenses in advance, obtain a competitive fee and save your descendants a great degree of anxiety.

Whereas death is inevitable, most of us want to ignore this possibility. In the meantime, consider the problems outlined in the adjacent chapters, including loneliness, and the need for mental, physical and material support. Identifying these potential hurdles enables you to plan how to address and combat the challenges of ageing, while active citizenship enables you to utilize these same skills to help others.

Chapter **3**

Social Isolation and Vulnerability

The prime social **problems** and **challenges** that need support for the aged are:

1 Lack of companionship; loneliness; and depression

2 The need for **mental**, **physical** and **material** support:

- Mental – motivation; stimulation; encouragement; reactivate/revitalise; inspire
- Physical – dressing; hygiene; mobility; foot care
- Daily activity – shopping for food and clothing, cooking, feeding; cleaning; sewing; mechanical – heavy lifting, repairs; decorating; electrical – TV, IT; organisation of diary, bills and finances.

Vulnerability

There can come a time when you need support, and you should consider the vulnerable position of such individuals. The elderly, living on their own, are easy prey to exploitation and abuse (page 335), particularly if this is accompanied by decreasing awareness and problems of mobility. Vulnerability, is becoming more of a problem as the number of clever scams (page 263) that target older people are increasing, everyone needs to be very aware of this. Particular threats include:

- Personal safety and security
- Addiction: alcohol/drugs
- Community ethnic and gender issues
- Poverty, Illiteracy

- Homelessness

- Physical/domestic violence and abuse

- Environment/climate

- Crime (including scams).

Abuse presents under many guises and is not limited to a physical and sexual nature – it is easy, even for close associates, to miss problems of omission and neglect, when victims are incapable of personal toiletry and feeding, and possibly presenting risk of flood, electrical and fire hazards. Older people are particularly vulnerable to scams from house and telephone callers, and also if they have access to the Internet. It is sad that scammers seem better at identifying the vulnerable than the community they live in. One good principle is never to respond to anyone cold calling by any means, such as the door, telephone or computer.

Emotional and psychological abuse may go unnoticed. Controlling and coercive behaviour may present in Institutions as well as within families, while in the latter financial and materials abuse may be concealed, and the victim may be unwilling to bring any form of action or charges against those they depend on for future support.

You may want to live alone and also to be left alone. This decision must be respected, but be aware that with total isolation you are at risk of the problems listed above: don't drift into self-neglect – wishing to live alone should not be synonymous with social isolation.

Management considerations

The Care Act 2014 addressed these problems by requiring Local Authorities to establish a statutory Safeguarding Adults Board (page 331), equating to what already existed for child protection. Some problems need Health and Social Professional help, but charities and volunteers deliver a large amount of care.

The public also needs education to recognise the existence and signs of abuse, and know of the local authority helpline and how to access it. Awareness and engagement help you to ensure safety of subjects at risk. It is everybody's responsibility: share your concerns – if you care, share; if you are not sure, pick up the phone so others can check, and take forward and escalate any proven abuse.

Living alone can leave you vulnerable in the event of falls and injuries: shared accommodation, organised through a fully monitored system, is one solution to provide a helping hand, to monitor your safety and to address loneliness. Local authorities usually run a **pendant scheme** that you can wear at all times: if you are in trouble you can press the alarm and the operator rings a designated relative or other key holder.

UK local communities have usually found local solutions through neighborhood watches to identify and watch over those in need: movers and shakers, and volunteers preventing social isolation. To plug into these movements, go out shopping to your local supermarket and launderette, visit a park or join the community of a church or mosque. Similar help can be obtained at the local library and other social public spaces where communities assemble; addressing local needs and breaking down barriers.

Participate and be **involved** in activities: clubs – literature, music, art, photography, cooking, gardening, bingo; meetings; talks; individual/group outings/visits to – places of interest, films, theatre, sports, libraries, hairdressers, lunches, shopping sprees; and arranging holidays.

Learning basic **media skills** promotes independence, as they enable you to do your own shopping on line, and keep in touch with your relatives and friends: competence in these skills prevents isolation.

In each geographic area there are many other **facilities and services** for the older resident, and it is important for you to be aware of what is available. They include **befriending** services, often with a very individual flavour. Consider your own skills and explore how these can be used to help community wellbeing; failing this, skills can be acquired enabling you to be part of a voluntary team, visiting and helping those in need. In some areas **credit schemes** are in operation, volunteers gaining credits for helping elders: the credits can be used on other local authority facilities, such as theatre tickets, gym and sports activities.

Organising older people to sort out problems that are bothering them becomes empowering and satisfying, however, they should not be viewed as passive recipients of advice and services, but encouraged to help themselves to the maximum of their potential.

There is no single answer to the problems of ageing, everyone has to be treated as an individual and requires a personal approach. It is a two way learning experience and help delivered with a smile may be rewarded with a smile of appreciation, reminding you that you are a valued member of society. The U4U project is designed to provide understanding, education and training, and to foster and enhance research in social wellbeing.

Chapter 4

Loneliness

Sasha Sikdar

Loneliness is a condition that can affect all regardless of status and age and is essentially a strong emotional response to a sense of isolation. It can strike a variety of groups such as mothers, carers, children, refugees, as well as older people. It is so pervasive that it can hide in plain view and be overlooked by close friends and family. Therefore most people have not treated it as a top priority. According to data collated by various charities, Campaign to End Loneliness, Age UK, Action for Children, Co-op, British Red Cross, the Royal Voluntary Service and Sense, over 9 million people in the UK, say they are always or often lonely. Almost 2/3 of these people are uncomfortable to admit this. Loneliness is so endemic in our society that a commission to tackle it was due to be launched early 2017 by a couple of MPs.

Considering their circumstances, naturally the over 65s, fall in the high-risk category. However, older people should not berate themselves for finding themselves under such a situation since most people cannot anticipate it occurring to them. Its causes can also arise from wider societal trends. People no longer pass the time of day on the street and services have become so depersonalised that there are fewer contact points in the community, for instance like a friendly postman, looking out for you.

According to research by Age UK 1.7% or 200,000 older people (over 65), have not had a conversation with friends and family for a month. 360,000 or 3.1% of older people have not had such a conversation in a week. The fact that some councils are still only commissioning 15 minute social care visits can only exacerbate the sense of loneliness. There is also an increased risk of falls, hypertension, heart disease, depression and drinking. Research from Harvard Medical School has equated the health risk of loneliness to smoking 15 cigarettes a day.

There are various causes that are unique to older people that can precipitate loneliness. Chief among these is housing. There is a greater concentration of single person households amongst the elderly caused by loved ones dying or families moving away. Astronomic rents and house prices means that older people cannot afford to have spare bedrooms to invite over friends and family. A lifetime of accumulating possessions can add clutter to a person's accommodation, which could also make them reluctant to entertain.

The world of employment is not age friendly and retirement can lead to a loss of previously held social networks. Services such as banking are now so automated that technology has reduced personal contact. This can lead to disenfranchisement and only further increase a sense of isolation. Lack of cultural amenities and a perception of high crime can dissuade older people from leaving the building. Increasing frequency of disability and infirmity also play their part.

Remember that loneliness is a natural feeling that signals that important needs are not being met. Simply changing your mind set and deciding to be more sociable is often the first step to discovering and cultivating a new circle of friends. It also has to be noted that solitude does not equate to loneliness. Do not deny yourself simple pleasures like watching a film or going for a nice meal just because you have no one to share them with.

There are several resources to combat loneliness and hence increase resilience.

According to Age UK, 3.9m of elderly people rely on the television as their main form of contact. As an alternative to this, the Internet and social media (Facebook, Instagram, Twitter and Snapchat) can be far more interactive and stimulating. However, this must be done in moderation as social media can increase a sense of loneliness as it amplifies how connected other people seem or even pretend to be. There are also specialised sites for online dating. Although this used to be a taboo subject, it is much more commonly used and has proven to be very successful in finding companionship.

However, interacting with the web requires a basic level of IT literacy. Courses are run at local libraries and community centres on how to use a computer, together with the use of mobile phone, Face Time and Skype. This makes it much easier for you to keep in touch with your friends and family as you can talk and see each other at the same time, and it is for free. You can also use social media to access health related information, and engage in patient/patient and patient/doctor forums. A negative aspect of this development is that your personal data is more freely available and is at risk of misuse, but understanding this puts you in control. It is very important, that your personal details are kept safe and you must never give out your password to anyone or your credit card details on any sites. In addition, several retail banks such as Lloyds and Barclays have Internet accessibility schemes for the elderly, which aids with the sense of alienation brought about technology.

Age UK offers Befriending Services. These offer older people companionship and emotional support. These can be face-to-face visits or regular phone calls. The Silver Line launched by Esther Ranzten is open 24 hours a day, 365 days a year and aims to offer information, friendship and advice, link callers to local groups and services, offer regular befriending calls, and protect and support those who are suffering from neglect and abuse. Their contact number is 0800 4 70 80 90. A search on the Internet will enable you to find a raft of similar such services including the lost art of letter writing on offer for the over 65s.

Other ways to battle loneliness include taking up a new hobby to find other likeminded people or acquiring a pet to assist with the need for companionship. There are also specialised holidays for the over 65 year-olds, organised by the group SAGA.

It is very important to understand that loneliness is a very common problem and **you are not alone**, so it is important to speak to someone today.

Further reading

http://www.ageuk.org.uk

https://www.thesilverline.org.uk

https://www.theguardian.com/politics/2016/dec/28/jo-coxs-campaign-to-tackle-loneliness-lives-on-with-help-of-friends

http://www.health.harvard.edu/staying-healthy/loneliness-has-same-risk-as-smoking-for-heart-disease

http://www.health.harvard.edu/ageing/5-ways-to-fight-loneliness-and-isolation

http://www.telegraph.co.uk/news/2017/01/10/around-16000-people-still-receiving-flying-visits-carers-despite/

http://www.barclays.co.uk/DigitalEagles/P1242671738729

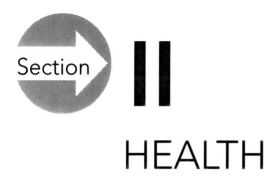

Section II

HEALTH

Chapter 5

Health Assessment

You can obtain a lot of information about your fitness by your response to exercise – and you are fairly certain to have thought this through:

1   How breathless (breathing deeply and rapidly) are you after going up one flight of stairs

2   How fast were you going and how many stairs can you do without stopping

3   Is your breathlessness getting worse

4   Are you getting more tired over the course of the day

5   What is happening to your weight (*Table 13.1*, page 76): emphasis is given elsewhere to a reliable, possible impedance, weighing machine on a noncarpeted surface (page 79)

6   Are your joints getting stiffer, or painful at rest or on exercise

7   What happens to your pulse after mild, moderate and severe exertion?

You are also prompted under each system when you should go to your doctor for a check.

Doctors have other skills and ways to assess your general state of health, such as anaemia, nutrition, hydration and muscle mass. They also have at their disposal many tests to screen your systems and may refer you for a specialist opinion:

1   In their discussions with you, a doctor is not only taking note of physical and metal problems, but also personal details that indicate your management of financial matters and your social integration, i.e. your total wellbeing

2   A doctor checks your pulse to find if your heart is beating regularly at a normal rate and pumping out a normal volume of blood

3   Checking pulses around the body may detect arterial disease, abnormalities are further assessed with pressure measurements and occasionally arteriograms – radio opaque fluid is injected into your circulation, outlining your arteries on a simultaneous series of X rays

4   Varicose veins are superficial dilated tortuous veins, possibly linked to previous deep venous thrombosis, and they can initiate skin changes around your ankles – they are assessed by clinical examination and ultrasound scans

5   Measuring your blood pressure is part of a routine health check – it is important to detect and treat a raised blood pressure before it gets out of control and damages structures, particularly the brain

6   An electrocardiogram (ECG) checks the electrical activity that maintains the heart beat, and can detect any irregularity (fibrillation) and other defects, such as damage from a heart attack

7   If you have had a history of a heart attack or other heart problems, imageing machines of varying complexity, may be used to scan your heart and check its function

8   The capacity and efficiency of your lungs is measured by blowing into various bits of apparatus, and also measuring the concentrations of gases in your blood and in what you breathe out

9   Shortness of breath and abnormal gas results may also be due to poor circulation through the lungs from a failing heart, rather than just lung disease

10 A chest X ray shows the heart size and identifies most lung diseases

11 Bone and soft tissue X rays and scans may be indicated for local pain and discomfort, and following injuries

12 A Dual Energy X ray Absorption Meter (DEXA/DXA) is used to determine the percentage fat in your body

13 Fat distribution and your nutrition can also be assessed from skin thickness, using a skin caliper at set reproducible sites, such as the abdomen, the back of your upper arm and your thigh.

Urine tests may be abnormal because of diseased kidneys (e.g. protein may leak out) or the kidneys may excrete abnormal chemicals from the blood into the urine (e.g. a raised blood sugar level in diabetic patients may also give rise to sugar in the urine).

Blood tests provide information on both the blood cells and the chemicals in the blood, a number are carried out routinely to check for anaemia, and diseases of the kidneys, liver and endocrine glands:

1   The number of red blood cells in the blood and/or their haemoglobin content is reduced when you are anaemic – haemoglobin is the chemical in the red blood cell that carries oxygen to all the cells of the body to keep them alive and healthy

2 White blood cells may be abnormal when inflammation is present in the body, and also in primary blood diseases (e.g. leukaemia)

3 Blood clotting can be tested (e.g. if you are on blood thinning drugs)

4 High or abnormal levels of some chemicals are present in kidney disease (e.g. blood urea and proteins)

5 Jaundice is an important clinical marker for liver disease, but bilirubin levels and those of a number of enzymes provide important information on the type of liver disease and its severity

6 Endocrine disease may be assessed by specific hormone levels (e.g. thyroid) or by abnormalities of the chemicals they control (e.g. blood sugar in diabetes)

7 Dietary abnormalities may be shown by high levels of some chemicals (e.g. raised cholesterol and lipids) or deficiencies (e.g. nutrients such as iron and magnesium).

Whereas many of the above tests are carried out on routine health checks, if you present to your doctor with specific problems, specialist referral opens the pathway to complex imageing studies and endoscopic examination (e.g. passage of viewing tube into either end of the gut, the lungs and joints), and specific blood tests for tumour-markers if certain cancers are suspected.

It is essential to discuss all your health problems and anxieties with your doctor – it is important to identify treatable disease early on, and equally important, to be reassured that you do not have a condition you are worried about.

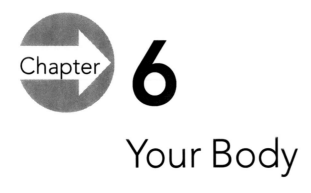

Chapter 6

Your Body

Humans, like all animals, are made up of living **cells** (billions of them). As animals get larger, cells are modified and grouped into active units, called **organs**, e.g. the heart, and all the bits performing a specific function are collectively called a **system,** an example being the respiratory system, concerned with breathing

Cells have a retaining **cell membrane** and most have a central **nucleus** where the majority of your deoxyribonucleic acid (DNA) is situated. **DNA** is a substance found in all living organisms: it contains the coded biological information about your form and function.

The DNA in the nucleus is organised into your 46 **chromosomes** – the long strands that contain your **genes**, i.e. the bits that you inherit from your parents that determine such things as whether you are a man or a woman and the colour of your eyes. There are an estimates three billion pieces of genetic information in your chromosomes.

The unique nature of every individual is reflected in the use of DNA fingerprinting in **forensic** identification. DNA analysis can also detect switched-off sequences, which become molecular fossils that can provide information on **evolutionary history.**

For organism to **grow**, cells have to divide and multiply, and DNA **replicates** by splitting and then reproducing the two parts of its double helix; the appropriate parts then reuniting. Sequences along the DNA strands can be used as templates and copied onto RNA (**transcription**) to be reproduced (**translation**). This process is of particular importance for the DNA concerned with mitochondrial function – **mitochondria** are cellular structures outside the nucleus that are concerned with energy production.

DNA can also be **cut up, joined up** and **corrected**. All these processes are under the influence of **enzymes**, and these cascading processes can be influenced by external influences, such as **toxins,** and **dietary** factors – these processes of **methylation** and the effects of **oxidants** are further considered with the diet (page 70).

DNA **damage**, abnormal sequencing and changes of gene expression may also occur with **ageing**, and it is variously estimated that DNA decreases by 40–90% by the age of 80. These changes may be responsible for many diseases, including a reduction of immune responses and the development of **cancer**. Developments in molecular biology pave the way for producing **recombinant DNA** and medications to influence abnormal DNA in body functions.

As well as the **respiratory system** (that takes in oxygen from the air and blows off waste carbon dioxide); you have a **circulatory system** (the heart and blood vessels that pump blood and its goodies to all parts of the body); the **alimentary system** (the teeth, gut, anus, that takes in food, digests good bits to get them into the blood and discharges what you don't want); the **genitourinary system** (the kidney, that gets rid of waste blood products in the urine, and the sex and reproductive parts); the **musculoskeletal system** (the bones, joints and muscles that move you about); and the **nervous system** (the brain, spinal cord and nerves that enables you think, receives sensation, including special senses such as vision and hearing, and directs movement); the **skin**, that covers and protects your body.

The **endocrine system** deposits its **hormones** directly into the blood stream, and these regulate many body functions, as do the numerous **enzymes** that facilitate the chemical reactions of the **metabolic system** that is the industrial factory that services all body activities.

Normality

When considering anyone's health and fitness, you are usually relating it to someone of a similar age, and are asking 'fit for what'. You assess their **mental state** (whether alert, well orientated in time and place, any memory problems and hearing or visual loss).

Physically, you note any over or under **weight**, their **strength** and **mobility**, whether they can get out of a chair unaided or touch their toes; whether they are **breathless** after climbing a flight of stairs, or can blow out a candle held at arms length, and note whether their **skin** is firm and smooth.

A **doctor** asks additional questions about recent and past **illness**, eating and bowel problems, aches, pains or other problems, and sleep patterns. Examination includes pulse, blood pressure, height, weight, basal metabolic index and possibly skin thickness.

Investigations may include a full blood count, haemoglobin, and where indicated dietary markers (HbA1c, homocystine, vitamins B_{12} and D, folic acid and minerals).

It is estimated that by not smoking; drinking only moderate alcohol; and eating a diet containing at least seven helpings of fruit and vegetables a day, you can add 14 years to your life (but a difficult figure to confirm!).

Disease

We will be looking at the systems to see how they work, what happens to them as you get older and what can go wrong with them: certain diseases, that affect more than one system, are also considered separately.

Diseases can be looked at as **congenital** (present from birth) or **acquired**. If you suffer from one of the former, you already know a lot about it, and hopefully it wont suddenly give you a lot more problems as you age. Acquired diseases can be divided into **inflammation** (the body reacting to infection and nonyou material getting into the body); **trauma** (accidents, but also poisons and chemicals); **neoplastic** (cancer); **degenerative** (bits wearing out or being mistreated); **metabolic** and **hormonal** (the chemistry of the body not working properly, as in diabetes).

Sometimes we do not know the cause of a disorder (**idiopathic**), or problems can be caused by the treatment given to improve them (**iatrogenic**).

Causes of Death

Heart attack and stroke are the largest killers in the developed world, followed by malignancy/cancer (lung, gut, genitourinary and blood). Infection may be due to flue or other epidemics, or the more common chest disorders. While liver disease relates to national as well as individual alcoholic habits.

In the UK, deaths from Alzheimer's disease (dementia) are higher in women (6%) than in men (3%). Worldwide infection has an increased incidence, from diarrheal, HIV, TB and tropical illness, together with diabetes and road traffic accidents.

Deaths from ageing slow after 90, but loneliness and neglect remain prime problems that have to be addressed.

Common Problems

A doctor has to decide what is wrong with you to be able to help – to make this **diagnosis**, he or she is looking for abnormal symptoms or signs, and may then request some investigations.

Symptoms are messages from your body about physical or mental problems. Some may be due to chronic disease, while others are short-term worries – all require an explanation. Common symptoms are **pain**, **fatigue**, **stress** and **shortness of breath**.

Signs are abnormal things you can see or feel, and which doctors are looking for when they examine you – they are concerned with excluding, as well as finding, abnormal signs (such as odd lumps and bumps, or unusual noises in your chest)

Pain is the most common and the most disturbing symptom. It is also the most helpful to the doctor when trying to work out what is wrong with you, and what to do about it. Therefore give some thought about what the doctor may want to know:

- Where is the pain situated; does it move or spread, if so where to

- When did it start; can you think of anything that brought it on; have you ever had it before

- How bad is it (on a scale of 1–10); is it sharp/stabbing/burning/throbbing

- How does each episode start and finish (gradually/suddenly); is it constant or come in waves; are you ever free of it

- What do you do when you have it (stay still/walk around)

- What makes it better/worse (position/tablets)

- How does it affect your life (carry on/sweat/feel sick/lie down)

- Is it getting better or worse?

If the information is complicated, keep a diary of events

Fatigue is expected after strenuous activity, or the morning after a heavy celebration. It can be more difficult to explain fatigue, weariness, weakness and frailty as unheralded symptoms. They can occur at any age and, on detailed assessment, are usually linked to a life event. If the symptoms are severe enough to take you to a doctor, they should take a full history and examine you, and arrange some screening tests.

If these are all normal, the doctor will give you firm reassurance and perhaps a prescription for their favorite 'pep pill'. The problem arises in the elderly; as such symptoms may also be attributed to 'old age'. While this is partly true, it is important to address underlying causes, and these include, poor diet, mental and physical inactivity, and above all, loneliness. Dealing with such problems on your own is difficult: consider and plan for them in advance and be willing to accept help when it is offered.

Stress produces a wide spectrum of emotional states: such as anger, tension, frustration, hostility, anxiety and depression, sleep disturbance and fatigue, and feelings of being overwhelmed and out of control. It may be precipitated by failure in personal circumstances and relationships, or can relate to environmental factors, alcohol and medication.

Stressed individuals are distracted and out of their comfort zone, they are not listening to or not understanding what they are being told, are often hyperactive but ineffective, dropping things and prone to accidents: they may resort to eating, smoking or drinking, and are not managing.

Signs include nail biting, clenching and grinding of teeth, dry mouth, muscle tension, weakness, sweating, shortness of breath, palpitations, diffuse pins and needles, and itching.

The first step is to recognise the condition, followed by removal of any cause. Someone has to take over and initiate focused, achievable and rewarding activity, enabling you to relax, and gradually take back and direct your own life. Longer term solutions are addressing each problem in turn, and introducing a healthy life style, with attention to diet, exercise and an active life, matching your desires and abilities. Programmes must be individually tailored and include training in slow deep breathing and addressing problems by concentrating your thoughts on the good things in life.

Shortness of breath The oxygen in the air you breath is used to convert food into energy: without this energy the cells of your body die, for example, without oxygen, the cells of the brain start to die within a few minutes.

With exertion you need more oxygen and you breath deeply and more rapidly, but you can still get short of breath and have to rest to get your breath back. The medical term used when you notice and complain of shortness of breath, is dyspneoa, and certain diseases (page 51) can bring this on with minimal exertion, or even at rest. When you are stressed you may also notice you are breathing deeply and are out of breath. In this case the approach is directed at relaxing, slow deep breathing through an open mouth, and directing attention to the cause of the problem.

These general symptoms are found in many diseases: subsequent chapters consider each system in turn, its structure and function, and common problems, particularly those encountered in the elderly. Emphasis is given to symptoms that you should not ignore but discuss with your doctor. As any medical student will tell you, on reading about an abnormality you are soon convinced you already have it: nevertheless, it is better to be assessed and reassured by your doctor than to miss early treatable disease.

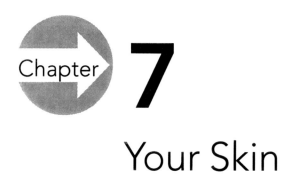

Chapter 7

Your Skin

The skin covers an area of about two square meters, and is the largest organ in your body. It provides a supple, elastic envelope protecting you against the elements and external trauma. It can be observed and abnormalities are easily detected: this is a valuable property, as many conditions, including ageing, have associated skin abnormalities.

Pallor is a feature of the cold, when small blood vessels in the skin contract down to prevent heat loss, but it is also a sign of a reduced haemoglobin level (**anaemia**), this is more difficult to detect in a black skin, but look at the palms and under the nails. **Jaundice** (page 60) colours the skin yellow – this is more easily detected in staining of the whites of your eyes. **Kidney failure** gives the skin a washed out colour while exposure to the elements give a healthy glow and a **suntan**.

If you are loosing weight, there is loss of the fat layer under the skin, with the development of lax skin folds. **Dehydration** produces a dry skin and sunken eyes. Excess tissue fluid can occur in heart, liver, kidney and some endocrine diseases: it is termed **oedema** and you can detect it by pressing and producing a dent in the skin above your ankles.

Your skin starts to age from your mid twenties; cellular changes are loss of supportive (collagen) and elastic fibres, fat, melanocytes (pigment cells) and sebaceous (lubricating) glands. The gradual changes of dryness, lack of elasticity and firmness, and slower healing are unlikely to be noted for a further twenty years, when wrinkles begin to form on the outer margins of your eyes (crow's feet), mouth and across your forehead.

After a further twenty years others will join you in noticing deeper wrinkles, sagging folds on the side of you face and under your chin. Skin folds also develop elsewhere, such as the axillae, breasts, groins and perineum (the region containing the scrotum, vulva and anus). The skin becomes thin, fragile and easily bruised. Hair is less greasy and more brittle, mostly grey and much of it is thinned out or lost: while hair is receding on your brow, in other areas, such as eyebrows, nose and ears, it is increased. Your **nails** become brittle and ridged, through years of trauma, and some may be deformed.

At this age individuals start to pay more attention to their skin, with creams, vitamin lotions and stronger sun barrier creams: botulin injections and face lifts are considered, together with plastic surgery to other unsightly folds. It is easy to develop extreme views for or against such procedures, or **bariatric** surgery (removal of excess fat) around the body. Such decisions are very personal, but always remember that no surgery is without any risk, and many of the procedures are only short-term fixes – discuss all these factors with you doctor and the surgeon.

Sensation may be reduced or lost with ageing, particularly in diabetics, and this makes you more susceptible to skin damage: infection can then set in. As your inflammatory response is also reduced with age, infection is more difficult to overcome: this is also a particular problem in diabetics. So pay particular attention, and give time for everything you do, to avoid knocking, catching or cutting your hands or other exposed areas.

As your skin gets older still, expect other changes: patches of hard skin (senile **keratoses**) are common, together with lots of small skin tags or protuberances, red blotches and pigment patches. If any of these keeps growing to over a 5 or 6 mm, **changes colour, itches, bleeds** or **ulcerates**, show them to your doctor, as changes of apparently innocuous abnormalities may be early curable cancers and they are easily neglected.

You may have had skin problems all your life, common examples are **eczema, acne** and **psoriasis** – hopefully you have tried everything and found out the best way to manage these problems at a much earlier age. This has to continue and new **allergies** identified and avoided. Show all new and persistent rashes, colour or other skin changes to your doctor, who can usually give reassurance of their nonserious nature.

Looking after your own skin, and the skin of others, starts with plenty of soap and water to remove dirt. Reserve the scrubbing brush for your nails, as it may damage fragile skin: instead, use soft sponges to apply soap and also to wash it all off, as soap is an irritant if left on a surface. Dry the skin fully by gentle towelling, as soggy skin folds are vulnerable to fungal and bacterial infection.

Talcum powder can be gently applied to dry skin to smooth it and allow cloths to move freely over it. Decide whether your skin would benefit from moisturising creams or oils by testing them over small areas. Vitamins A and C are both beneficial to skin, and can be applied directly as, like other vitamins such as E, they are absorbed through the skin and are available as creams and lotions.

Exposing the skin to the sun, is an essential source of vitamin D production, but **sunburn** is very harmful to skin that is not usually exposed to the elements. Fortunately you can produce your daily need of vitamin D with 15 minutes of sun exposure, after which you should apply the appropriate strength of barrier sun cream.

As well as vitamins A and C, the skin benefits from some healthy fats, such as provided by oily fish and olives, together with nuts, seeds and a diet containing plenty of fruit and vegetables.

Skin is particularly vulnerable in a number of specific situations, and these include urinary and faecal **incontinence**, and when bedridden. Urinary incontinence (page 295) is a problem for men and women of advancing years. Sufferers must never miss an opportunity for having a wee, but urgency and dribbling cannot always be controlled. Awareness of the problem allows planning, stocking up with appropriate pads and protective appliances, to avoid soiling cloths and odours

Faecal incontinence carries the same problems as urinary leakage, of soiling and odour. Carrying pads and spare undercloths is advisable, and showering whenever feasible, washing with soap and water, washing away all soap residue, followed by careful drying to reduce potential skin infection.

Skin management of bedridden individuals is a very difficult problem for carers. Lying on a pressure point (buttocks, hips, ankles, heels, sides of feet, toes, elbows, back of head) compresses and empties the fine skin blood vessels. If unrelieved, these white bloodless (ischaemic) areas can undergo irreversible damage. When the subject is moved, blood floods back into these areas, with a temporary red glow (hyperaemia). However, if there has been permanent damage to the blood vessels during the ischaemic phase, they will leak. This bruising leaves a purple stain and further damages the skin. Subsequent pressure can cause blistering, allowing bacteria in and infection to start, with further skin damage and potential ulceration – **bedsores**.

In individuals with good skin, a good blood supply and some movement, this sequence is unlikely, but if the subject is malnourished, with arterial disease and immobile, such as after a stroke, the changes may start within two hours. The responsibility of a carer is high; usually a trained nurse has this responsibility, but occasionally the task falls to a relative. The skill is to roll or turn the subject into a different position every two hours and gently massage the pressure area with the flat of your hand for two minutes. It is easier if the subject can move himself or herself or if two helpers are available.

Consider how pressure can be reduced for immobile subjects. In a chair or wheel chair rubber rings and foam cushions help, Special beds include water and air filled, and ripple mattresses. It is essential the sheets are drawn flat in all bed making to avoid ridges that could produce their own pressure lines.

Bed baths are again the province of a trained professional, but you may be asked to help. The technique is to lay a plastic sheet flat along the length of the bed alongside the subject, and then roll them onto it while it is extended over the rest of the bed. Bathing is with sponge, soap and water; catching excess water with towels; drying the subject carefully; followed by massage to pressure points, moisturisers and appropriate lotions; and ensuring smooth, clean dry sheets to roll back onto.

Ensure the subject is kept warm and, areas not being washed, covered. Use warm towels for drying whenever possible. Breasts and perineum require full toilet, if the subject is mobile enough, they can do these areas themselves, but otherwise undertake with appropriate cover and delicacy. For hair, use a plastic covered pillow and a neck towel: position the subject's head downward over a bowl so that water flows downwards during washing and rinsing. Dry with warm towels and a hair dryer.

Carers must take care of their own health and hygiene, wearing aprons or overalls for bathing or dirty jobs. Gloves are appropriate, particularly if there are infected areas being dealt with. Nails must not be sharp and rings are best removed; hair should be retracted. Consider your own dietary habits as discussed in this text, regular exercise and time away from someone you are looking after permanently: do not allow circumstances to interfere with your personal hygiene, and changes of undercloths and socks.

Chapter **8**

Wounds and Chronic Ulcers of the Skin

Carol Forde-Johnston

Your skin is an amazing sense organ that can make you aware of pain, heat, cold and touch. It forms a robust, water-resistant, flexible outer covering, which protects the soft structures underneath from injuries, bacterial attack and dehydration.

Wound Assessment

A wound is a break in your skin that may be **acute**, e.g. a cut from broken glass or a surgical incision, or **chronic**, such as a lower leg ulcer: the latter has a high prevalence in the population over 65. When you have a skin wound, any of these properties may be affected. The nurse, or doctor, will initially need to assess your wound to establish the following:

1 **The type of wound:** the cause and whether it is acute or chronic

2 **How long your wound has existed and whether it is improving or worsening:** you will be asked whether the wound has increased in size, length, width and/or depth

3 **An initial review of the wound:** observing the site, size, odour and the colour of the wound site and surrounding skin: if there are signs of infection a swab may be taken

4 **Related signs and symptoms, your current health and medical history:** acute or chronic pain, fever, other chronic conditions, such as diabetes or arterial disease

5 **The best treatment option:** the type of dressing required and how often your wound needs to be redressed.

Different types of skin wounds/ulcers

- **Surgical incisions** are usually produced by a scalpel under sterile conditions; they can be sewn together and expected to heal

- Other **acute injuries** may be clean enough to suture, but if there is doubt suturing may be delayed or the wound left open to heal; an antibiotic may be prescribed. [In the acute phase, press on any bleeding point and call for help: if excessive, call 999 and ring for an ambulance]

- **Venous ulcers** occur particularly on the inside of your lower leg, associated with varicose veins and previous deep vein thrombosis (that you may never have known about). They need leg elevation to reduce swelling, and appropriate dressings and bandageing under the care of a skilled nurse

- **Arterial** (ischaemic) **ulcers** are due to narrowing of the arteries to your legs; the ulcers occur in the feet, where the circulation is worst affected. The condition needs specialist attention to prevent progression

- **Mixed ulcers** occur when venous and arterial disease coexist

- If you are a **diabetic** patients you are more at risk from leg ulcers, since you develop arterial disease earlier than the rest of the population, are more subject to infection, that aggravates the condition, and have reduced sensation in your feet and are thus less aware of injury and developing ulceration

- **Pressure sores** are due to prolonged pressure on a localised area of skin, occluding its blood supply: the lack of oxygen leads to death of the skin, producing a bedsore. You are especially at risk if bedridden or immobile in a wheelchair. Skilled nursing care is required to prevent their occurrence

- **Malignant ulcers** are due to cancer breaking through the skin: they require urgent specialist attention

- **Burns** can produce extensive skin loss, the immediate management is to gently run cold tap water over the area for 10 minutes and cover with a clean pad of whatever material is available: if severe call 999 and ring for an ambulance.

Wound dressings

During your lifetime you will have seen many changes in the type of dressings. Gradually they have reduced in size and are designed to shape around different part of the body, usually with an adhesive border around the edges. Dressings may be **passive**, just covering a clean dry wound or **active** retaining a moist environment to support healing, while **interactive** dressings include factors that promote wound healing.

- **Gauze** dressings are cheap and highly absorbent and can be easily changed if discharge seeps through, but may stick to a dry wound if left in place too long. **Film** of thin polyurethane, combined with an adhesive coating is elastic, conforming to the body contour. Its transparency allows observation of the wound, but if allergic reactions are noted alternate dressings must be used

- **Hydrogel** are glycerine-based dressings that are permeable to gas and water, but need a second dressing to keep them in place. **Foam** is very absorbent for discharging wounds but must be removed once saturated; some forms are available with sticky borders and/or a transparent film that acts as a bacterial barrier. **Alginate**, derived from seaweed, is highly absorbent and retains a moist environment. It requires a secondary dressing to retain it in place, but is easily washed away during dressing changes

- Many other **composite** dressings are available as well as a changing market, your nurse specialist will decide on the most appropriate. **Maggots**, digest and remove dead tissue from a wound, and are a time-honoured dressing, but less aesthetically pleasing to some recipients.

Dressing Technique

Meticulous hygiene is essential in all clinical practice. In hospital, all staff in clinical areas must adopt the 'Bare below the elbows dress code'. Effective hand washing is acknowledged as the most important measure to reduce the infective microorganisms that are transient or resident on the hands. Some microorganisms are known to survive on the hands for a number of hours if the hands are not adequately cleaned: they are responsible for most hospital-acquired infections.

Sources of transient microorganisms include: Direct skin to skin contact, contact with contaminated surfaces, contact with contaminated environmental sources, e.g. dust on furniture, and contact with infected body sites and/or body fluids.

Resident skin organisms: Resident microorganisms are also referred to as normal skin flora or commensals. Resident microorganisms live within the epidermis, e.g. in skin crevices, hair follicles and sweat glands, where they are not easily removed. Their primary function is to protect the skin from more harmful microorganisms. Resident microorganisms have the potential to cause infection when introduced into the body, e.g. during surgery.

N.B. Techniques for hand washing are laid down and must be adhered to.

The Treatment of Post Surgical Wounds

Acute surgical wounds vary in size, depending on the surgery you have had, and they normally heal on an orderly time line. If your surgical wound fails to heal within 6 weeks, it can become a chronic wound, and you will need to alert your doctor to advise appropriate treatment. Always find out from the surgeon what type of sutures you have, for example they may be thread, staple or dissolvable sutures. If you receive stitches that need to be removed, you should be given an approximate date for removal and clear instruction for taking care of your wound:

- Always keep your wound clean and dry, for at least the first 48 hours. Seek medical advice as to whether you must keep your wound completely dry (i.e. no showering) for longer than 48 hours

- Showering is usually allowed after 48 hours as long as the wound is waterproofed as much as possible. You must never soak post operative wounds as bugs grow in moist places. Soaks in the baths are generally not advised if you have lower limb wounds until your sutures are removed and the wound has completely healed

- If sutures loosen or break contact your GP immediately for further advice as there is a risk of your wound becoming infected

- The approximate date for suture removal should be advised before you leave a hospital ward or clinic. You need to make a suture removal appointment in advance with a professional; at your GP surgery, or a District nurse may visit you if you are immobile

- If your post operative wound starts to look red, inflamed, or is hot to touch, is oozing pus or blood, or starts to become raised or painful, seek an urgent medical referral. If an infected wound is left it can lead to serious complications, such as a limb amputation or septicaemia (infection in the blood). If in doubt it is always better to have your wound checked out by a professional to be sure

- Times for suture removal vary, depending on the part of anatomy involved. You must check your suture removal date with a professional, however, approximate post-operative suture removal are: **Face:** 3-5 days; **Scalp:** 7-10 days; **Trunk:** 7 – 10 days; **Arms and legs:** 10–14 days; **Joints:** 14 days.

The Treatment of Chronic Ulcers

The treatment of a chronic ulcer depends on a comprehensive physical assessment to determine the cause of the ulcer and to allow for treatment. Chronic illness, such as unstable diabetes, heart disease and renal failure need to be treated, as they may affect the circulation and blood supply to the related limbs. The doctor decides whether you need rest, or whether your limbs need to be raised up, e.g. on a stool to improve the circulation. Ulcers require tailored therapy appropriate to you and your exact diagnosis. If you have a 'diabetic foot' you may need an urgent referral to a diabetes foot clinic and further referral may be required to the vascular department. Gangrenous feet/limbs need to be assessed by a specialist vascular doctor.

Observation of Wounds

Every time your dressing is changed a wound assessment should take place until your wound has completely healed. If you are at home it helps if you keep a diary to note any improvement or worsening of the wound and new signs and symptoms:

Are the edges of a stitched wound stuck together?

Has the size of the wound got bigger or smaller? Does the wound smell any different? If yes, in what way has the smell changed?

Is there a discharge or bleeding from the wound site? If yes, what colour is the discharge and how much discharge is there?

Is the base of an ulcer red and clean (granulating – a good sign), or is there yellow infected material or black dead material present?

Is the surrounding skin red, inflamed and hot, and is the wound painful?

Your overall physical and mental health is assessed as part of your care, as the healthier you are, the quicker your wound will heal. It is very important that acute and chronic wounds are correctly assessed by a health care professional to ensure the correct wound dressing can be prescribed.

Factors Delaying Wound Healing

A number of factors can delay your wound healing; they include:

- Poor hygiene and wound care, e.g. leaving dressings off for too long and not using a sterile technique

- Unrelieved pressure – you should move position every hour to promote blood supply to bony areas around the body

- Malnutrition and unhealthy diet, e.g. lacking protein, vitamins and minerals

- Obesity, as it decreases tissue perfusion (decreases blood supply to tissues)

- Chronic conditions that reduce blood supply, e.g. cardiovascular disorders

- Underlying diseases such as diabetes mellitus and autoimmune disorders

- Other infections in the body that depress the immune system and weaken the body

- Medications, e.g. steroids that make the skin thin and paper-like

- Alcohol and drug abuse which will lead to general poor health and effect wound healing

- Chemotherapy, as it suppresses the immune system and inflammatory response

- Radiotherapy, as it can cause cell damage

- Psychological stress, depression and lack of sleep.

Wound Infection

All wounds contain bacteria but are not necessarily infected, therefore routine wound swabbing is not always recommended. A wound swab will only be taken and sent to laboratories if you have clinical signs and symptoms of infection and antibiotics are being considered. Note: wound swabs should be taken before antibiotics are started, otherwise the signs of infection may be masked.

Localised infection causes deterioration of the wound and surrounding skin. The treatment aim is to reduce bacterial infection, promote healing, reduce odour and minimise pain. Infected wounds should always be swabbed to determine the pathogen, which allows for the correct antibiotic to be prescribed. The **key signs and symptoms of wound infection** are:

- Swelling, redness, or bleeding at the wound site

- Increased temperature around the wound site – it will feel hot to touch in comparison to other areas of skin

- Discharge of pus or fluid

- Unusual or offensive smell

- Tiredness, general feeling of unwell, increased temperature, sweating, fever and worsening of your medical condition

- Delayed healing and unexplained wound deterioration.

Dressing the Wound at Home

- When a nurse or doctor is preparing to clean and redress your wound they must always wash their hands using soap and water and use gloves to dress your wound. They should review your notes and talk to you about your symptoms, any improvement or worsening, and any signs of wound infection

- Health care practitioners must always use a clean dressing trolley and sterile dressing pack when redressing your wounds in hospital or a GP practice

- In your home, practitioners will ask for a stable table or alternative place to ensure their dressing pack does not fall off or become accidentally contaminated

- It may help you to take analgesics 30 minutes before your dressing is removed if you suffer from pain during the dressing procedure

- If you are having your wound dressed at home make sure that pets are kept away and out of the room to prevent cross infection, e.g. pet hair or pets jumping on the clean dressing

- Your dressing should be removed with gloves. The soiled dressing should not touch any of the prepared clean area. The soiled dressing is placed in a plastic bag and this is usually present within the sterile dressing pack used. After removal of the dirty dressing, these soiled gloves are taken off and the practitioner washes their hands rigorously again

- A new pair of sterile gloves should be worn if the wound needs to be touched to ensure there is no cross infection. This is called **Aseptic NonTouch Technique (ANTT)**. The dressing pack will be opened and all equipment will be prepared, including a wound swab if there are signs of infection

- Once the wound site is satisfactorily cleaned, the appropriate dressing can be placed and secured

- All waste materials should be discarded in a plastic clinical waste bag and a final hand washing takes place. You should always document any changes linked to your wound, as you will have had the opportunity to observe the site with the dressing off. You may use a mirror to view wounds in awkward places.

Dressing Supplies and Ordering

Dressings either come from the hospital main stores, the Pharmacy dispensary or your District/ GP nurse. Before you leave hospital you should be given at least a week's supply of dressings until your community team of practitioners take over. The community team will need to take over the ordering to ensure that you have enough until your wound is completely healed. If you are immobile, District Nurses may visit your home to redress your wound, but if you are mobile you are expected to visit your GP to have your dressing changed at regular prescribed periods. It is important that you check that you have enough supply of your dressings to ensure your continuity of care, and sometimes more obscure dressings can take a few days to order. Some dressings are expensive or rare and are called *nonformulary.* They will only be supplied for you if approved by a Medicine Advisory Committee (MAC).

Further reading

Briggs, M and Flemming K (2007) Living with leg ulceration: as synthesis of qualitative research. *Journal of Advanced Nursing.* 59 (4): 319-28.

Damani, N (2012) *Manual of Infection and Prevention Control.* Oxford: Oxford University Press.

National Patient Safety Agency (2008) *Clean hands saves lives.* NSPA Alert 2009-09-02 accessed on line: http://www.npsa.nhs.uk/clean your hans/resource-area/

WHO (2009) *World Health Organisation guidelines on hand hygiene in health care.* Geneva: World Health Organisation Press.

Chapter 9

Your Heart, Arteries and Veins: the Cardiovascular System

The **cells** of the body require nutriment and oxygen to work: these are carried in the **blood** and delivered throughout the body by the **circulatory** (cardiovascular) **system**. The system is made up of the **heart** and **blood vessels** and can be looked on as a figure-of-eight circuit: blood passing through the lungs (**pulmonary circulation**) at one end and the rest of the body (**systemic circulation**) at the other.

Some blood passes through **additional loops** on the systemic circulation – to pick up food from the gut, to collect hormones from various glands and to be cleared of waste products in the kidneys.

The heart is the **pump** at the crossing point of the two circulations, it has two separate sides: the **right** for the pulmonary and **left** for the systemic circulations, there is **no mixing** of the blood in the two systems. The vessels leaving the heart are termed **arteries** and those returning **veins**.

Each side of the heart has two compartments: the **atrium**, receives the blood returning to the heart in the veins, and passes it onto the **ventricle**, and this pumps the blood out into the arteries. A one way **valve** at each end of the ventricle ensures the direction of flow (*Figure 9.1*).

Figure 9.1 Diagram of the circulation

1. Right atrium.
2. Right ventricle.
3. Left atrium.
4. Left ventricle.
5. Blood circulating through the lungs, to receive oxygen from the air you breathe.
6. Blood circulating around the body, delivering oxygen to where it is needed.

Understanding this circuitry defeated scientists for many centuries, as the joining up of the arteries to the veins throughout the body is through an unbelievably large network of very narrow **capillaries** that are too fine to see with the naked eye. Also, the complex **folding** of the heart during development, in order to produce a pump that drives both systems as a **single unit** means that the arteries from the two ventricles leave the heart in the **same direction**, and blood returns to each atrium through more than two veins.

The **capacity** of the two sides of the heart must be the same, but the bulk of the **muscle** in the walls of the atria is much smaller than that of the ventricles, as they only pump blood into the adjacent ventricle. The muscle of the **left ventricle** is largest, as it has to pump blood around the whole body (*Figure 9.2*).

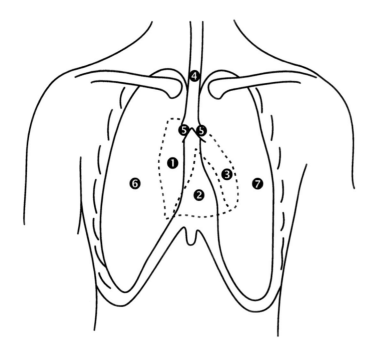

Figure 9.2 Position of the heart (dotted line) and lungs in the chest

1. Right atrium.
2. Right ventricle.
3. Large powerful left ventricle.
4. Windpipe (trachea).
5. Right and left bronchi passing to their respective lungs.
6 & 7. Right and left lungs: the bronchi repeatedly divide, each final division ending in an alveolar air sac, which make up the substance of the lungs.

Before birth, blood does not need to go through the lungs, as they have no air in them. To overcome this problem the pulmonary circulation is short circuited through a **hole in the heart** between the two atria. At birth this hole closes, but a variety of **congenital defects**, relate to this closure and the folding of the heart – these problems are not a concern of the aged.

The heart has an inbuilt ability to contract. This is through the **conducting system**, made up of modified heart muscle. Electrical impulses pass along the system, ensuring the atria and ventricles contract in a cyclical sequential fashion. Damage to the system produces abnormal contraction (**arrhythmia**) and this can markedly affect the efficacy of the heart as a pump.

The cardiovascular problems of old age relate to high blood pressure (**hypertension**): hardening of the arteries (**arteriosclerosis**) and its complications, including **heart attacks, heart failure** and **strokes; venous thrombosis** and **varicose veins**. Most **risk factors** are common to all arterial disease: in view of this, they are considered first.

Risk Factors in Arterial Disease

Many of our enjoyments and excesses in life unfortunately have a cumulative detrimental effect on many of our systems, the cardiovascular being at the top of this list. Arterial disease starts at about the age of 20, but the effects are cumulative, due to narrowing of your arteries from then on. In this list particularly consider familial, smoking, alcohol, diet, exercise and hypertension.

Familial: you cannot choose your parents, but you can take note of any familial health problems. Should they exist, consider ways of avoiding them, consider regular health checks and consult your doctor if you note any related symptoms. Familial problems are accentuated by environmental factors, but take particular note of hypertension, heart attacks and strokes. Cardiac problems in relatives before the age of 55 fall into this category.

Consider how you can address other factors in this section to reduce your personal risk. This is particularly so if you are male. Your **health checks** should include at least an annual blood pressure measurement and an eye check. Consider also an ECG and scans of your arteries, including your carotid arteries, your abdominal aorta and the arteries of your legs.

Smoking: this is the greatest preventable cause of death across the world. The effects of smoking are the same whether using cigarettes, cigars or chewing tobacco. Tar inhalation is reduced, but not abolished with filters, but another important factor is the risk of passive smoking to those around you. This is partly addressed by stopping smoking in pubic places.

Smoking is closely linked to cancer of the lung, larynx, mouth and pancreas; prominent in the cause of chronic chest disease; and an important cause of vascular disease, increasing the risk of heart attacks by five fold, as well as the incidence of strokes, hypertension and renal artery disease.

Other reported problems relate to stress, anxiety, depression, impotence, loss of taste and smell, loss of energy and poor skin. It increases both clotting and the level of cholesterol in the circulation, thus having a further harmful effect on the cardiovascular system.

It is estimated that smoking shortens life in men by 14.5 years and 13.2 in women. Stopping smoking at 30 increases life expectancy by 10 years, and even after 60, there is an increased life expectancy of three years. In spite of these powerful messages, giving up smoking is difficult, on account of physical and psychological dependence, and you are advised to get external help if you are in this situation.

Diet and **alcohol** are considered on pages 70 and 73.

Other serious **risk factors** for cardiovascular disease include **hypertension**, although this is also a disease in its own right and is considered in the following section. Prolonged **stress,** and poor sleeping patterns can affect both your blood pressure and heart, while **inactivity** in a stationary employment does not supply the stimulation required to keep your body efficient. **Exercise** has beneficial effects on the vascular system and is considered on page 245. **Renal disease** is often an asymptomatic companion of cardiovascular disease; the urine should be monitored for any trace of protein. **Diabetes** has marked effects on the circulatory system and is considered on page 84.

Hypertension (Raised Blood Pressure)

The **contracting phase** of the heart is termed **systole,** and the **relaxing phase** diastole. During systole, the powerful left ventricle forcibly ejects about 70 ml of blood (**stroke volume**) into its main outflow tract (the **aorta**) reaching a pressure of 120 mm Hg (**systolic pressure**). As the heart relaxes, reverse flow from the aorta closes the ventricular outflow (**aortic valve**), preventing reflux: the pressure falls, but only to 80 mm Hg (**diastolic pressure**).

This **pulse pressure** of 80–120 mm Hg can be felt in all the major arteries of the body, this pressure not reducing until it reaches the smaller **arterioles** near the organs they supply. Arterial pressure can be measured in many ways. The usual noninvasive method is with a **sphygmomanometer**.

The cuff of the machine is wrapped around your upper arm and blown up above the expected systolic pressure; the pressure in the cuff is measured by means of a monometer. When listening over an artery beyond the cuff with a **stethoscope,** one can hear the **appearance** of a thud of a pulse as the cuff pressure is slowly allowed to fall below the **systolic pressure.** On further letting down the cuff pressure, when the blood flows without resistance, i.e. when the **diastolic pressure** is reached, the sound changes and then **stops.**

The blood pressure of 80–120 mm Hg remains fairy constant throughout your life and if above **90** mm Hg diastolic or **140** mm Hg systolic, it is considered abnormal: the term hypertension, or **arterial hypertension** is applied.

Hypertension is both a **risk factor** for other forms of vascular disease, including heart attacks, stroke, heart failure and renal disease, as well as being a disease in its own right: more than a billion people suffer from the condition worldwide. An increase of over 20 mm Hg systolic or 10 mm Hg doubles the incidence of cardiovascular disease, justifying the name of the **silent killer** that is sometime applied.

In 90% of cases no underlying cause can be found for hypertension, and it is then called **essential hypertension.** The condition has a familial tendency, but this is accentuated by other factors, including obesity, stress, smoking, alcohol, increased salt intake, low potassium, high cholesterol diets and vitamin D deficiency.

Secondary hypertension occurs in a number of conditions, these include hormonal (Cushing's, acromegaly, pheochromocytoma, hyperthyroidism, hyperparathyroidism, diabetes), immunological (lupus erythematosis, polyarteritis nodosa), coarctation of the aorta, renal disease and drugs (indomethazin, ibuprofen, aspirin): smoking and alcohol may give rise to secondary hypertension, while at a younger age it can occur in pregnancy, without recurrence after delivery.

The primary **symptoms** of hypertension are often nonspecific and easily missed; they include headache, light headedness, vertigo and fainting. An important sign is change in the ocular vessels, seen on ophthalmoscopy (**hypertensive retinopathy**). Acute elevation of blood pressure can cause brain swelling and an altered conscious level (**hypertensive encephalopathy**) that must be controlled to prevent cerebral haemorrhage.

Although mild hypertension is usually asymptomatic, potential serious complication make it imperative to undertake **routine checks** at 55 and over, and before this, if there is a familial or other history of vascular disease. It is also important to diagnose the causes of secondary hypertension, as many are treatable, but fatal if not controlled.

The many feature of hypertension described above are unlikely to be relevant to the elderly, however even a sm**all lowering** of a raised blood pressure has been shown to have beneficial effects in this age group. Treatment starts with a low dose of a thiazide-based diuretic, progressing, if necessary, to a calcium-blocking agent. Sudden or large falls are to be avoided, as they could precipitate some of the effects they are intended to prevent.

Cardiac Disease

If heart muscle cannot get enough oxygen to work, it tells you with pain across your chest; a symptom known as **angina**. This happens because the coronary arteries, that supply blood to the heart muscle, are **narrowed** with atheroma, and there may be associated arterial **spasm**.

Angina typically occurs during **exercise**, when the muscles of the body require more oxygen and an increased blood flow to deliver it: the diseased heart is unable to increase its workload to meet this extra demand. Angina gives the warning sign to stop whatever it is that you were doing to cause the problem.

The pain is situated on the lower left side of your breast bone, over your heart: it is a gripping severe pain that makes you stop. The pain not infrequently extends into the upper chest and into your left arm, and may also be felt in your shoulders, both arms, your neck and jaw, and your upper back.

When the pain starts in the chest on exercise, the diagnosis is not usually in doubt, but it can start in the other sites mentioned, and until this pattern is recognised, other conditions have to be excluded, particularly indigestion.

Mild **stable angina** does not usually progress, and if it is not markedly limiting to your normal activity, does not necessarily require treatment. You should discuss this with your doctor who may prescribe nitroglycerine (**GTN**) tablets to pop under your tongue, to relax the coronary arteries, increase blood to the heart muscle and speed recovery of an attack.

Your doctor will also check your pulse and blood pressure and advise on any further management. An **ECG** will probably be undertaken and indicate whether other cardiac events had been going on unnoticed or the heart is normal.

You may have been aware of the beating of your heart (**palpitations**) during the angina, or at another time: note whether this was a regular or an irregular beat. Irregularity (**auricular fibrillation**) is another common cardiac symptom that should be discussed with your doctor. A single ECG may not show irregularity and in suspected cases, a portable ECG can be attached to you to check the heart over a longer period.

Occasionally angina may not go away for more than 15 minutes, it may occur spontaneously without exercise or it may persist with increasing intensity. This form of attack is termed **unstable angina (crescendo angina, acute coronary syndrome)**: such attacks are much more serious, and may herald a heart attack.

Such an episode requires **urgent medical attention. GTN** is required to relax the narrowed arteries, **oxygen** to ensure maximal availability for the ischaemic heart, and medication to **lower the blood pressure** and **reduce the load** on the heart; such as a beta-blocker and a calcium-blocking agent. There are no ECG changes in half these cases, but a 24-hour ECG recording may be needed and any **arrhythmia** (irregularity of the heart beat) treated.

Unstable angina is subject to the **risk factors** described above, and those of heart attacks as described below; but it is also important to identify and remove contributory or **precipitating factors**. These include: extreme exercise; extremes of temperature (both hot and cold, including a hot or spicy meal); all causes of **hypoxia** (reduces available oxygen such as chest disease); drugs (vasoconstrictors, vasodilators, illicit); thyroid disease (hypo or hyper); polycythemia; and anaemia.

Once the acute attack has been treated (and before if this has not been possible), **angiography** is considered to assess the state of the coronary vessels. Every attempt must be made to **prevent unstable angina progressing** to a heart attack, with death of heart muscle, and possible death of the subject.

Narrow vessels can be **dilated** (a balloon is threaded into the stenosis and blown up); **stented** (a metal coil is inserted across a dilated segment to keep it open); **endarterectomised** (the disease is surgically cored out); or **bypassed** (a length of vein or a synthetic tube is used to take blood from the aorta to one or more vessels beyond a block).

Myocardial Infarction (heart attack)

Heart attacks are the greatest annual cause of death worldwide and, apart from the great flue epidemic in 1918, this has been so since the beginning of the twentieth century: the current combined incidence of heart attacks and strokes is higher than all the next seven major causes of death put together.

Heart attacks differ from angina in that a segment of heart muscle is permanently deprived of its blood supply, and is dying. The term **ischaemia** is applied to any tissue when this occurs and, unless the blood supply is reestablished, the tissue dies – a condition known as **infarction**. Infarction takes place in the brain within minutes of being deprived of its blood supply, but in peripheral muscle ischaemia, some recovery can still occur if the blood supply is returned within twelve hours. Ischaemic heart muscle may recover if the blood supply is reestablished within about 90 minutes.

Heart attacks are influenced by all the **risk factors** considered above, particularly a family history of early vascular disease. In spite of this, death is **unheralded** in about 60% of cases and many other attacks go **unnoticed**. Death is not inevitable, but depends on the amount and the position of the heart muscle damage, and how this affects the rhythm of the heart and its ability to maintain the circulation.

When **symptoms** do occur, the pain is similar in distribution to that of angina, but severe and unrelenting. There is shortness of breath, sweating, weakness, nausea and vomiting. There is often marked anxiety, together with a sense of impending doom. There may be pallor and irregularity of the pulse, but often no specific signs. The **diagnosis** is made from this history, the ECG findings and cardiac markers in the blood.

An **ECG** (electrocardiogram) is a measurement of the electrical activity of the heart, recorded through electrodes placed at set positions on the body: gel is applied to ensure good skin contact. In a normal heart, the beats are regular and produce a well documented, and characteristic waveform, traditionally labeled the **PQRST complex**. After a heart attack there is immediate elevation of the ST segment, indicative of ischaemia, while other changes help the doctor interpret the severity of the damage.

Ischaemic cardiac muscle has no oxygen reaching it, this affecting its normal activity. Abnormal products from this area, and the partly damaged areas surrounding it, pass through unaffected veins into the blood stream: these products can be detected in a blood sample. Useful **markers** include creatinine kinase and troponin.

In any patient with severe chest pain, the doctor also has to consider and exclude other diagnoses. These include gut problems: such as severe indigestion, gastrooesophageal reflux and a ruptured oesophagus; a tension pneumothorax and pulmonary embolus; and aortic dissection and pericardial tamponade.

When a heart attack is diagnosed, **treatment** depends on the expertise of those present and the available facilities. If the subject has no pulse, a shock from a defibrillator is given. Oxygen is supplied through a mask; a nitroglycerine tablet is placed under their tongue, to reduce any spasm in the coronary arteries; and medication to reverse any abnormal cardiac rhythms or failure of cardiac output.

Consideration is given to treatment of the blocked artery. This may be by **thrombolysis**, i.e. dissolving the clot, or dilating, clearing or bypassing the disease. To reverse ischaemic muscle changes, measures have to be immediately available and implemented within two hours.

Bad prognostic signs include a cardiac arrest, cardiac failure, cardiac shock, uncontrolled abnormal cardiac rhythms and multiple blocks in the coronary arteries: patients with underlying renal disease and diabetes also do less favourably. Other complications include ventricular aneurysms and rupture, and damage to a papillary muscle, producing valvular incompetence.

Stroke

Stroke is death of a part of the brain due to vascular disease. This is usually arterial in origin, an artery being blocked by local clotting (**thrombosis**) or blocked by clot from elsewhere (**embolism** – from the heart or a carotid artery) and, less frequently; **haemorrhage** (about 13%).

Sustained **low cerebral blood flow**, as in cardiac arrest and major extracranial occlusive disease, is a rare cause of stroke; while **venous thrombosis** as a cause of stroke (e.g. pregnancy) is rare in the aged.

Cerebrovascular disease is one of the commonest causes of death world wide, being second only to heart attacks. It is subject to all the risk factors considered above, particularly hypertension, which if controlled can reduce these problems by as much as 50%, and sources of embolism, such as carotid artery stenosis and auricular fibrillation.

The incidence of stroke doubles over the **age** of 55 in men and 65 in women: the increased incidence of death in women probably reflects the later onset. The incidence is at least double in **diabetics** and there is an increased incidence of stroke in black **African** races.

An important feature of stroke is the common prodromal warning sign of a transient ischaemic attack (**TIA**). This a temporary stroke produced by a small embolus that breaks up and disperses before producing permanent damage. The symptoms of these attacks depend on the areas where the emboli land.

The usual distribution is in the middle cerebral artery producing temporary disturbance of **speech**, **sensation** or **motor** function. The symptoms last for a few minutes to a few hours with complete recovery. Emboli may also end up in the ophthalmic artery, giving temporary blindness, or spots passing across the visual field of an eye (**amaurosis fujax**).

It is essential that TIAs are recognised and embolic sources identified and removed, as recurrent episodes may produce a completed stroke. The commonest source is disease of the **carotid bifurcation**; this can be identified by ultrasound scanning, and dilated or cored out to eradicate the problem.

The cardiac irregularity of **auricular fibrillation**, where the two auricles beat independently of the ventricles, is often well tolerated by the heart, but there may be some associated stasis and turbulence, that can lead to thrombosis. The thrombi are usually small, but when small pieces embolise to the brain, they can easily be big enough to block a major brain artery. Once the problem is identified steps must be taken to regularise the rhythm, prescribe anticoagulants to reduce clotting and occasionally, surgically remove a part of the left atrium where clot can form.

The symptoms of a completed stroke depend on the artery involved: this is usually the middle cerebral artery that supplies areas controlling movement and sensation in the opposite side of the body. Extensive brain damage is usually immediately fatal, but survivors are subject to long-term disability with devastating implications on the subject and close associates.

In the **acute phase** of a major completed stroke, the subject is dependent on others getting them to hospital: preferably to a stroke specialist team. Decisions are made as to whether the problem is due to **haemorrhage** or occlusion and whether imageing is necessary. Occasionally a large collection of blood needs surgical evacuation.

Blood pressure must be retained within normal limits, and confusion and anxiety treated with sedation. Treatment with **anticoagulants**, to 'clot bust' and reduce progression of thrombosis, may be appropriate, current anticoagulants include recombinant tissue plasmin activator (**rtPA.**) This must be initiated within three hours as some changes are irreversible and anticoagulation at a later time carries the risk of bleeding into these areas.

In the acute phase, the subject may be **unconscious** and unaware of their surroundings, and incontinent: this may take one or two days to settle. It is only then that the full damage of the stroke can be assessed and long term management planned. The subject may be aware of their surroundings, and the appreciation of any disability, and its implications on future lifestyle, are likely to produce great anxiety and future depression.

Headache occurs with haemorrhage, but otherwise is usually absent. Severe stroke effects include paralysis (**hemiplegia**) on the opposite side of the body to the brain injury. The paralysis may include the lower half of the face; there may be associated loss of **sensation** and speech disorders. The latter may affect mainly the formative aspect of language (**expressive dysphasia**), language appreciation (**sensory aphasia**, or **jargon aphasia**, producing meaningless phrases) or both aspects (**global aphasia**).

Long term treatment is directed at rehabilitation of mobility, through **physiotherapy** and exercise (page 245), **speech therapy** and **occupational therapy** (reeducating towards future activity): a stroke affects **reemployment** in 75% of subjects. Fits (**seizures**) occur in 10% of cases and require recognition and medication. In an effective unit these measures are in place from the time of admission.

Peripheral Vascular Disease

Atheroma affects all arteries of the body, and although heart attacks and strokes deservedly gain most attention, the disease can be quietly destructive to the kidneys and produce severe symptoms in your legs.

The main femoral artery enters the leg midway between the prominence on the front of your hip bone (anterior superior iliac spine) and the midline: this artery can be felt in your groin. It descends down the inside of your thigh to the back of your knee, where it becomes the popliteal artery. The popliteal artery divides into smaller arteries just below the knee, and these can be felt around the ankle.

Active muscles, e.g. when you walk or run, need more oxygen and this is carried to them in the blood. If the arteries are narrowed by disease, they are unable to deliver this extra blood, and muscles working without enough oxygen produce painful byproducts. The resultant pain on exercise is termed **claudication** and this is an indicator of arterial disease. When you rest the additional demand is stopped and blood can take away the painful products; the usual presentation is therefore **intermittent claudication.**

If the disease progresses, there is inadequate oxygen to keep the skin of the foot alive, and severe disease can present with pain even at rest, and areas of **gangrene** on the foot. Areas of **ulceration** occur particularly over pressure areas, such as the tips of the toes, the side of the foot and the heel.

If any tissue is not getting enough oxygen it is termed **ischaemia**, if the blood supply is returned, the condition is reversible. If this tissue dies it is termed an **infarct**, and this is irreversible (the term myocardial infarct means death of some heart muscle). Gangrene indicates that anaerobic bacteria (those not requiring oxygen to exist) have got into the dead tissue, and started the rot, turning it black.

Whereas intermittent claudication can be treated by exercise to improve the blood flow, rest pain and gangrene need treatment to dilate or to surgically bypass the blocked parts of the system, to avoid the need for some form of surgical amputation.

Health Screening is considered on page 17.

Veins

Veins return blood to the heart, they are thinner walled and usually a little wider than their associated artery, but they can contract, and therefore provide a reservoir of blood should you need it, e.g. a sudden bleed. In a few instances veins travel to another organ, rather than the heart: this is known as a **portal system.**

The prime example of the latter is the **portal vein** that takes blood from the gut, loaded with absorbed nutrient, to be 'manufactured' in the liver. If there is **cirrhosis** (page 60) in the liver, backpressure in this vein produces **portal hypertension** and blood tries to find an alternate way back to the heart. Your body develops **varicose veins** (thin walled, dilated and tortuous veins) for this purpose, and in this case they occur around your umbilicus, anus and lower oesophagus. **Oesophageal varices** can bleed and cause severe problems in late stages of liver disease.

Varicose veins in your legs may be a familial occurrence, but they may also develop to bypass blockage in the deep veins caused by **deep venous thrombosis**. Thrombosis (blood clotting in a vessel) is due to an abnormality of a vessel wall (as in atherosclerosis), altered clotting factors in the blood and stasis. It is particularly the latter that occurs in your legs when your muscles are still and not helping to pump blood along the veins in and around them: as when sitting still in long air flights, being confined to bed and when under anaesthesia.

Deep venous thrombosis is a particular problem in hospital, and you may have been prescribed an anticoagulant during a recent hospital admission. One of the problems of the condition is that a length of thrombus in your leg can break off, pass through the heart and on into the lungs. This **pulmonary embolus** in the system can upset the heart enough to produce a fatal arrest.

Another problem of leg venous thrombosis is leg swelling and the stretched skin is easily damaged and heals slowly. A late consequence therefore is **ulceration** of your lower legs requiring lots of careful bandageing – keep your legs up to the level of your waist when sitting, to reduce these effects.

10

Your Blood

Blood is a fluid with many remarkable properties: it has to flow through the arteries and veins to supply oxygen and food to every part of the body, and to remove waste, yet if you cut yourself it has to stop flowing so you do not bleed to death. To stop bleeding, blood **clots**, but if this happens inside the body (termed **thrombosis**) blocking an artery or a vein, the result can produce severe problems (as in a deep vein thrombosis) or can even be fatal (as in a heart attack, when the thrombosis is in an artery supplying the heart muscle). Blood also transports your defensive cells and immune complexes to any place where invading organisms, such as bacteria are trying to enter the body.

Blood is made up of cells (**red** and **white** blood cells, and **platelets**) and **plasma**. Measurement of the substances dissolved or suspended in the fluid plasma provides a great deal of information on how well your body is working. Examples are: food products (glucose, fats and proteins); minerals (sodium, potassium, calcium, magnesium, iron, chloride and phosphate); waste products (urea and creatinine); liver products (bilirubin and liver enzymes); hormones (measures for all endocrine glands); fibrinogen and other clotting factors; immune complexes; and markers for some cancers.

The red blood cells have no nucleus; they contain **haemoglobin**, a substance that combines with oxygen and transports it around the body. The cells of the body use this **oxygen for** the **energy** they need to survive. Carbon dioxide is the byproduct of this reaction, and it is taken up by haemoglobin and transported to the lungs, where it is exchanges for fresh oxygen and the cycle repeated. When the number of red cells in the blood is decreased, the level of haemoglobin available for oxygen transport is reduced resulting in a condition known as anaemia.

Anaemia has a number of possible causes and can have a marked effect on your health. The symptoms include tiredness, weakness, fatigue, faintness and breathlessness. It puts a strain on your heart that has to pump blood around the body more rapidly to get the oxygen to where it is needed. You may feel the fast heartbeat, known as **palpitations**, and you may be very pale, particularly noticeable in your nail beds and beneath your lower eyelid.

Although there are congenital causes of anaemia, if you were born with one of these conditions (e.g. **sickle** cell disease, **thalassemia**) you will have been under the care of your doctor and know the problems. The anaemia that is more likely to affect you as an elder is due to slow unsuspected blood loss and dietary deficiency.

Blood loss (**haemorrhage**) can occur from your gut gradually over many months, possibly be due to an unsuspected cancer that is otherwise not producing any symptoms. Overt bleeding from trauma and frank blood loss in vomit, stool and urine, or from gynaecological causes is easily identified and then managed. Nutritional **deficiencies** are usually due to severe malnutrition and not common in the UK, but **iron** deficiency and low B_{12} and **folate** in the diet are still potential causes of anaemia.

Iron is present in green vegetables, liver, eggs, meat, flour and milk; additional symptoms of iron deficiency anaemia are dry hair and skin, brittle nails, soreness in the angles of your mouth and, rarely, difficulty in swallowing. Vitamin B_{12} is found in meat, eggs, milk and fish but not in vegetables, whereas folate in present in green vegetables (particularly in spinach), liver and kidneys, it is destroyed on boiling. Dietary problems are accentuated by gut problems, alcohol abuse, and some drugs (e.g. phenytoin).

Destruction of red blood cells can occur in advanced kidney and liver disease, and with some drugs and cancers of the blood and elsewhere. With all anaemia it is your doctor who has to sort out the cause, but you must remain alert to the possibility; if you are getting fatigued for no specific reason discuss this with your doctor who can eliminate this worry with a blood test.

White blood cells are one of your defences against **infective** disease. Different organisms produce different responses, some are engulfed (phagocytosed) by a white blood cell; the outcome of this battleground is the production of **pus** and collections of pus are termed an **abscess**. Other organisms stimulate white blood cells to produce **antibodies** to resist the invasion. Blood tests help your doctor find if you have an infection that is not obvious on the outside, and can monitor the progress of a disease.

The **spleen** has not gained attention elsewhere: in early development it produces blood cells, but this function is taken over by your bone marrow before birth. The adult spleen is housed at the back of your upper abdomen on the left side under the ribs. It is the size of a bread roll and is very vascular: it is a useful blood reservoir and is involved with the body's immune responses. The ribs provide protection against damage, but if they are fractured their broken ends can tear the spleen, producing troublesome bleeding.

Cancers of the blood, such as leukaemia, are commoner in the young, but lymphomas and some other blood malignancies do occur in later life. The symptoms may be mild initially, similar to the anaemia that usually accompanies them, and you should pay similar attention to this possibility.

Platelets are involved in the **clotting** process, as are **fibrinogen** and **calcium** in your plasma. Thrombosis is related to these **various factors** in plasma, but also to **abnormalities of the**

vessel wall, as in arterial disease (page 37) and trauma. The third major factor is **stasis** of blood in a vessel. The latter is an important consideration in venous thrombosis, where increased capacitance can slow flow as in **varicose veins**. Stasis occurs when the muscles of your legs are inactive, such as sitting down on long flights, with enforced bed rest or having surgery under anaesthetic. There is also an increased incidence of **venous thrombosis** in the elderly, the obese, and if you have a family history of the condition or if you have had a previous thrombotic episode.

From the previous paragraph you can see there are things you can do yourself to reduce the possibility of venous thrombosis, i.e. keeping **mobile**, getting up and walking around during a long flight, **stretching** your ankles up and down for a minute every half hour at other times, and when confined to bed. Full length compression **stockings** also reduce the capacity of the veins in your legs, and keeping your legs raised to the level of your waist when sitting down.

When undergoing surgery you will probably be asked to wear compression stockings and prescribed low molecular weight **heparin** while in hospital. If you have suffered a venous thrombosis it is usual to be prescribed a longer course of an **anticoagulant**, such as warfarin: it is important to follow the instructions about dosage control, as excess can lead to bleeding. Other bleeding problems can be seen after major transfusion, when your clotting factors have been diluted, and in liver disease, where **vitamin K** (an essential component in the clotting reaction) is not being adequately absorbed from the gut.

When you are very anaemic, or have lost a lot of blood, **blood transfusion** can be life saving. Great care is taken in matching this to your own blood group. The precautions taken when obtaining blood from UK donors, also ensures that there is minimal risk of introducing infection during transfusion.

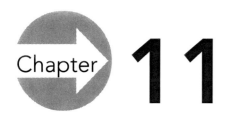

Chapter

11

Your Lungs: the Respiratory System

Respiratory disease tends to receive less media attention than heart attacks, cancer, obesity or diabetes, yet it as a major cause of mortality in the UK (in the region of 20%), probably the most frequent call for a doctor's visit and a substantial cause of disability.

The airway passage extends from your nose, through the pharynx and larynx into your **trachea** (windpipe). The trachea divides into two **bronchi** (*Figure 9.2*, page 38) that pass to the right and left **lungs**. Subsequent divisions into smaller tubes (**bronchioles**) end up in multiple small air sacs (**alveoli**). The fact that you can breathe through your mouth emphasises that the alimentary and respiratory tracts have a common pathways in part of their course, enabling food to go up into your nose, and down into your lungs, if your muscle control is inadequate. The lung and adjacent chest wall are covered by a thin membrane (**pleura**) and there is a potential cavity outside the lungs, between these respective coverings (**pleural cavity**).

Expansion of your chest and flattening of your diaphragm draws air into your lungs: when these muscles relax the lungs empty by elastic recoil. Each alveolus is rather like a balloon on the end of a pump. It has been estimated that the combined surface area from all these sacs, and available for oxygen transfer into the blood stream, is the size of a tennis court (although disease may reduce this to a tramline!).

The symptoms of respiratory disease include a **cough**. This may be productive, in which case, the **sputum** may be clear mucus, but if infection is present in the tract this may become thicker and yellowish-green. Traces of blood may be indicative of cancer, whereas coughing up larger quantities of blood (**haemoptysis**) is more likely to be due to severe infection.

Shortness of breath (page 24) is a common symptom: it may also be a symptom of cardiac disease, as heart failure produces back pressure on the lungs with resultant copious frothy white sputum. Shortness of breath may progress to being present at rest and not being able to lie flat in bed (**orthopnoea**). **Sleep apnoea** is another nocturnal symptom, when every so often a listener hears a sufferer of chest disease stop breathing for a short period. It is commoner when the sufferer is sleeping on their back: they need to be turned onto their side. Wheezing when you breathe out is a feature of asthma in the young; it is due to spasm inhibiting normal airflow. In the elderly, wheezing may also be present in nonasthmatic **bronchial disease**.

Pain is not a prominent feature of chest disease, but if present can be unremitting as it occurs with every breath. This pleuritic pain can be due to infection (**pleurisy**); it is most severe with a broken rib, when the pain is also from the fracture. Pain may occur if a cancer grows into surrounding structures. Tears of the lung allow free air into the chest (pleural) cavity (**pneumothorax**) and this can collapse the lung, it may occur in trauma and more rarely disease of the lung itself.

Pleurisy can produce fluid in the pleural cavity (**pleural effusion**), when this occurs, pain can be reduced or abolished, as the two layers of pleura, that have been rubbing against each other and producing the pain, are separated. Effusions may have blood in them (haemothorax), e.g. after trauma, or become infected, termed an **empyema**.

Smoking is a common companion of chest disease. The link to cancer of the lung is well established, but it also plays a prominent role in damageing the lining of the respiratory tract, making it susceptible to all forms of infection. Smoking is also a risk factor in vascular disease (page 39), and cancer of the bladder and prostate. Giving up does have a long term success rate of about 20%, but it is essential to keep an eye open for possible complications.

Your doctor can listen to your chest to make sure there is air entering both lungs, and hear crackles and signs of infection. There are also a number of tests to assess your **lung function**. These include blowing hard into a devise that shows how much air you can expel in a forced expiration and other instruments that measure flow characteristics. A **chest X ray** is still the key method to screen for lung disease, and where indicated, this can be supplemented with CT and MRI scans. In the management of severe disease in hospital, a sample of blood is taken from an artery to measure the amount of oxygen and carbon dioxide the blood is carrying.

When cancer is suspected **malignant cells** are looked for in the sputum, and a fibreoptic tube passed down the trachea, or into the pleural cavity to see and sample any suspicions areas.

The respiratory tract diseases that you might encounter in old age include the common cold with nasal discharge and infection of the adjacent nasal sinuses. Inhalation of food is more common, particularly after a stroke, where control of the muscles of the pharynx and larynx is reduced: coughing may also be impaired and inhaled food particles then act as a focus for infection.

The commonest chest problem in old age is **chronic bronchitis**. This is aggravated by smoking, recurrent winter infections and recurrent bouts of flue over many years. Healing is less complete and the walls of adjacent alveoli fuse and break down, producing a larger sac with a reduced surface area for oxygen exchange – a condition known as **emphysema**. The chest becomes barrel shaped and breathlessness increases. The combination of chronic bronchitis and emphysema is also referred to as chronic obstructive pulmonary disease (**COPD**).

If severe infection sets in, the bronchial walls also undergo permanent damage and dilate, a condition known as **bronchiectasis**: this is accompanied by an increased quantity and infected sputum. This progressive destruction of lung tissue reduces your respiratory reserve, and a severe infection, such as a bout of flue, may require a hospital admission, with more substantial respiratory support. In view of this increased risk, an annual **flue jab** is advisable. Infection and consolidation of a segment of lung is known as **pneumonia**. This may be secondary to chronic bronchitis, flue or inhalation of food; it is commoner in smokers and alcoholics.

A severe problem in hospital is infection with organisms that are resistant to common antibiotics: these can flourish in an already diseased respiratory tract. Other hospital problems are protecting the airway in an unconscious patient to prevent stomach contents being inhaled. Deep vein thrombosis may occur due to immobility in hospital. One of the complications of this condition is a large thrombus from the leg breaking off and being carried by the blood stream into the lungs (**pulmonary embolus**). The resultant blockage of the blood supply to one or both lungs can be fatal: the reason why prophylactic heparin is commonly prescribed.

Chronic conditions, requiring skilled medical help, include tuberculosis and prolonged industrial exposure to toxic dust and chemicals, or irradiation (pneumoconiosis, silicosis, fibrosis); exposure to asbestos produces a cancer over the outside of the lung (asbestosis). The above conditions can progress to respiratory failure, when the lungs cannot provide enough oxygen for your tissues to survive; additional oxygen is required through various appliances at home or in hospital. In extreme conditions a tube can be passed into your trachea (tracheostomy) and respiration taken over by a machine.

Lung (bronchial) cancer is the commonest cancer in the UK, amounting to nearly 35,000 new cases every year. It also has the lowest survival rate of any cancer, largely due to a late diagnosis in two third of individuals: the initial presentation of cancer of the bronchus is the same as bronchitis, with cough sputum and breathlessness, so it is easily missed. Suspicion should be raised by traces of blood in the sputum, and pain from invasion of various structures around the chest wall. There are general changes of weight loss, anaemia and a general unwell appearance.

Other signs include swelling of the nail beds (clubbing). Spread of the disease into nerves can cause hoarseness of the voice, and weakness in the arm: spread to the liver can give jaundice and into the bones, bone pains and fractures.

Secondary spread to the lungs is common in a number of other cancers, including breast, kidney, prostate, ovary and gut. With all these cancers the presentation may be insidious perhaps only being detected by a routine chest X ray. The management of cancers is by skilled clinical teams.

SO – what can you do to help yourself?

If you are a smoker, the first, and the most difficult task, is to give it up; avoid smoking environments (you may have to persuade your friends to give up as well, or ask them to smoke outside).

If you suffer from chronic chest problems, work closely with your doctor in its management. If you get a new infection or a change in your symptoms consult your doctor early on, so that the cause can be identified and managed before it has a chance to progress.

You may end up with a large number of **drugs**, e.g. cough suppressants; mucolytics (to thin your sputum and help clear it); antispasmodics/bronchodilators (possibly as a spray); nonsteroidal antiinflammatory (to reduce harmful action of infection on the lining of the respiratory passages); steroids (also for their antiinflammatory effect); and antibiotics.

Be sure you take all the medicines prescribed by your doctor: if these include antibiotics, a full course must be taken to avoid the development of resistant bacteria. Additional infections must be avoided, so be sure to have an annual flue jab, delay contact with friends who are suffering from acute chest infections, or confined crowded spaces if you know there is a lot of infection around. Do not venture outside in cold or foggy days if you can avoid it.

You must pay attention to your **general health**; this particularly means matching your diet to your optimal weight (page 76). Exercise is considered on page 245. Your chest may not enable you to carry out an active full body programme, but regular chest exercise helps clear sputum, and improves your chest expansion and respiratory reserve.

Chest exercises are designed to improve use of your diaphragm in breathing. They can be carried out sitting, sitting at a table with your elbows on the table, and your hands supporting your chin or lying on your back, with bent knees. With your lips pursed, breathe in deeply through your nose. Feel your belly expand through decent of your diaphragm, rather than chest expansion. Hold your breath for two or three seconds. Blow the air out through your open mouth, taking twice as long as the in breath. As you get used to the exercise, you can lengthen and increase the pressure on your expiration.

These exercises should last for five, increasing to fifteen, minutes, and carried out four times a day. If you are coughing sputum during them, arm yourself with plenty of tissues. Physical activity is important, and if you are fit enough you should carry out other exercise for 30 – 40 minutes a day, e.g. stretching, walking, cycling (real or in gym) and lifting small weights (dumbbells or full soup cans) – sideways initially to your shoulder level, gradually progressing to above your head.

An acute blocked nose is usually due to a cold, sinusitis or flue, but if this is persistent and progressive, it should be discussed with your GP, and steps taken to exclude a cancer. Nosebleeds are not uncommon in the elderly, particularly if you are on anticoagulants, or if your blood pressure is raised. You can usually control it by pinching your nose and holding this for at least four minutes (by the clock!). Relax, sit down with your head over a table, after preparing an icepack to put over the back of your neck. If bleeding persists you need professional help in an A&E department, but make sure you have given the nasal pinch a full trial, as the bleeding is usually from a vascular area near the front of the nose that responds to this treatment.

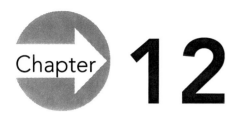

Chapter 12

Your Gut: the Alimentary (gastrointestinal) tract

The alimentary tract (your gut) is a tube extending from your mouth to your anus. Food passes from your mouth into your throat (pharynx), on through your gullet (oesophagus), stomach, duodenum, and small and then large bowel to reach the anus (*Figure 12.1*). Various glands along the way deliver digestive juices (**enzymes**) to break down the food into a form that can be absorbed into the blood stream.

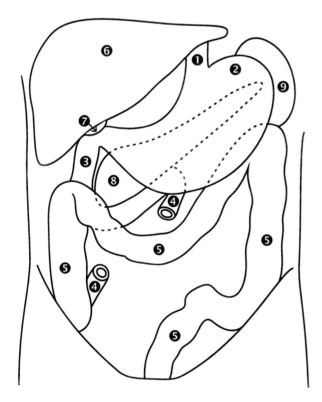

Figure 12.1 Position of the Abdominal Organs

1. Oesophagus.
2. Stomach.
3. Duodenum.
4. Cut ends of small bowel loops that have been removed.
5. Parts of the large bowel.
6. Liver.
7. Tip of the gallbladder.
8. Pancreas.
9. Spleen.

Initial digestive juices (saliva) are produced by the **salivary glands** and drain into your mouth. The **stomach** adds enzyme and acid to the gut content. **Bile** is produced in the liver and is concerned with digesting and absorbing fats and fat soluble vitamins: it also contains some unwanted waste products. Bile reaches the gut through bile ducts, and pancreatic juice, rich in enzymes, joins the common bile duct to reach the food channel in the **duodenum.**

The wall of the **small gut** adds further enzymes: it is coiled up in your belly giving extra length for the food to be digested and absorbed. The **large bowel** reabsorbs excess secretions and collects unwanted waste (faeces, stools, motions, number two, shit, poo) ready to be evacuated.

The blood flow to the gut is increased after a meal, stimulating the manufacture of enzymes, and also facilitating the absorption of digested foodstuff across the gut wall into the blood stream. The gut blood passes to the **liver** on the way back to the heart: the liver is the body's factory for turning the absorbed food into forms that can be used by the body for growth, repair and energy.

Food requires chewing, and you should visit a dentist to sort any difficulty. If you have always had a bit of indigestion, abdominal discomfort or a chronic problem with your motions, you should discuss these with your doctor at a convenient time. If, however, any of these problems is of recent origin, it is essential that you obtain an early opinion, as they can be than early sign of a cancer that needs sorting.

Teeth

The current older generation grew up without the benefit of a National Health Service or free dental care, and only some benefitted from fluoridated water. Tooth extraction was preferred to tooth conservation, and so edentulous members of this population are not infrequent.

Although normal nutrition can be maintained without teeth, with soups, purees and blended meals, you need to be able to chew to enjoy the flavour of a good meal. Chewing also stimulates saliva production from the salivary glands (parotid, submandibular and submaxillary glands), starting off digestion, and teeth are needed for a nice smile.

Bone resorption continues in the jawbones, even after all your teeth have been lost. Thus dentures tend to loosen and should be checked every year, even in the absence of pain or ulcers. Poorly fitting dentures do not allow you to bite or chew efficiently, and can make eating a miserable, rather than a pleasurable, occasion. Dentures need changing at least every five, rather than every 30 years!

New dentures take a number of days to feel your own, particularly the bottom set. While they are still an unaccustomed mouthful, eat soft, well chopped up food, and eat slowly. If there is pain from a poor fit or a sharp edge catching your tongue, put in your old set and return to the dentist as soon as possible, for their adjustment. It is better not to try your own DIY: the dentist can see what needs doing and has had training in this area! Always take your full current set of dentures with you to every dental visit.

Always keep an old set of dentures for an emergency, and take good care of the new one. Dentures should be cleaned at least twice a day, and whenever food gets under them, and is causing discomfort. Use a firm brush for cleaning dentures, use mouthwashes when they are removed, and gently brush your gums, tongue and the roof of the mouth. Keep your dentures out for 20–30 minutes each day: they can be kept in place overnight, unless they are loose, and could block your airway. When dentures get loose and can be inadvertently coughed out, discussing products that fix and prevent food collecting under them, with your dentist or pharmacist can prevent embarrassment.

Old age is not synonymous with *no teeth*, but neither does longevity of a few teeth guarantee their perpetuity. All teeth need an annual check: **decay** (**dental caries**) needs to be removed, holes filled and crowns replaced. **Implants** may be appropriate (although not a cheap adventure).

The dentist checks for **gum disease**, poor **oral hygiene**, and identifies any other oral or systemic disease. Dental **plaque** and tartar contain bacteria, and can give rise to gum inflammation, ulceration and overgrowth: they require removal by your dentist.

Although the amount of saliva reduces with age, there is still enough to lubricate your food and initiate digestion – reduction below this level is usually due to your medication, or another disorder, and if this becomes a problem, it should be discussed with your doctor.

Furring of your tongue is usually a benign hygienic problem; it may also cover your palette and elsewhere in your mouth: you should include these areas in your brushing.

Tongue furring is very occasionally the start of a cancer. Medical students are taught that this can be initiated by the 5 Ss – sharp teeth, smoking, sepsis, syphilis and spices, although the latter is probably only relevant to the betel nut chewed in Asia, where **cancer** of the mouth is more common. If you find an area of furring that does not come off, whether it is painless or painful, show it to your doctor who can advise: an adherent coating termed leukoplakia is a precancerous condition.

Other diseases and conditions also influence oral hygiene. Excess sweet products rot teeth, and acute and chronic illnesses alter diets, and are accompanied by infection, notably in diabetics. Salivary gland disease alters salivary flow, and may introduce infection into the mouth, while liver diseases reduce the uptake of vitamin K: this increases bleeding tendencies, such as from your gums.

Some diseases can affect your ability to hold a toothbrush – these include mental and neurological problems, and physical disability, such as rheumatoid arthritis.

Cleaning your teeth ideally should be after every meal, but if this is not possible, it should be undertaken at least in the morning and before going to bed. There are a confusing number of types of toothbrush; they are probably all capable of cleaning your teeth effectively, at least when new. Your personal choice can be discussed with your dentist.

The shape of the **handle** is again a personal choice, but if you have difficulty in gripping examine all available types to find the most appropriate form. **Electric toothbrushe**s are very effective, but need a steady hand to control and prevent damage. Persistent junk between your teeth should be cleared with a toothpick, dental floss or fine dental brushes.

The direction of brushing should be up and down, to clear food from between the teeth and massage the gums; the latter improves blood flow, as well as removing debris from the gum margins. The force should not be enough to produce bleeding or to damage the mouth if the toothbrush slips out of control.

When cleaning someone else's teeth, use a soft brush, up and down movements; gently lift the lips to reach and massage the gum margins. Ensure you remove all food from between the teeth, and brush the roof of the mouth and the tongue: avoid brushing too far back in the mouth, as this can cause gageing.

It is probable that you had addressed any tooth grinding, or **clicking-jaw** problems earlier in life, but rheumatoid arthritis can produce pain in the temporomandibular joint on chewing. This should be discussed with your dentist who may be able to advise remedial exercises or refer you to your doctor for appropriate management.

At all times, in your mouth and tooth care, aim to enjoy your food, retain a clean mouth, good looking teeth and avoid bad breath, that could affect your companions.

Swallowing

When your food has been chewed and mixed with saliva, you need to swallow it. To do this, the muscles of your tongue, cheeks and throat work together to direct the food into your gullet: this initial part of swallowing is under your conscious control. However, during this manoeuvre other muscles close off the airway – so that food does not go up into the back of your nose or down the windpipe into your lungs.

If your muscles are weak (as with some rare muscle disorders), or the nerves controlling them are not functioning properly (e.g. when coming round from an anaesthetic or a head injury, or after a severe stroke) food can go the wrong way, into your lungs: the same is true if these individuals vomit. This can give rise to a lung infection and the problem must be avoided: unconscious people must be nursed on their side, with their head lower than their feet, and expert guidance about feeding is needed in other situations.

Once food has reached your **gullet** (**oesophagus**), further advancement is by the muscle in the gut wall, and is no longer under your control. The gullet enters the **stomach** at an acute angle, reducing the chance of food refluxing in the other direction, The junction is also surrounded by parts of the diaphragm that help to close it off. Occasionally a bit of stomach can slide though the diaphragm into the chest – known as a **hiatus hernia** – and reflux of the stomach acid can then occur, particularly when you are lying flat. If the symptoms disturb you, use extra pillows and discuss possible management with your doctor.

Indigestion

Ageing does not protect you against poorly prepared food: ensure you maintain high standards of cleanliness, fully cook meat and only eat carefully washed fruit and vegetables. These standards should also prevail in your choice of restaurants. Episodes of acute infection are usually termed **gastritis** or **gastroenteritis**, and typically affect more than one person eating the same meal. Fortunately such outbreaks of nausea, vomiting and perhaps diarrhoea usually subside over a few days

The gullet does not like acid, as this makes it inflamed and gives you discomfort behind the lower part of your breastbone; described variously as heart burn or indigestion. Any swelling or irregularity, such as a cancer, of the gullet wall can produce discomfort or difficulty on swallowing (**dysphagia**), and this should be discussed with your doctor.

The **stomach** is a reservoir where food is churned, mixed with acid and enzyme, digested and stored for a few hours. The narrow outlet is surrounding by muscle that serve as a valve, controlling passage of food into the duodenum. The duodenum, like the gullet, doesn't like acid, and can become inflamed and ulcerated (**duodenal/peptic ulcer**). Stomach ulcers usually give pain soon after a meal, whereas duodenal ulcers give you similar discomfort a few hours later when digested food leaves the stomach.

Pain from the stomach and duodenum is in the midline just under the ribs, it is usually referred to as indigestion, but is not always linked to meals, and has to be differentiated from heart pain – because of its position, indigestion is often referred to as 'heart burn'. It is frequently accompanied by feeling sick and occasionally vomiting. If the symptoms are of recent origin, it is wise to discuss them early with your doctor, as cancer of the stomach can present in this way and should be excluded.

A major step in the management of stomach ulcers was the discovery that many were initiated by a specific bacterium (*Helicobacter pylori*) that can be tested for (breath, stool or blood tests) and eradicated. Another important step was the introduction of medication that reduces acid production, rather than just neutralise the acid produced.

Checking the cause of indigestion that is persistent or of recent origin, is with X rays and/or a flexible viewing tube (gastroscope/gastroscopy) passed through your mouth and on into your stomach and duodenum to look and exclude anything serious: ulcers can be sampled and sorted before they give rise to complications. Your doctor will also take the opportunity to exclude other causes of chest pain, such as gallstones or heart problems.

Liver, Gallstones and Jaundice

The **liver** is a large solid organ situated high up on the front of your belly on the right side, under your diaphragm and behind your lower ribs. It is the body's factory. It receives the blood from the gut, with its absorbed foodstuff, and turns this into usable forms, such as glycogen, for stored energy, proteins and hormones. Factory waste is excreted in the **bile**, which has been described as the fluid that 'launders the liver'.

A number of conditions cause inflammation of the liver (**hepatitis**). These include infection by a series of viruses. **Hepatitis A** virus is transmitted in food and through poor hygiene. It usually produces mild debility, with nausea and vomiting, recovery takes a number of weeks, but is full recovery and there is lifelong immunity. However, occasionally, and particularly in the elderly, it can progress to liver failure.

Hepatitis B may be sexually transmitted or through shared drug needles: symptoms may be mild or progress to liver failure and the sufferer may be a lifelong carrier. **Hepatitis C** has similar features to B with chronicity. The liver is also subject to a number of tropical infections, including schistosomiasis and malaria, often accompanied by marked liver enlargement.

The liver detoxifies harmful products, but in so doing can be damaged: it has the power to regenerate, but the scars interfere with its cellular organisation and function. If the toxic challenge persists, as with excess **alcohol**, the outcome is a shrunken scarred liver, known as **cirrhosis.** The scarring also compromises the liver blood flow producing **portal hypertension,** and this progresses to terminal **liver failure**. Other examples of toxins are poisonous mushrooms and susceptibility to some drugs.

Primary cancer of the liver is unusual, but the liver is a common site for secondary blood stream spread of cancer from other sites, particularly the gut. In the early stages these **secondaries** are not symptomatic: very occasionally solitary lesions can be surgically removed, once the primary cancer has been dealt with.

Bile produced in the liver, is collected into a network of fine tubes that converge into the **common bile duct**: this is joined by the **pancreatic duct** just before in opens into the duodenum. The alkaline bile serves to neutralise gastric acidity and usually prevents duodenal ulceration.

Bile is stored in a pouch, known as the **gall bladder**, arising from the side of the common bile duct: by this means, bile is always available when food enters the duodenum. However, this efficient arrangement is not without problems, as bile is loaded with a lot of waste products, and when stagnant in the gall bladder, the contents can be precipitated to produce gallstones.

Gallstones may be lifelong companions, without you ever knowing. Unfortunately, when the gallbladder contracts to discharge bile into the duodenum, a stone may get lodged in the narrow opening of the gall bladder into the common bile duct. The resultant pain is variable. There may be vague indigestion as considered above or a stone may block the exit and contraction of the gall bladder may give spasms of pain (**biliary colic**): this may be more to the right side than indigestion, and occasionally felt in the back.

Two other serious complication of gallstones are infection around them (**cholecystitis**) and secondly, if a stone passes into the common bile duct, it can block the opening into the duodenum: the backlog of bile in the bloodstream stains the tissues of the body producing a condition known as **jaundice**: The effects of these complications are usually severe and quickly get you to a hospital for emergency treatment.

Jaundice is the yellow colouration of your skin when the waste pigments from broken down red blood cells that are carried in the bile (a continuous normal process), cannot be fully discharged into the gut. The pigments stay in the blood stream and stain the skin and your urine goes dark, as the kidneys try to remove them, Meanwhile your stools are deprived of pigment and are pale, clay coloured. Any suspicion of jaundice should be reported to your doctor.

This form of **obstructive** jaundice can also be produced by disease of the pancreas, as a **cancer of the pancreas** can grow into and block the opening of the common bile duct into the duodenum. Pain from pancreatic problems can produce indigestion, but also present with pain in the middle of your back. A **nonobstructive** jaundice occurs in the severe destructive diseases of the liver described above, and in certain congenital blood disorders, where an excessive number of red blood cells is broken down.

Pancreas

The pancreas is a gland lying across the back of your belly, extending between the two kidneys: it has a head, body and tail. The head lies on the right, within the C-curve of the duodenum, the body lies behind the stomach and the tip of the tail reaches the spleen. The pancreas produces digestive enzymes and the hormone **insulin**. Reduced production of insulin produces type 1 diabetes (page 84) and reduces sensitivity to the hormone type 2 diabetes (page 84).

Cancer of the head of the pancreas can produce obstructive jaundice as described above. Symptoms from cancer of the body of the pancreas are more difficult to diagnose, as they are ill-defined upper abdominal pain that eventually becomes unrelenting and goes through to the back. Once the diagnosis has been considered, it can be confirmed or not by imageing. The diagnosis of **pancreatitis** has similar difficulties. The condition may be acute or chronic, and is usually associated with biliary problems: blockage in the duct system causes pancreatic juices to leak into the tissues and start a little autodigestion. The conditions require hospital management.

Acute Intestinal Obstruction

The small bowel does not usually cause many problems. You will know if you have had lifelong allergies to dairy products or have an **inflammatory bowel disease**. However, because this part the bowel is mobile and slides around in your belly, it is the part that occasionally twists, gets stuck down on old operation scars (**adhesions**) and slides easily into openings, producing a **hernia**.

In any of these situations the passage of food, fluid and wind is blocked off – a condition termed **intestinal obstruction**. Your belly distends, you start vomiting, you stop passing any stool or wind and you experience spasms of pain (**intestinal colic**) as waves of bowel wall contractions try to push food through the blockage.

A **hernia** is a defect in your belly wall that has often been with you for life, and you may have noticed a bulge in your groin when you coughed. Only occasionally does gut get stuck and twist (**strangulate**) in one of these areas. Internal hernias and mechanical problems may arrive unexpectedly, but all **obstructions** need skilled management, usually in hospital and some need surgical intervention: seek medical help as soon as possible if you experience colic, distension, vomiting or stop passing stool.

Large Bowel Problems

A number of large bowel problems present in old age and require medical attention. Conversely, the commonest abdominal problem – appendicitis – is uncommon in the elderly: but not unknown, and acute pain down your right side needs medical assessment at all ages. **Constipation** is a frequent problem in the elderly and this may be improved by dietary or medical means.

There are a number of inflammatory conditions that attack the wall of the large bowel. They are collectively termed **inflammatory bowel disease** (IBD), but may be individually termed, such as Crohn's disease and ulcerative colitis. They are chronic conditions usually starting at an earlier age. They can produce any type of bowel symptoms diarrhoea, constipation, bleeding, abdominal pain, obstruction and, in some, the possibility of later cancer). When your symptoms suggest these problems, your doctor will refer you for specialist management.

As you get older pouches develop along the large bowel, and these can get inflamed (**diverticulitis**) and cause acute appendix-like symptoms on either side of your belly: they require an expert opinion on management. The main concern, however, is of a **cancer** of the large bowel, as if detected early enough, this is curable. Consequently, any **change** in your bowel habit must be reported to your doctor who will decide on the best way forward.

The presentation may be with constipation, diarrhoea, blood mixed with stool or there may be belly distension. The latter indicates an element of obstruction: the symptoms are not so acute as with small bowel obstruction, the constipation may not be absolute, but if vomiting starts it is of brown foul smelling material. Blood that has arisen from bleeding in the stomach and duodenum gets digested, and produces black stools (**melaena**).

As described for the stomach, a viewing tube (**colonoscopy**) can be inserted into your tail end to observe the wall of the large bowel and exclude serious problems, or identify and sample problems that need sorting.

Anal conditions

Piles (**haemorrhoids**) are common in the elderly, and are accentuated by constipation and straining at stool. They are protrusion of the lining of the anal region through the anus, due to reduced tone in the anal sphincter muscle. This mucosa differs from your skin, which is dry, as it secretes mucus and is moist, and difficult to clean with toilet paper. The first symptom is fresh blood on the toilet paper, but as the condition progressed the piles protrude, initially they can be pushed back, but eventually remain outside, as soft, fleshy protrusions.

Protruded piles bleed easily, are uncomfortable, soil clothing and interfere with your control of wind and stool, and this may cause embarrassment. The manoeuvres that many people have to go through to get rid of hard stool do not usually reach a medical textbook. They are undertaken in the seclusion of the toilet: use paper to push up around an obstinate stool. Disposable gloves can be bought from a chemist, but should be disposed of in a sealed plastic bag, rather than risk blocking the toilet.

The availability of a shower, rather than a bath after going to the toilet, to attain the comfort of cleanliness, is rewarding. Be sure that the shower has rails or other devices to hold onto, that you can walk in, or climb in without risk of a fall, and that you can easily adjust the temperature. Soap and water are great cleansing agents, but be sure you wash all the soap away, as if left it is an irritant.

When **bleeding** and **protruding** piles interfere with your life style they should be discussed with your doctor who may send you for a specialist opinion on management. Very occasionally prominent piles may twist and strangulate, producing severe pain needing a hospital admission.

As a child you may have experienced the supposed irritant nature of soap, when you had a small piece of soap pushed into your bottom to relieve constipation – a **suppository** is the modern equivalent – discuss these and constipation medicines with your pharmacist or doctor. Diet is also important, as you need bulk in the diet to produce a stool; this includes fruit, vegetables, oat products and plenty of fluid.

A **fissure** is a longitudinal crack/chap in the lining of the anal margin. It is often brought on by a hard stool and is very painful every time you open your bowels. Ask your pharmacist for a soothing lotion and to advise on constipation. If a fissure persists, or you develop any abnormality around the anus that is not settling within a few weeks you should discuss it with your doctor

An anal **discharge** is uncomfortable, soils your clothing, and is unhygienic and distressing: it can cause soreness, irritation and itching (**pruritus**) of the skin. There are a number of causes, including constipation, when a very hard stool is blocking the passage and you are leaking around it, or possibly taking an oily laxative that is not working. Piles can soil and a condition known as a **fistula** is an abnormal passage from the bowel to the skin passing outside the muscular anal sphincter that usually prevents any leakage.

All these factors must be discussed with your doctor who, if necessary, will refer you to a rectal surgeon with considerable experience in this area. This enables you to get advise on the best management: it may include a minor or a more extensive surgical procedure.

13

Food, Diet and Obesity

Why you need food

At any one time there are many thousands of chemical reactions taking place in your body, directed by your DNA, and ensuring you live a long healthy life. Many of these relate to the efficient use of what you eat and drink.

Food is essential for everyone: it produces and maintains the **tissues** of the body, and provides the **energy** that makes them work. Without food you waste away, but if you eat too much, it is turned into fat and obesity kicks in.

Eating habits

When you are young, fit and healthy, and exercise regularly in a sporting pursuit, you can eat what you like and pay little attention to what is 'good' and 'bad' for you. A happy **balance** is usually in place: **hunger** tells you when you need more, and you begin to feel sick if you overdo it. Some unfortunate people have eating problems, but for most of us, eating is a pleasure: you learn what you like and avoid the rest.

In your **working life**, you develop an efficient pattern for meals and match what you eat with your activities. Things can change in **middle age**, women finish childbearing, and affluence allows both sexes extravagances in their choice of food and drink, often with a resulting trend towards being **overweight**.

In **retirement**, more time is available, and unless you have planned otherwise, there may be reduced activity, accompanied by boredom, all of which lead to **overeating** and **drinking**.

Overeating has a detrimental effect on the cardiovascular system. It promotes arterial disease (**arteriosclerosis**); **fat** is deposited in the arteries, they become more rigid, furred up and narrow (**atheroma:** the condition being **arteriosclerosis**), there is also an increased tendency to **clot**. Eventually the arteries **block**, resulting in death of the tissues they supply (**heart attacks, strokes, kidney disease, leg problems**).

You may also suffer a **reduced** or **damaged DNA**, increasing the potential for cancer. It is therefore wise to consider what can be done to prevent this trend at an early stage. Your resistance to infection (**immunity**) weakens with age – some foodstuffs may improve this reaction, they include: onions, olives, turmeric, root-ginger and fish oils.

Food allergies such as to nuts and shellfish are usually obvious and worrying when severe, but mild ones can be missed, with lifelong minor malaise – if you suspect this is so, you have to meticulously remove and replace dietary items in documented sequences over a number of months, until food or foodstuff and symptoms are linked.

Foodstuffs

The food you eat is derived mainly from plants, with a variable animal content; the animals themselves have also had a predominantly plant diet.

Most parts of a plant are made use of in your food: vegetable roots supply, potatoes, carrots, beetroot, parsnips, yams and cassava; bulbs produce onions; stalks, celery, asparagus and bamboo shoots; and examples from the leaves and their florets are lettuce, spinach, artichokes, cabbage, broccoli and cauliflower.

Fresh fruit provides essential food for most societies, and include olive and cocoanut oils. Seeds are the most nutritious part of the plant, providing the staple diet (i.e. the major food components and essential minerals) for most civilisations across the world. Prime examples are the grains of rice, wheat and maize; others include legumes (beans, peas, lentils), pulses (dried legumes), and the oils of flax, sunflower and safflower.

The most nutritious part of the seed is within the kernel and the outside husk, it is therefore important to retain these parts, for example, using brown rice and brown bread from wheat.

Meat is obtained from the muscle of animals and fish, while animal products include milk, dairy products (cream, butter, cheese), eggs and honey. Nonplant or animal food sources include fungi (mushrooms), plankton (that are the main diet of the fish you eat) and various minerals, such as salt additives.

Food is made up of carbohydrates, fats and proteins, with small amounts of vitamins and essential minerals; you also require **fluid**.

Carbohydrates (carbs) provide over half of the energy (**calories**) you require for the normal working of your body, such as in breathing, moving about and for the lifelong working of your heart. Carbohydrate-rich foods include **cereals**, **bread** and **rice**, and also more **refined sugars**, such as in cakes, biscuits, pastries and chocolate.

These products are digested in your gut and when absorbed into your blood stream raise your blood sugar. The raised **blood sugar** stimulates the release of **insulin** from your pancreas, and this turns the sugar into **glycogen** that is stored in your liver and muscle. Glycogen can be quickly used for energy whenever you need it. Excess blood sugar, however, is turned into fat. This can also be used as an energy source, but through a less efficient pathway, and continuous **overloading of your body with carbs makes you fat.**

More complex carbs are digested and absorbed at a slower rate, avoiding a sudden rise in blood sugar and insulin levels. A measure, the **glycaemic index** (GI), has been devised to assess the relative amount of complex and refined sugars in your food. This estimates the rate at which your food raises your blood sugar, compared with the same weight of pure **glucose** (the simplest carb). You can also calculate another food measure, the **glycaemic load** (GL), by GI x carb weight (g)/100. As a general rule GI>50 and GL>20 are less desirable in a foodstuff.

Although some foodstuffs carry these measures on their wrapping, for most of us it is best to ignore the last paragraph. Nevertheless, what you must never forget is that chronic overload with carbs can reduce the efficiency of your insulin, and the resultant **insulin-resistance** leaves you with a persistent high blood sugar, a condition known as **type 2 diabetes** (secondary, late onset diabetes), the complications of which are considered later.

Some carbs are indigestible, but are still valuable foodstuffs, as they contribute to the **fibre** in your diet, and this **roughage** helps with digestion and the evacuation of waste. The amount of fibre in different foodstuff is usually written on the packageing. High roughage is present in bran, legumes, berries, apples and nuts, but some fibre dissolves in water, producing more wind than solid, and you have to find out for yourself the effect of different foodstuffs on your bowels! Increased roughage limits the cholesterol load, and reduces type 2 diabetes and colon cancer.

Fat is present in foodstuff as **triglycerides, cholesterol, phospholipids** and some free **fatty acids**. High levels are present in **fish oil, dairy products, nuts, seeds, egg yolk, fatty meat** and **poultry skin**. Fat is essential for the integrity of cell membranes, and these control the material coming in and out of a cell, keeping it healthy. It is essential for normal brain development and maintenance, and plays an important role in your immunity. Fat is also the packing tissue of the body, providing insulation against adverse conditions. It provides an important energy source: weight for weight fat has twice the calorie value as a carb.

While most of your fat is eaten as triglycerides, your digestion breaks this down into free fatty acids that can be absorbed from the gut into the blood stream, they are then taken to the liver and recreated into the form that the body needs. While it is an essential foodstuff, different types of fat have a varying effect on your health, as considered in the following sections, and excess produces obesity, which is becoming a worldwide challenge.

Proteins are essential for building the tissues of the body, and their smaller elements (the **amino acids**) carry our genes, promoting growth and reproduction. They are the only source of some chemicals, such as nitrogen and sulphur and are important components of enzymes and hormones. Proteins, like carbs, are found in wheat, maize and nuts, but also in many low carb foods, such as **fish, meat, poultry** and **dairy products.** It can be an energy source, but through different pathways than carbs and fat, and primarily through muscle breakdown and wasting.

Vitamins

Vitamins are a diverse group of dietary products that, although only required in small quantities, the body cannot adequately reproduce. They are essential for the normal development and growth of the tissues and organs, and later for their maintenance, replacement and normal function.

Although their name is derived from vital amine, this was revised when proteins were not always found to be present. Vitamins are **named by the capital letters** of the alphabet; these reached from A – U, but as research progressed, there was found to be overlap and repetition, leading to reclassification: B became a complex of eight vitamins and, with the single exception of K, the titles from F onwards were dropped.

Identification of the vitamins has taken a number of centuries, as this is based on the development of deficiencies in a population, and these do not occur with a normal varied diet, also the body store of most vitamins lasts for many months. A classic example of a deficiency was that of vitamin C in sailors on long voyages; they developed scurvy – a disease of the skin and gut lining that leads to bleeding and death – this was prevented by an allocation of citrus fruit, resulting in the British sailor being called a limey.

The diversity of vitamins is seen in both their actions and properties. Vitamins A, D, E and K are fat soluble, and require bile for their digestion and absorption into the body; B_2 and K can be produced by the action of gut flora; and D can be produced in the skin, but requires sunlight to do so. The **absorption** of vitamins is adversely affected by smoking, excessive alcohol, medications and gut disorders.

Fresh fruit and **vegetables** are a rich source of many vitamins, but their quantities diminish with storage and cooking. Some foodstuffs are **fortified** with additional vitamins and minerals (check the packet!), and inexpensive synthesised **vitamin supplements** are widely available both individually and as multivitamins. These are valuable when deficiencies exist, or when restrictive diets are in place, but there is no evidence that the normal body requires additional vitamins, and excess can give rise to gut and other complications: consult with your doctor if the label does not give a full answer.

Vitamin A is important for your healthy skin and normal vision, particularly in low lighting. It is a powerful antioxidant (see below) and deficiency reduces your immunity. Vitamin A exists as **beta-carotene** in plants and is converted to this from the **reservatol** form in animals. It is present in fresh fruit and vegetables, particularly in carrots, spinach and broccoli. Animal products rich in vitamin A include liver, cod liver oil and dairy products.

The **vitamin B complex** encompasses a wide variety of compounds; deficiencies are most striking when part of severe malnutrition in children, often with lethal affects on the heart and brain (e.g. beriberi/B_1 and pellagra/B_3). In adults deficiency may go unrecognised, with slow generalised deterioration, accompanied by skin changes, anaemia and mental slowing. They are linked to low food intake.

Vitamins B_9 (**folic acid**) and B_{12} (**cyanocobalamin**), deserve special attention in the UK. Folic acid deficiency can produce birth defects, but more relevant to this text, are the **anaemia** (pernicious/megaloblastic) and disturbances of the nervous system that deficiency of these vitamins can produce in the elderly. This deterioration may go unnoticed unless your blood is examined for the typical changes to be identified.

Folic acid is present in leafy vegetables and cereals, but cyanocobalamin is only present in animal products and your diet may be low in meat and your digestion less efficient to deal with it. Possible vitamin deficiencies, such as this, are an important reason for **annual checks** by your doctor, and discussing any change in your health, or worries you have – vitamin deficiencies and dietary problems can usually be very effectively sorted.

Vitamin C (ascorbic acid) promotes healing, the integrity of small vessels, preventing bleeding, it is an antioxidant and is also concerned with immunity. It is present in fruit and vegetables, particularly peppers, gooseberries and blackcurrants: nonhuman animals can manufacture their own vitamin C, and their liver is a rich source.

Vitamin D (ergo/cholecalciferol) is concerned with the management of calcium in the body and deficiency may lead to more fragile bones (osteomalacia and osteoporosis). It can be manufactured in the skin, but this requires exposure to the sun (recommended 15 minutes 3 times a week), and this may not be available in the UK! It is not widely distributed in foodstuffs, but oily fish is a good source, many cereals are fortified with the vitamin and it is available in the form of supplements.

Vitamin E encompasses a group of chemicals that have various roles in the body, these include the nervous control of your muscles and your immunity, and it is a powerful antioxidant (see below). Deficiencies are rare, but present with a mild anaemia and muscle weakness. A high level of the vitamin is found in the oils of nuts and seeds, and it is available as supplements.

Vitamin K comprises a number of chemicals and is concerned with blood clotting. It is derived from leafy vegetables (such as spinach and cabbage), animal liver (particularly goose pâté) and produced by gut flora. Digestion and absorption are dependent on its fat solubility; this is interfered with in liver disease, the deficiency resulting in a bleeding tendency. The action of vitamin K can also be interfered with by various medication; supplements are available, both as capsules and an injectable form, for more rapid effect.

Minerals

Your food contains essential chemicals that have various roles in the working of your body. Carbohydrates, fats and proteins are made up of **carbon**, **hydrogen**, **nitrogen** and **oxygen**, but a foodstuff is rarely limited to just one of these components. **Sodium** and **chlorine** are prime constituents of your body fluids and are provided in table salt, while **potassium**, an important cellular element, is present in bananas, legumes, grains and leafy vegetables

Calcium is essential for your bones and for normal blood clotting; it is present in nuts, seeds and dairy products. **Phosphate** and **magnesium** are also important in bone formation, the former being present in animal products and grain, while the latter is present in a wide spectrum of vegetables.

Iron is important in the production of haemoglobin, the compound in red blood cells that carries oxygen around the body. Iron is eaten in the form of red meat, leafy vegetables, walnuts and dark chocolate, and in fortified products, such as cereals. **Zinc** plays an important role in your immunity and is present in shellfish and grain.

Iodine is concerned with thyroid function and found in shellfish and dairy products; if sources are low in a location, iodised salt has been introduced.

Traces of a number of other elements are present in your body, having essential functions, such as enzyme activity; they include **sulphur**, **copper**, **cobalt**, **manganese** and **selenium**, they come from diverse sources, but are often added as supplements.

Diet

From the above preamble, you have either been totally bemused, and switched off, or you have rushed out to buy a weighing scales and a book on calorie counts.

For most people, just eat what you enjoy, i.e. what you always have done!

Unfortunately, there are a few individuals with eating problems: certain foods may upset them; they are underweight; or they are gaining too much weight. The latter is considered below. You should discuss food allergies and indigestion with your doctor, particularly if of recent origin. Being underweight has many causes; it also needs a full discussion with your doctor, and possibly referral to other professionals to determine the cause and to sort it out.

Having got this far, it would be a shame not to give some advice on what is meant by a '**balanced**' or a 'healthy' diet! This varies with different cultures and different locations.

The low level of arterial disease in **Mediterranean** countries has led to much study of their **diet**, together with the **DASH** (dietary approach to stop hypertension) diet in the US: the latter was initially introduced to reduce hypertension but shown to be effective in controlling cholesterol levels. Other diet watching schemes have been set up, and you will not be short of advice (often conflicting) worldwide.

These diets usually start with cereals, fruit and vegetables; fish is common in the Mediterranean, and red meat and sweet products are always taken in regulated quantities. The Mediterranean diet also includes a daily modest allowance of alcohol.

In view of the variation in approaches, and the conflicting opinions, no attempt is made to be prescriptive, but some rules are worth considering:

1   A typical diet supplies 57%carbs; 30% fat; and 13% proteins

2   Avoid excess carbs, keep refined sugar to less that 10% of this figure, and favour whole grain, and brown bread, brown rice and bran

3   Avoid excess fats, particularly fries, preserves (trans fat) and saturates

4   Include plenty of soluble fibre (oats and barley)

5   Plant proteins are recommended, but add two portions of lean meat and one of an oily fish each week – branched chain amino acids (BCAA), in meat, eggs and beans, improve insulin sensitivity

6   Include at least seven portions of fruit and veg a day

7   The above should provide you with all the vitamins and minerals you need

8   If you are a vegetarian you will already have explored additional supplements

9   Pharmacies give excellent advice on supplements, but if you have followed the above regimen and have no eating problems, just get on with your life

10 If you wish to follow green and pasturised pathways, and to resist force-feeding of animals (considering the harm of antibiotics and hormones in animals, and pesticides in plants), then search the net for reliable suppliers, although these can be difficult to monitor

11 Drink plenty of water and, if you enjoy it, occasional alcohol

12 Guidance on quantities are to be found on foodstuffs (many of which are fortified with vitamins and minerals), typical daily figures (usually related to an adult woman) are:

Calories 2000 kcal; Carbs 230g (refined < 90g); Fat 70g; Protein 45g; Fibre 24g; Salt 6g (NaCl < 2.4g)

Baddies – headline hitters

The increasing worldwide incidence of obesity has triggered widespread interest in foodstuffs by Governments as well as individuals. This has resulted in extensive research initiatives by universities and the food industry, together with a plethora of books and education programmes in all forms of media.

Regrettably the advice is complicated and frequently contradictory. Nevertheless, certain foodstuffs have been found to give rise to health problems and have received particular attention: this may initially have been the chance finding of a harmful product, be related to a specific disease or linked to a chemical that can be easily measured.

It seems to be easier for the public to complain about food manufacturers, than to take matters into their own hands and to choose a healthy diet, i.e. one that is varied and predominantly fresh from local sources.

Here we focus a few of the foodstuffs that can reduce your long term survival, and more importantly, ones that you can do something about, they relate to **homocystine**, **oxidants**, **glycation**, **alcohol** and **harmful fats**.

Methylation is a common chemical reaction in the body, related to protein and DNA function. It is important, as there is a measurable byproduct, **homocystine,** produced when methylation malfunctions. A raised blood homocystine level has been linked to cardiovascular disease, a raised blood pressure, raised cholesterol and dementia.

Although this does not necessarily indicate it is the cause of these diseases, homocystine is an important **marker** of **DNA damage** and degenerative disease. It can also be used to measure the therapeutic effect of any treatment. Homocystine levels are raised by stress, smoking, excess alcohol and coffee.

Homocystine can be lowered with vitamins B_6, B_{12} and folic acid, available in milk, eggs, lentils and nuts. Two other products are powerful methylating agents: trimethyl glycine (**TMG**), found in spinach, grain and beef; S-adensyl methionine (**SAMe**) is present in many chemical sequences in the body and both products have been synthesised and are available as supplements.

Oxidants: oxygen is needed for cellular function (such as energy production) and after completing these reactions, the vast majority of the oxygen you breath is discharged in the harmless forms of carbon dioxide and water. However, a small amount of oxygen (perhaps 1-2%) remains as **free radicals** or combined in other forms, collectively termed oxidants.

Although oxidants can be of **value** to kill bacteria, neutralise toxins and to maintain vascular tone, if they accumulate, as occurs in **ageing**, they produce degenerative cellular changes, including damage to your DNA with the potential of developing **cancer**.

Oxidants can also be formed by **external factors**, such as smoking, air pollution from car exhaust, aircraft fuel and industrial waste; high temperatures, strong sunlight, ultraviolet, radiotherapy; and water pollution, toxic industrial and domestic chemicals; plant pesticides, and antibiotics and hormones in animal products.

Sadly oxidants are also present in a number of **foodstuffs** that you probably enjoy: deep fried food, such as chips, batter and crisps; trans fat (that includes processed food and soft margarine – see below); red meat; dairy products (that include cream, ice cream, milk chocolate, cakes and biscuits); potatoes; white bread; white rice; pasta; and excess alcohol. Additional factors promoting oxidant production are stress, lack of exercise and obesity.

However, there is some good news! There are many dietary **antioxidants** that have **oxygen radical absorbing capacity** (ORAC); these scavenge oxidants, slow DNA damage and allow its repair. An important group is the multicoloured (**rainbow**; the darker the better!) **fruit** and **vegetables**: including strawberries, raspberries, blueberries, blackberries, apricots, grapes, oranges, citrus, pineapples, and tomatoes, peppers, carrots, beetroot, peas, beans, lentils, broccoli, spinach, asparagus and green tea. **NB** heating easily destroys the antioxidants in these products.

Other 'good' foodstuffs include whole grain products, spices, herbs, onions, nuts, seeds and **vitamins A**, **C** and **E**. Vitamin A is a powerful antioxidant. Other powerful antioxidants are found in greens, nuts and seeds and available as the supplements **CoQ10** and **glutathione**. Minerals also contribute antioxidants, and these include magnesium, zinc, copper, manganese and selenium, seafood being an important source of the latter. Red wine gets the go ahead, but only in moderation.

Glycation is the nonenzymatic union of excess blood sugar products with protein and lipid fats. Whereas **glycated haemoglobin** (page 48) is broken down within a few months with the death of the red blood cell in which it is contained, other **advanced glycated end products** (**AGE**) are not so readily removed and are harmful to the body. In diabetics, problems of the heart, kidney, eyes and neuropathy are all exacerbated by AGEs.

These products are raised in ageing, and they damage DNA and block the production of HDL ('good cholesterol' – see below). AGEs are raised in renal and liver disease, and in vitamin B_{12} and folic acid deficiency: they are also contained in some foodstuffs, particularly when exposed to high temperatures, and some flavouring and colouring additives. Foodstuffs that help to remove AGEs are cinnamon, ginger, black pepper and green tea.

Alcohol: this is not all bad news, as regular moderate daily alcohol is part of the advantageous Mediterranean diet – a much lower incidence of vascular disease is reported in this region.

Nevertheless, excess alcohol is harmful. It contains carbs but no additional nutrients. It is treated by the body as a prime energy source, in preference to burning off fat, thus adversely influencing blood cholesterol levels. Although alcohol is initially a stimulant, in larger quantities it depresses cerebral function, and the cravings and addiction can end up with depression.

The greatest concern is the toxic effect of excess alcohol on the liver. This reduces the ability of the liver to deal with toxins or metabolise drugs, with the potential of over dosage. An increase in body cortisol is accompanied by loss of muscle mass, increased fat and a raised blood sugar, with resultant insulin resistance, while fluid retention is a risk factor for hypertension. The final outcome is **liver failure**.

The **fat** you eat is as **triglycerides**, **phospholipids** and various forms of **cholesterol**: all are needed for normal nutrition, but are harmful in excess.

Hydrogenated fat is a synthetic product, produced by converting liquid vegetable oil into solid forms. These are easy to use in food production, but the process increases the fat content. **Trans fat** is a partly hydrogenated product that is a high fat source: it is found in junk food, cookies, cakes, crisps, doughnuts and sweets, and is used as a preservative in frozen foods. Because of its probable link to cardiovascular disease, it has been banned in some countries.

Cholesterol has proved easy to measure and monitor – it has thus become the target for many studies and receives most of the abuse from those having to adjust their dietary intake. Cholesterol is insoluble in blood and, for it to be transported around the body it is bound to a protein. It is lighter than protein and the different proteins carrying cholesterol have become defined by their relative weights. The two most easily measured, and reported, are low and high-density lipoproteins (**LDL** and **HDL**).

The liver recycles excess HDL, but excess of LDL, the major carrier of cholesterol, causes problems. The **macrophage** cells of the blood engorge **excess LDL** molecules, producing **foam cells**; these adhere to the arterial wall starting the process of **atheroma**. For this reason LDL has become known as **bad cholesterol** and HDL as good cholesterol. They are variously reported as mmol/L, mg/dl and as a ratio of HDL/LDL.

Your total cholesterol should be < 5.1 mmol/L (200 mg/dL); LDL < 2.6 mmol/L   (100 mg/dL); desirable HDL >1.5 mmol/L (60 mg/L).

Some families are unfortunate in having exceptionally high levels of cholesterol. These cases of **familial hypercholesterolaemia** are rare, and usually well recognised and cared for. Other families have a tendency towards high cholesterol and they, like the rest of the community, should keep a sensible approach to maintaining a normal weight (*Figure 13.1*, page 76).

A high level of **cholesterol** is found in eggs, liver and shellfish, and high fat levels in dairy products (whole milk, cream, butter, cheese), cooking oils and animal fats (pork, bacon, veal, beef). The latter may also be increased by use of hormones and antibiotics in animal husbandry, while poultry fat and skin contain high fat levels. **Saturated fats** are most harmful, and are present in coconut and cottonseed oils, and chocolate. Smoking, alcohol, and liver and kidney disease raise LDL levels.

But not all is lost! **Low LDL** levels are present in **mono** and **polyunsaturated fats,** as present in olive, safflower, corn, sesame and rapeseed oils, cereals, nuts, vegetables and fruit (particularly tropical and avocados). Oily fish contain long chain **omega-3**, and this, like the unsaturated fats, and the nonfat or low fat **sterols** of plants, serve to lower LDL in the body. Some plants, such as the pulses (dry beans and peas, and lentils) are rich in protein with no fat. Sterols may also be added to butter substitutes, soft cheeses and yoghurt. **Exercise** increases body HDL.

As well as specific diets, there are **lipid-lowering agents**, such as statins, cholesterol-absorbing inhibitors, nicotinic acids and bile acid sequesters. A large practice of weight-reduction (**bariatric**) surgery has developed, but before you try these, be aware that no surgery is without risk, and self discipline is a safer and cheaper alternative. Removal of cholesterol from the blood (**aphoresis**) is limited to severe familial forms of the disease.

Statins are the current preferred cholesterol lowering drugs. They are usually well tolerated, with minor gastrointestinal symptoms or headaches, but liver function must be monitored, and a mild myopathy occasionally progresses to lethal muscle destruction. Particular care is needed in the older, female, and sufferers of liver disease, diabetes, hypothyroidism, or following trauma, surgery, or heavy exercise.

Nevertheless, doubts have been raised about taking statins prophylactically, if you have not had a heart attack or a raised cholesterol level. They lower your antioxidants (see above) and supplements of CoQ10 are advised. Some minor side effects are also not always appreciated or reported; these include alteration of your mental state, with memory loss and depression, fogging of vision and loss of libido.

The interaction of multiple drugs needs careful monitoring by your doctor, as combinations can cancel their effects or even be harmful; effects variously described as **drug-muggers** and **drug-busters**.

Obesity

Although obesity can have a genetic predisposition, and there are mental, physical and hormonal conditions that are linked to it, these are specific medical problems, and the focus of this text is the obesity accompanying the changing lifestyle in later life. You can check your own status by referral to the graph in *Figure 13.1*; this compares your height with your weight, together with the following table, this classifies obesity in terms of your **body mass index** (BMI). A BMI of over 40 is morbid (dangerous) obesity: always remember you are what you eat.

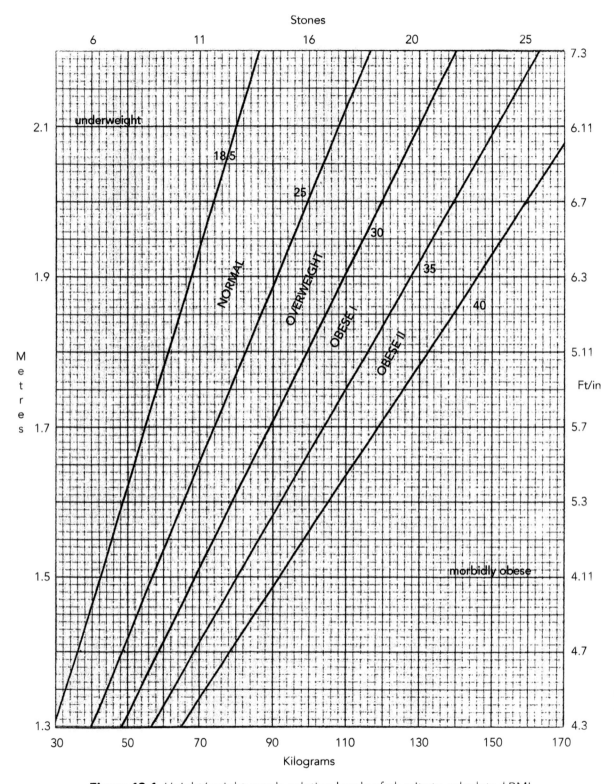

Figure 13.1 Height/weight graph, relating levels of obesity to calculated BMI

Body Mass Index

$$BMI = \frac{Weight~(kg)}{Height~(m)^2} = \frac{Weight~(lbs)}{Height~(in)^2} \times 703$$

< 18.5	Underweight
18.5–24.9	Normal
25–29.9	Overweight
30–34.9	Obese (class I)
35–39.9	Obese (class II)
> 40	Obese (class III)

SO – you are a bit too heavy! Your excuses are probably already in place:

- I am big boned
- I have always been this size
- I always will be
- It is too late to do anything about it
- I barely eat anything
- I just have not got time to exercise
- I need to eat
- I like eating
- I enjoy my food (and drink)
- Eating has become a habit and a great pastime
- I have cravings when I smell food
- I have to eat when I see food
- Food is sitting in the fridge/freezer
- I am very content when stuffed
- I can give up whenever I want to – have done many times
- I have been a bit down; depressed; bored; stressed; sad recently
- Not eating makes me sad
- Giving up food makes me irritable and unlivable with.

Your excuse is probably a lot more original – but you are kidding yourself – emotional excuses are the expression of emotional and psychological hunger – fat people eat until they are full, while slim people eat when they are genuinely hungry.

What are you going to do about it? Your body is your responsibility, and only you can decide to change your eating and drinking habits.

Perhaps you think you do not need to – perhaps you accept what you look like – perhaps you just do not bother. If it is yes to all of these, you will fail in any effort to change, and you will end up disappointed. In this case, you would be wise not to try, since you have to build in an acceptable life long eating pattern. Although this is possible for everyone, it can be hard work and you have to want it.

But before you say 'Fine, then I'll leave it', just read the next few paragraphs that recap some of the consequences of obesity!

Problems of Obesity

The prime concern with late onset obesity is its link with **arterial disease**: this is accompanied by heart attacks, strokes and dead legs. It is also associated with the onset of insulin resistant, **type 2 diabetes**, itself a risk factor for arterial disease, with additionally, hypertension, infection and impotence. Your lower limbs are more susceptible to swelling, **varicose veins**, and the subsequent problems of skin changes and **ulceration**.

The effects on your chest are **shortness of breath** and alteration of your **sleep** patterns. Extra weight places an additional burden on your musculoskeletal system, the load increasing wear and tear of your joints, promoting **osteoarthritis, low back pain, muscle weakness, fatigue** and **reduced mobility**.

The effects of obesity on your gut are to predispose to **a hiatus hernia**, with acid gastric reflux, **indigestion, gallstones** and a **fatty liver**. Your skin sweats more, promoting scaling and **infection**, particularly in skin folds.

Psychologically, obesity carries **antisocial stigmata** and discrimination that can influence reemployment and social networking. These factors lead to loss of self esteem, **anxiety** and **depression**, all of which affect your quality of life. Your cerebral function is reduced and you are probably more prone to **dementia**.

At a cellular level, repair of any DNA damage is impaired, and this reduces your resistance to **infection** and increases your susceptibility to **cancer**. Overall, obesity **reduces your life expectancy** and, of equal importance, it can lead to **disability**.

SO – what can you do?

If the last section has failed to provided a wakeup call, or convince you that you are too fat, you do not need to read on! BUT if it has, you need to set your mind to doing something about it.

Firstly you have to build a mutual respect with you body, to love it and talk to it – thank, congratulate and complement it on getting you to this age, and apologise for imposing a potentially lethal eating programme. Explain things are going to change: it will not change overnight (after all, it took years to get to this state), and it may be heavy going, but the reward will be a new look and a healthier body.

SO where do you start?

For starters, audit your current state: be sure you have reliable weighing scales and place it on a flat noncarpeted surface. An impedance machine also determines the resistance to a weak current passed through you body, and calculates your percentage fat. Note your waist, collar or dress size; take photos of yourself from the front and side, in light clothing, and document your usual diet for a week (no cheating!).

The latter will show you what you eat and drink in routine meals, eating out, in snacks, when raiding the fridge and in grazing. This is likely to show you where the carbs that sustain your bulk come from. People vary, but possible sources include: fried food, crisps, preserved foods, fast foods, sarnies, butties, bread and butter, pizza, pasta, brownies, cakes, biscuits, milk, cream, cheese, ice cream, dates, raisons, sweats and chocolate, together with fruit juices, smoothies, sweet drinks and alcohol.

None of these products are harmful on their own, nor should they be excluded from your diet for the rest of your life, but it is the combined load that needs to be addressed. To achieve a substantial weight reduction and bring you into the normal range (*Figure 13.1*), many words spring to mind, such as the need for resolve, dedication, willpower and determination.

At home you can set off in a number of ways. Eat regularly two or three times a day, and avoid snacks at other times. Use small helpings (small plates help) and take small mouthfuls. Think about what you are eating, and chew it slowly and thoroughly: be aware of, and appreciate its taste and smell, and savour its flavour. Enjoy each mouthful as if it was the first time you were being exposed to this foodstuff. Placing your cutlery on your plate between mouthfuls helps chewing and allows you to savour.

If you are to concentrate on your food, it is not the time to be reading, watching TV, or accessing a social media, and avoid eating when walking, running or exercising. Although your savouring must be developed, there is no need to finish every morsel on the plate. Drink plenty of water, two or three glasses with a meal; this helps fill your stomach and is essential for your digestion. Avoid all alcohol in your initial diet.

Eating at home, rather than a restaurant, is preferable in the initial reduction dietary phase; although many restaurants now indicate calorie values, the alternatives offered can weaken your resolve. You may also be hooked into a conversation with a friend and not focus on the food, as suggested above, and add alcohol.

To slim, you have to be motivated (hopefully this is not because of a recent heart attack) and you need help. You wont be short of advice: there seem to be more experts in this field than any other! However, when the advice is from an overweight individual who tells you they have 'succeeded' on many occasions, their credibility is suspect – slimming must be for life. Once you have 'succeeded' you will also want to tell everyone how to do it – but keep it brief!

There are many good books on dieting, sadly they often tell you different things. They explain how straightforward slimming is, but frequently describe the difficulty the author had: remember the programme they now propose was usually developed after they had completed the hard bit. What is perhaps not adequately addressed is that individuals differ, and you have to find the programme that best suits you, and the one you think you can stick to. Sooner or later you have to learn a bit about carbs, calories and food weights – the writing on the packageing is a good place to start.

In view of the variety of approaches, and the conflicting opinions, no attempt is made to be prescriptive, but some general comments are worth considering: calorie restriction (CR) can leave you cold and hungry, but go for soluble fibre (oats, barley) rather than refined sugar; low fat diets can lead to a craving for extra carbs and be unsustainable. The branched chain amino acids (BCAA), in meat, eggs and beans, improve insulin sensitivity and palatability. However, if used as a calorie source, protein is broken down in a different way from carbs, and can give your body a noticeable (ketotic) odour.

One of the many **slimming classes** can provide help, advice and the camaraderie of a group of like-minded individuals, and most importantly, routine documentation of your progress. A strategy is needed, and regrettably, if you are aiming to lose many stones, rather than a few pounds, this involves what you had previously considered 'near starvation'. The most important question is how to lower your carbs without feeling starved, and one factor is to stay hydrated, as thirst can be interpreted as hunger (but make sure your drinks are sugar-free).

Smoked salmon, grapefruit and celery can become a bit repetitive and a key factor of joining an established class is the advice they give you on the variety of food that is within your calorie target. It also takes into account your choice of flavours and your budget. The programme literature provides a wealth of new nutritious and enjoyable recipes and copious ideas on food presentation.

In your early weight reduction you may need some form of rescue system in place to deal with unmanageable cravings. It is wise to consider acceptable, satisfying snacks that are of low carb value. At home this may include humus for a celery or carrot dip, outside a small tin of low sugar mints may help. Make sure your journeys do not pass bakeries, food stalls or your favorite restaurant.

Consider introducing activities that can detract from your mental and physical food cravings. These need not be as extreme as a cold bath, introduce a new recreation or hobby (unrelated to food!), phone a friend or join a media group, and consider walks and outings. Exercise (page 245) is often suggested as a way for 'melting off' the weight – probably not so – but it is a valuable detractor; it is a good health measure and does increase your longevity.

You have probably been told that dieting makes you look and feel good, improves your wellbeing, increases your fitness, strength, energy and mobility, and improves your self confidence and self esteem. Do not give up if these factors do not match the effort you are putting in; slimming does not happen overnight. What you will note is the slight change in you belt size and the laxity of your cloths.

After four to six months of your chosen diet you may find the weight is coming off in the wrong places, such as your face, rather than your belly or bottom. This is the time to reassess your rate of weight loss, and perhaps reassess over-ambitious targets; you do not necessarily want to end up as a scraggy youth. If you have reached this form of decision time, congratulations! You are now in a position to consider your body image and plan a future **exercise programme**. Consider joining a gym to add muscle strength to flagging areas.

Your long term eating plan

You must continue the dialogue with you body once you have reached your target weight. After hearty congratulations and rewards (cloths, rather than food and drink), decide how you are going to retain your new image. **It is your responsibility**, and you should not need to be tied to a class for the rest of your life. Yet, as has already been hinted at, slimming is more easily reversed than introduced, and you must avoid the need to become a repetitive practitioner.

Your strict dietary regimen has to be gradually relaxed and give way to a **sustainable** long term eating habit. You now know the relative value and the importance of different foodstuffs, their calorific value and how they affect you. Although you can eat anything you like, this must always be in moderation and within planned calorie and nutritious limits. Some suggestions link with those already given above:

1 Your calorie need relates to your activity, and starts about 2000/day

2 In your carbs go steady on the fried, fast, preserved, bread, pasta, white rice, pastry and the sweet stuff

3 Include plenty of fibre

4 Fats are fun but limit the saturates; grill>fried

5 Include oily fish and poultry each once a week, and red meat twice

6   Include at least seven portions of fresh fruit and veg a day – i.e. about half a plateful at each meal – best raw, but otherwise steam

7   Use plenty of herbs to provide flavour; lemon>sauces; avoiding added salt

8   Alcohol is best to average not more than a unit/day; don't forget water.

These basic foodstuffs should provide sufficient vitamins and minerals without the need for supplements. Currently the 2/5 'fasting' diet (reducing intake to 500 kcal/women and 600 kcal/men every third or fourth day) is popular, this allows unrestricted diet for the other five days in a week. You may find the severe restriction on two days unachievable (to be effective, you must not cheat) and there are many alternative ways of reducing your calorie intake, choose one that you can maintain. Don't eat if your not hungry or between meals (i.e. don't graze), and avoid second helpings.

You may eat with your eyes, but you enjoy with your taste and smell; aim to relish your food, while eating **small helpings, slowly** from **small plates**.

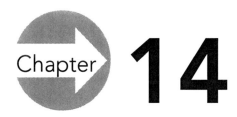

14

Diabetics, Thyroid and other Glands: the Endocrine System

The endocrine system is made up of **glands** that discharge their secretions (**hormones**) directly into the blood stream. The **pituitary gland** is often referred to as the leader of the endocrine orchestra as a number of its hormones influence other endocrine glands, while some have direct influence on body functions.

The pituitary gland is a pea sized structure situated in the depth of your brain. It produces a hormone that influences growth (overproduction in the adult gives rise to a prominent jaw and facial bones, together with large hands and feet – **acromegaly**); another pituitary hormone controls what is excreted in your urine,

The **thyroid gland** is situated in the front, lower part of your neck, around the windpipe. It regulates the rate at which your systems work: over activity (**thyrotoxicosis**) raises your heart rate and places a strain on your heart; makes you hyperactive, burning up energy, with resultant loss of weight; other effects are prominent eyes, a tremor and sleep problems. Under activity (**myxoedema**) slows the heart rate and the rest of your activity, including your mental state, and you gain weight; the skin is thickened with extra fluid. Tablets can help both problems, but surgery or radiation therapy may be advised for overactivity.

Tumours can occur in all the endocrine glands, they may be cancerous or noncancerous, but even noncancerous swellings in a limited space may compress vital structures, such as the nerves to the eyes in the case of the pituitary, and the windpipe in the case of the thyroid. Tumours may also be actively producing additional hormones. As with all endocrine problems an expert team is advised to decide the best treatment. A thyroid swelling is termed a goitre.

The two **adrenal** (suprarenal) glands lie adjacent to the upper part of each kidney at the back of your belly. Their hormones include steroids: **cortisone** excess from adrenal over activity (**Cushing's disease**), or over treatment, causes weight gain, particularly in the face (moon face) and trunk, raised blood pressure, secondary diabetes, fatigue, weakness and mental changes. There is an increased incidence of infection, as steroids reduce your immune response – thus their use in the treatment of many inflammatory conditions.

DHEA, another steroid, is one of the most abundant hormones in youth, and is a precursor of both male and female sex hormones. Levels fall to about 20% of these values by the age of 65, accompanied by loss of drive and motivation, sleep problems and inability to cope. Much research has been undertaken to see if DHEA could be a way addressing ageing: regrettably replacement has not proved easy or effective for rejuvenation.

A different part of the adrenal gland secretes **adrenalin-like** substances that are involved in your fight or flight responses: over activity produces a very high blood pressure, a raised heart rate and strain on your heart.

Insulin is produced by parts of the **pancreas**, situated at the back of your belly. It is the best-known hormone as it is abnormally low in **type 1** (primary, congenital) **diabetes,** or if the body becomes less sensitive to its effects – type 2 (secondary, late onset) diabetes. The consequent raised blood sugar makes you very thirsty, with resultant drinking and excess weeing; there is tiredness, weakness and weight loss, in spite of an increased apatite.

Acute uncontrolled rises in blood sugar can lead to a lethal coma. Insulin injections can control these effects, but doses must be monitored to avoid equally dangerous low blood sugar levels. **Type 2 diabetes** can usually be managed by weight reduction and, for this reason, it has also been termed noninsulin dependent diabetes (NIDD).

The major complication of diabetes is **arterial disease**: this produces the arteriosclerotic problems of heart attacks, stokes and lower limb disease (page 37) about ten years earlier than in the rest of the population. In type 1 diabetics, disease of the smaller arteries may be severe and can lead to kidney failure, blindness and nerve damage; the latter producing numbness of your extremities. The coexistence of arterial disease and insensitive feet make them vulnerable to injury, added to which diabetics have reduced resistance to infection – a combination that may lead to lower limb amputation. **Foot care** is therefore an essential part of diabetic management.

Blood sugar measurements are used to manage acute problems of sugar control. However, **glycated haemoglobin** (HbA1c) is a valuable marker for long term management of diabetic medication. Sugar products are broken down by enzymes and used to produce energy, but excess sugars, especially fructose and sucrose, may be chemically linked to protein and lipid fats, a nonenzyme process termed glycation (see also page 73). These products accentuate heart, kidney, eye and neuropathic complication of diabetes.

The male and female sex hormones are considered with the genitourinary system (page 88).

The effects of hormone deficiency in ageing are multifactorial, but their general effects include reduced muscle mass, loss of energy, mental changes; abnormal sleep patterns; skin wrinkles, pigmentation, bruising, thinning, slow repair and hair loss; and loss of libido.

15

Your Waterworks and Sex: the Genitourinary System

The genitourinary system is made up of the organs of excretion (kidneys, ureters, bladder and urethra) and reproduction (testes, ovaries and uterus).

The two **kidneys** are situated on either side of your backbone, at the back of your belly. They remove waste products and excess water from the blood, producing urine: this in turn passes down two narrow tubes (the ureters) into your bladder. The **bladder** is a muscular reservoir, situated within the pelvis: when you want to pass water (micturate, number one, wee, pee) it contracts, forcing urine through another tube (the **urethra**) out of the body. Valves (muscular rings termed sphincters) are situated at various places in the system to make sure urine only goes in one direction, and you do not leak.

If your **kidneys fail**, there is a build up of waste products, particularly urea and fluid that eventually are a lethal combination. Excess fluid in your tissues is called **oedema**, it can also occur in heart failure, when your heart fails to pump blood efficiently around the body, and liver failure, where this food factory can no longer keep the food and water balance right. **Excess fluid** in and under the skin can be dented by pressure, particularly around your ankles: it can also collect in your lungs and make you breathless, or collect in and swell your belly.

Kidney failure can be treated by being attached to a kidney machine, for a number of nights each week, or by a renal transplant, but unless the latter is from an identical twin, you need to be on tablets long term, to prevent your body reacting against the foreign organ.

In men the urethra passes through the middle of the **prostate** gland: this is situated just below the bladder, and is about the size of a walnut. In later-life the prostate enlarges, compressing the urethra, and producing a range of problems collectively termed **prostatism**.

Initial effects of urethral compression are hesitancy on starting, a poor stream, prolonged time to empty your bladder and terminal dribbling. Incomplete evacuation means frequency of peeing, getting up at night (**nocturia**) and having a repeat pee within the hour after the first of the morning. More disturbing are superadded infection, urgency, soiling and incontinence: you should never miss an opportunity to pee. Extreme problems are levels of narrowing that damage your kidneys from backpressure or completely block the outflow (acute **retention**).

Progressive prostatic enlargement is not usually due to cancer, but to benign swelling and increase in size of the middle zone of the prostate. **Cancers** of the prostate start in the outside of the prostate and usually do not give any symptoms until quite late. Furthermore nonlife-threatening cancer cells are commonly present after the age of 50 in every man, which is why more than two thirds of patients diagnosed with cancer through PSA blood test screening go through a period of surveillance to try to distinguish the slow growing "Pussycat" from the fast growing aggressive "Tiger" cancers. The latter are far less common, though they are far more frequent if there is a family history. As these cancers are so lacking in symptoms it is important that you do see your doctor if there is pain on peeing, any blood in the urine, if you are anxious about anything or if the problems are interfering with your lifestyle.

Although there are drugs that help reduce the size of an enlarged prostate, surgery is often needed for progressive enlargement. A skilled multidisciplinary team should manage prostatic cancer, in order to obtain appropriate treatment. Evidence of renal damage and acute retention need emergency medical management.

The **testis** (testicle) is subject to infection, trauma and cancer, but all of these conditions are commoner in the young, related to indiscriminate sex, contact sports and two types of cancer that are rare in old age, Nevertheless, if you experience pain or swelling of a testis you should discuss this with your doctor.

A common condition in the scrotum is a collection of fluid around the testis, known as a **hydrocele**. Provided a normal testis can be felt within the swelling, and it is not causing you any discomfort or inconvenience, it can be left well alone: see your doctor if you are worried about it.

In women, multiple pregnancies can damage the muscles forming the floor of the pelvis. These muscles also control the outflow of urine and damage may cause urgency and leakage of urine on straining, such as with a cough (termed **stress incontinence**). Regular emptying of the bladder and use of sanitary pads are usually sufficient to control these problems, avoiding surgical intervention. As with men, talk to your doctor if these problems interfere with your life style, if there is blood in your urine or any pain on passing it (the latter, termed **dysuria**, commonly accompanies infection of the urinary system).

The female womb (**uterus**) and **ovaries** are subject to disease. The womb is subject to benign tumours (**fibroids**) and **cancer**, both may present with discomfort in your lower back or belly, or vaginal bleeding. The latter can be confused with menstrual bleeding before the menopause, but if there is change in your menstrual pattern, you should consult your doctor. Removal of the womb (**hysterectomy**), with or without the ovaries, may be required for any condition that interferes with your life style, or is life threatening.

The **ovaries** are also potential sites for a **cancer**. They are enclosed in your pelvis, and the presentation is not easy to identify in the early stages. You may not feel one-hundred percent, with loss of energy and motivation, or have mild indigestion: at a later stage there may be lower back pain and abdominal swelling, both of which should be reported to your doctor, who will decide further management.

Breast lumps are common in women of all ages, the majority are simple, but in the region of 10% are **cancers**. In the UK, breast is the commonest cancer in women, amounting to 48,000 new cases each year: they require early diagnosis so that the optimal treatment can be started. Breast cancer is a hundred times less common in men, but still requires urgent management.

Although no 'cause' has been identified, the extensive research on breast cancer has identified a number of **risk factors.** High oestrogen levels throughout life is one, and this can be related to an early menarche, a late menopause, nonchild bearing, not breast feeding and prolonged hormone replacement (HRT), particularly with a high oestrogen preparations. A family history doubles the incidence and is also linked a presence of ovarian cancer: the gene BRCA 1 has been implicated.

A few of the usual health hazards have been linked to breast cancer and these include smoking, excess alcohol, inactivity and obesity, whereas you can address these factors, this is not so for others, such as being tall or having radiation for a childhood disease.

The **diagnosis** is usually made by you personally finding a breast abnormality (90%). These changes include an alteration of the breast contour, a lump, a thickening of breast tissue, or changes in the skin over the cancer: including discolouration, thickening, puckering, swelling and, in the late phase, ulceration. The nipple may be altered, retracted or have a surrounding rash. Nipple discharge is due to a number of causes, but it should be investigated, especially if blood is present. Pain and tenderness may be present, but they do not differentiate breast cancer from other lumps.

Self examination involves looking in the mirror for changes, especially new asymmetry that could be due to tethering to an area of breast tissue or to the nipple. Move your arms out, above your head and press on your hips, during this observation. Examine the breast with the flat of your hand rotating each area onto the underlying chest wall, feeling for firmness, a lump or any change. Gently feel each quadrant of breast tissue, and behind the nipple between you thumb and fingers for abnormities. Lastly feel for any abnormality in your axilla: be sure to examine both breasts.

Spread of a cancer may produce a lump in the axilla and arm swelling, and symptoms from spread to the lung, bone or liver, or produce general debility. If you suspect a breast problem you must go straight away to your doctor who will refer you to a **specialist breast clinic**. They will make a definitive diagnosis screening by examination, possibly a mammogram (a special X ray of the breasts) and a biopsy of the abnormality.

If a breast cancer is confirmed there are set protocols for its management, depending on the stage it is at: this may include breast surgery, radiotherapy and hormonal or chemotherapy. Discuss the various options, but remember that these clinics are staffed by experts, and you are receiving the best available management. Current NHS guidelines suggest that every woman between the ages of 50 and 70 should have a mammogram every three years and on request after that time.

Sex

Traditionally, **sex** and masturbation made you deaf, and the subject of orgasm was as difficult to discuss as hard porn – medical students were taught to have an innocuous backup question ready to use when embarrassment set in. However, in recent years even older people are willing to discuss, as well as enjoy sex.

Secondary sex characteristics, such as facial hair growth in boys and breast development and periods (menstruation) in girls, start at puberty. These changes are under hormonal control: the pituitary gland (in the brain) stimulates production of testosterone in the testes in boys, and oestrogen in the ovaries in girls. Hormones also regulate pregnancy.

In women, at about the age of fifty, oestrogen production from the ovary stops because of running out of eggs. This condition is termed the change or the **menopause**. This is accompanied by stopping of periods, and commonly hot flushes, mood changes, headaches and insomnia. There is loss of glandular tissues in the breasts, which droop, reduced lubrication and shrinkage of the vagina, and weight gain. These effects are variable and unpredictable as many women continue to produce oestrogen from the adrenal gland or adipose tissue, some of which is still driven by the pituitary gland.

Hormone replacement therapy (HRT) may be prescribed to combat these problems and reduce osteoporosis (page 94). However, your doctor must prescribe this, as it can increase the incidence of thrombosis and cardiovascular disease, and susceptibility to cancer of the breast, womb and ovaries, particularly if there is a family history of these diseases.

There is also a fall off of hormone production in men beyond middle age, but this is not so sudden as in women. There is a gradual change in prostatic secretions and the content and quantity of sperm. The angle of erection also gradually changes with age. In both sexes changes in hormonal balance reduces libido, but the prime stimulus of mental desire is not lost. The fear of unwanted pregnancy is removed and knowledge and experience in sexual relationships is a valuable asset. It is important to remember, at all ages, and whether your preference is vaginal, anal or oral sex, the risks of gonorrhea, herpes and HIV remain: **safe sex** must always be a key priority.

Changes in sexual activity may be related to physical and social factors as well as those of a physiological and psychological nature which can lead to a cyclical or periodicity of activity.

Chronic pain from any source has a profound influence on mood, sleep patterns and levels of anxiety and depression, inhibiting other mental and physical activity such as sexual desire. Disability can interfere with sexual activity, this including musculoskeletal problems and stroke: management of these problems requires exploration and adaptation to alternative positioning.

Cardiovascular disease and diabetes affect the arteries supplying the penis providing inadequate flow to produce an erection, while diabetes also has a profound effect on the nerves to these blood vessels; over half younger diabetics have problems with impotence. Surgery of any form can have a detrimental affect on vitality and interest, and specific problems are pain, urological procedures and stomas. Urinary incontinence and problems with hygiene can markedly affect the attitude towards sex, and require an understanding partner.

Drugs are a common problem interfering with potency and desire. Particular examples are antihypertensive drugs and cancer chemotherapy. Read the literature of any medication, and if you think it could be interfering with sexual relationships, discuss this fully with your doctor. Alcohol is another important 'medication' that may appear to increase desire, but can have a detrimental affect on performance due to "brewer's droop". Its effect is relatively easily reversible by alcohol free holidays that should be tried before trying any drugs. Smoking is not overemphasised in this text, as those addicted to it know the penalties; impotence is another to add to the list because of the damage smoking produces to the arteries supplying the sex organs. Stopping smoking can be as effective as stopping alcohol though it can take longer to repair the damage and perseverance helps to set up a permanent change.

Social standards and opinions change with time and between generations, but there are still many taboos about discussing sex among older people and even the young find it difficult to believe that granny is still actively seeking sexual satisfaction. Ignorance is mixed with misinformation, misconceptions and often blurred with moral and religious principles in this field.

The most damageing event is the loss of a lifelong partner, with the associated familiarity, affection, emotional understanding and trust. Finding a new partner with similar qualities is difficult, social networks are limited and the Internet is fraught with technical difficulties and scams, even for the young who are more experienced in these areas. Privacy and security are other serious problems unless you live alone in your own property,

Other physiological and psychological changes in sexual behavior do occur with age. It is estimated that over the age of 70, libido drops to 80% in men and 60% in women. In both, orgasms take longer to build up, are of shorter duration and decline more rapidly, but the pleasure is undiminished, and desire, sensitivity and enthusiasm for sex are retained.

The importance of sex relates to your lifelong experience and expectations; if it is disturbed, discuss this with your doctor who should direct you to an appropriate therapist. Avoid buying any medication over the Internet without medical recommendation, as they can have adverse effects on your heart and other systems. Specialist management is required on penile implants and other devices that may help you.

It should not be necessary to abandon sex on account of age or lack of an expert opinion. Ensure you persist until you have obtained professional advice on any sexual problems: sexual activity is an essential part of life at any age and must not be shrouded in mystery or social prejudice.

Chapter 15

Your Bones, Joints and Muscles: the Musculoskeletal System

The musculoskeletal (**locomotor**) system is made up of the **bones**, the **joints** and the **muscles** of your body. The bones support the body (as in the limbs and spine) and protect organs (as around the heart and brain), the joints enable you to move (as in walking and using your hands), while the muscles supply the power to move the joints, putting your feet, hands and head, where you want them.

Joint disease occurs throughout life, affecting about a quarter of the population: **congenital** disease, i.e. from birth, may continue to give problems throughout life; **inflammatory** joint disease commonly starts in middle age; and **degenerative** disease is added to these problems in later life. Throughout life you are subject to **accidents**, with peaks in your youth, due to accident-prone sports, and the risks taken at this age; and in old age, when you are unsteady on your feet, with stiff joints, weak muscles and neurological problems, all making you accident-prone: the latter problems are also slow in their recovery and **rehabilitation**. *Figure 16.1* shows a typical joint.

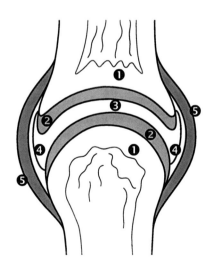

Figure 16.1 Typical joint

1. Bones on either side of joint, reciprocally shaped, to facilitate smooth movement and accurate placement of your hands and feet.
2. Cartilage covering the joint surfaces: it is subject to wear and tear.
3. Joint space, filled with a small amount of lubricating fluid.
4. Synovial membrane covering the nonarticular joint surfaces, and retaining the synovial fluid in place.
5. Ligaments holding the two bones together, but flexible enough to allow movement of the bones by the muscles attached on either side.

This chapter concentrates on inflammatory joint disease (**rheumatoid arthritis**); joint disease of old age (**osteoarthritis**); the fragile bones (**osteoporosis**) that occur in later life, and are easily damaged; and the common **injuries** of old age (see also page 97) and their **rehabilitation**: backache is considered on page 112 and fitness and exercise on page 245.

Rheumatoid Arthritis

The body responds to an injury of any kind with an **inflammatory reaction** – the cells of the immune system react around a broken bone or foreign material, such as invading bacteria. Occasionally, the body gets it wrong and sets up this reaction to its own tissues: these diseases are termed **autoimmune** and rheumatoid arthritis is one of them.

In the case of rheumatoid arthritis, it is not known what turns its proteins into **foreign material**, and a target for inflammation. Although the disease is mostly in the joints, inflammation is also present in other tissues, including the membranes covering the heart and lungs, the sclera of the eyeball and the skin.

The disease affects 1–2% of the population, it is commoner in women (3:1) and usually starts between the ages of 40 and 70; there is a slight familial tendency. The joints of the **hand**, **wrist** and **feet** are commonly affected, although larger joints are not immune, and the distribution is usually symmetrical.

The tissue changes are typical of inflammation: the joints are **swollen**, **red**, **hot** and **painful**, with **loss of function**; the tissue swelling is increased by fluid in the joints (**effusion**). The reaction destroys the synovial membrane, the capsular ligaments and the cartilage, making the joints unstable, and subject to **deformity**, tethering and fixation (**ankylosis**).

The **pain** in an acute attack can be extreme, the joints being very tender, and sensitive to contact as well as to movement. **Stiffness** is particularly marked after a period of inactivity, it taking at least an hour to mobilise in the mornings; this **immobility** leads to muscle **wasting** and **weakness**.

The **systemic effects** of a raised temperature, loss of apatite, nausea, weight loss, weakness, tiredness and feeling unwell, emphasise the general nature of the disease, and there is associated anaemia and osteoporosis (see below). **Skin nodules** are present in 15–20% of cases, and reflect a worse outcome. Progression of heart and lung disease is uncommon, but there is an increase in arterial disease, and the disease can shorten life expectancy by 3–12 years.

Joint symptoms occur in bouts and are often followed by a period of remission: but the frequency is unpredictable and **repeated attacks** and chronic recurrence lead to **disability**. The deforming effects in the hands are very **characteristic**, with bent, slim fingers turned sideways. The effects on **daily living** are cumulative, affecting getting out of bed, washing, bathing, dressing, walking, cleaning, shopping and driving. If this progression cannot be stopped it can result in loss of independence, although fortunately this is unusual.

Treatment must be early and prolonged to ease the pain of the attacks, reduce the destructive effects, maintain mobility and, by so doing, reduce deformity. Treatment of pain starts with simple analgesics. **Antiinflammatory drugs**, such as ibuprofen, are more effective, but they must be carefully monitored as they can produce gut ulceration and bleeding: similarly **steroids** must be prescribed with care. Smoking has a harmful effect on the progress of the disease. A balanced **diet**, with all possible allergic foods tested for and removed, is essential, together with regular sleep and a **safe environment** to avoid possible injury.

Heat and short wave diathermy applied to painful joints give some relief, and attacks are less severe in warm climates. Gentle **movement** of affected joints through their **full range** of movement must be undertaken as soon as the pain allows, and then followed by **active exercises** to maintain muscle strength. Acupuncture and reflexology may help, and with these **physiotherapy**, together with **occupational therapy,** to maintain useful movement.

Various splints and appliances (**orthoses**) serve to retain optimal joint positions at night and when deformity is appearing and progressing. None of these measures halt the progress of the disease, and disease modifying antirheumatic drugs (**DMARD**) may be needed when the progress is unremitting. These include a number of anticancer drugs, such as **methotrexate**, and must be monitored by experienced doctors to avoid damageing the rest of your body.

NB Although not of direct concern to an older generation, everyone must be made aware that these drugs can damage a baby in early pregnancy, and they must never be left around, or offered to help anyone else's symptoms.

If deformity is already present, consideration is given to **surgical** removal of diseased tissue, to avoid further progress, and other corrective maneuvers and joint replacement.

Rheumatism, rheumatics and rheumatic disease are terms that are in general use and to describe joint pain from any source. The terms may be applied to any of the headings in this chapter, and there are many other joint diseases, such as gout, ankylosing spondylitis and joint disease from a number of metabolic and congenital defects, that are not detailed. Thus, while they are useful lay terms to describe your aches and pains, if these are interfering with your life style, you should discuss them with your doctor who can identify and advise on any serious problems.

Osteoarthritis

Osteoarthritis is a degenerative joint disease; although it is not caused by old age it runs a parallel course, affecting the weight bearing (hip, knee, spine) and other 'working' (elbow of a baseball pitcher) joints, that gradually wear out.

Some degenerative change can be expected over the age of 60, and earlier, if there have been congenital problems, injuries or other previous joint disease. The cartilage covering the joint surface of the bones has been rubbed off, and new bone replacing it is rough, exuberant around the edges and not designed for smooth efficient joint movement – there may be frank deformity of the joint.

Movement is painful, stiff, restricted and may be accompanied by grating, clicking and possibly locking. Disease progression is usually slow, pain can be accepted, or treated with mild analgesics and morning stiffness worked off with a bit of walking.

Some modification of life style is advisable: obesity must be avoided, and regular exercise (20–30 dedicated minutes every day) undertaken to retain a full range of joint movement and muscle strength (resisted movement rather than impact running). Insoles, knee braces or other appliances may ease pain and enable you to partake in your favorite activities.

In a few individuals, pain, stiffness, deformity and disability are not manageable using the above measures. In these cases joint replacement can be considered. Remember, however, that no surgery can guarantee a perfect, uncomplicated outcome: to date, hip replacement has the most encourageing results.

Osteoporosis

The **bone mass** and **density** of your bones gradually reduces from the age of 30: this weakens the bone and increases the risk of fractures. When the bone mass reduction is markedly below the expected age-matched normal value, the condition is termed **osteoporosis**. The measurement is made using an X ray absorption technique known as a **DEXA scan**.

When osteoporosis is present, there is marked bone fragility and risk of fracture and deformity. The initial at-risk group is of women with an early menopause (the female to male age-matched ratio being 3:1). The next high risk group is of individuals over the age of 75 (female to male ratio is still 2:1).

As well as these two groups, there are a large number of diverse conditions, usually with a similar sex incidence, that put you at risk of osteoporosis, they include: individuals with a prolonged period of **inactivity**, such as sedentary or bedridden; **hormonal** problems includes diabetes, hyperparathyroidism, hyperthyroidism and increased steroids; **dietary** abnormalities include vitamin D deficiency, and high protein and high energy diets; **drugs** include lithium, anticoagulants and antacids; toxic **heavy metals** such as lead and cadmium; and **malignant** bone marrow infiltration.

Osteoporosis is usually **asymptomatic**, but there is progressive **loss of height** and a **hunchback** may develop. **Fragility fractures**, however, may be spontaneous, where the body cannot support its own weight, or occur after minimal trauma. It is therefore important to identify sufferers and protect them from these complications.

Treatment is initially identifying and addressing the cause. The main focus is on **fracture prevention**, ensuring a safe environment, and commencing an exercise programme to strengthen muscles and ensure stability. Plenty of **sunshine** should be encouraged, to supplement the formation of vitamin D, and a balanced **diet**, should include milk, yoghurt and fish oils. Drugs have not been as effective as expected, but may include vitamin D, bisphosphonate, calcitonin and, possibly most effective, recombinant **parathyroid** hormone. **HRT** is advisable for 3 to 7 years after the menopause, provided there is no history of breast cancer.

Fractures

Falls and fractures (broken bones) are a serious problem of old age, as **susceptibility** increases after 75. **Stability** is markedly diminished, because of reduced righting reflexes after stumbles, and from joint stiffness, muscle weakness and possible neurological problems, Obesity is more difficult to balance, while slight individuals are easily knocked over.

Hypotensive and antidepressive **drugs,** can accentuate the problem, while osteoporosis makes individuals vulnerable to fractures. Fractures through abnormal bone, such as osteoporosis or malignancy, are termed **pathological**.

Fractures of old age are not usually highspeed injuries, but commonly of the **hip**, **wrist** or **back**. The classical features of fractures are present: pain, deformity, swelling, local tenderness, crepitus (although you should never test for it) and, most importantly, loss of function.

Back (vertebral) fractures can be missed, and are further considered with backache (page 112), but hip and wrist fractures are obvious: the individual with the hip fracture is lying down (there is no way they can or should walk) with the great toe (or the shoe) on the affected side pointing out sideways; an individual with a wrist fracture holds it with the other hand, and does not want anyone to touch it, it is angled backwards at the fracture site.

These fractures do not usually have the **complications** of broken skin, with the risk of infection, or associated nerve or major blood vessel damage, but the bone may be a bit crunched, making setting more difficult. The individual with the hip fracture may have not been able to attract attention for some time, and be pale and in a state of **shock**. They both require surgical involvement, possibly with a general anaesthetic.

The complications of **surgery, anaesthesia** and enforced **bed rest,** carry the risk of **chest** infection, venous **thrombosis** in the legs and bits of these clots breaking off and causing chest problems.

The **rehabilitation** after these injuries is also problematic. The involved and other joints may already be stiff with related muscles weakness. The incident brings home to you your vulnerability, and makes you realise that, at least temporarily, you have **lost your independence** and have to rely on others. This can markedly affect your self confidence and self esteem, and requires a lot of moral support, as well as expert physiotherapy.

Rehabilitation exercises vary with your ability, and it is important that the exercise relates to your fitness: even with marked joint and mobility problems, you can gain great benefit from Tai Chi or chair exercise. Find out the leisure facilities supported by your Local Authority as most have exercise classes tailored for older people, where rehabilitation can continue. Consider the use of walking aids (page 298), and do not be embarrassed to accept a seat offered you on public transport or elsewhere.

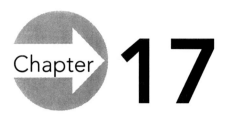

Chapter **17**

Falls Prevention

James Berwin

Falling over may sound innocuous, but as you get older falls can have a serious impact on quality of life. Falls can cause distress, pain, injury, loss of confidence, and loss of independence.

Falls are a common and serious problem for older people. The National Institute for Clinical Excellence (NICE), states that people over the age of 65 have the highest risk of falling, with 30% of people older than 65 and 50% of people over 80 falling at least once a year.

The primary aim in dealing with falls is to prevent them from ever happening, the secondary aim is to prevent serious injury should you happen to fall. The first step in preventing falls is to identify your risk of falling, and then to take steps to manage that risk. An assessment can be made by your GP to determine your risk factors for falling. These include:

- A history of previous falls

- An assessment of your gait, balance, mobility and muscle weakness

- An assessment of your osteoporosis risk (lack of bone density)

- An assessment of your perceived functional ability

- An assessment of your fear relating to falling

- An assessment of any visual impairment you may have

- An assessment of your neurological status including cognitive impairment such as dementia

- An assessment of whether you have urinary incontinence

- An assessment of whether you have any home hazards

- An assessment of your cardiovascular system

- An assessment of any medications you are on that can drop your blood pressure and cause falls.

As the above list suggests, the cause of a fall is often multifactorial. Fortunately, the majority of risks are modifiable through often simple interventions that can make a big difference.

Balance and Mobility

Recommended interventions include muscle strength and balance training that can be tailored to your specific needs. Your local gym may offer strength and balance training, which many find effective. There is some evidence to suggest that Tai Chi, a form of martial arts, can also help reduce the risk of falls through improving balance, coordination and movement. A professional should monitor any form strength and balance training.

Home Hazards

Home hazard assessment and intervention is an effective way of reducing your risk of falling at home and can be instigated by your GP. General advice includes removing clutter, trailing wires, and frayed carpet, using nonslip mats and rugs, and using high wattage light bulbs in lamps and torches so you can see. You should try to organise your home so that climbing, stretching and bending are kept to a minimum, and obstacles likely to trip you up should be cleared away. Always ask for help to do things you cannot do safely.

Never wear loose fitting, trailing clothes that might trip you up, never walk on slippery floors in socks or tights, wear well fitting shoes with good grip and take care of your feet.

Bathrooms are a common place for falls to occur and are a prime example of why home hazard assessments are useful. The installation of bars or railings in the bath can help you to get out safely. The installation of a personal safety alarm is highly recommended; it is an effective way of alerting your next of kin or carer that you have fallen and are in need of help. An alternative would be to have a mobile phone within reach at all times.

Medication review

Some medication, although necessary for treating many long term medical conditions, can produce side effects, which may increase your risk of falls. For example, if the dose of a medication required to treat your high blood pressure (hypertension) is too high, it can cause your blood pressure to drop to a point that you become dizzy and fall when standing up.

If you're taking regular medication on a long term basis, it is recommended that you ask your GP to review your medications at least once a year. This ensures you are on the correct medication at the correct dose. Your GP may recommend a lower dose; an alternative medication or it may be possible for a medication to be stopped entirely.

Sight test

Poor eyesight is a clear risk factor for falls. Even if you already wear glasses, it is always worth ensuring your lens prescription is up-to-date. There are many causes of deteriorating eyesight; not all eye conditions are treatable, but conditions such as cataracts are treatable with a simple day case operation.

Alcohol

As with most things in life, drinking alcohol in moderation is unlikely to do much harm. Drinking to excess however, can pose a real risk of falls. High blood alcohol levels affect your balance and coordination, leading to the inevitable, but alcohol can also alter the strength and effect of regular medications by dysregulating the way in which the liver metabolises them. The consequences can be disastrous.

Long term alcohol abuse can also have a dramatic effect on bone density (osteoporosis). Thus the primary effect of being intoxicated with alcohol is the increased risk of falling; the secondary consequence is that your bones are more liable to fracture should you fall.

Osteoporosis and Vitamin D

Osteoporosis is a condition that weakens bones, making them more likely to break. The most common sites for osteoporotic bone breaks, also known as fragility fractures, include your wrists, your hips and your spine. There are many risk factors for developing osteoporosis see page 94 for full details.

Vitamin D deficiency is a significant, but modifiable risk factor for the development of osteoporosis. Given that your main source of vitamin D is derived from sunlight, it's hardly surprising that a staggering percentage of the British population is vitamin D deficient. This is particularly the case during the winter months, and is prevalent amongst the elderly population as well as Asian and African communities. Recently, there has been emerging evidence to suggest that vitamin D deficiency can also impair muscle strength and function, leading to an increased risk of falls.

Thus, ensuring your vitamin D levels are in range will go some way to reducing your risk of falling, but will go a long way towards maintaining good bone health which is key to reducing your risk of fragility fractures should you happen to fall. Your GP can test your vitamin D levels via a blood test and your bone density via a bone density scan, known as a DEXA scan.

Deficiencies in vitamin D can be treated by supplementing vitamin D via your diet or with tablets, which can be bought over the counter in pharmacies and health food shops. Higher doses can also be prescribed by your GP.

The current recommended daily dose of vitamin D is 200IU for people up to the age of 50, 400IU for people aged 51 to 70 and 600IU for people aged over 70. Dietary sources of vitamin D are surprisingly hard to come by unless fortified with the vitamin itself. Wild mackerel, salmon and mushrooms are all good natural sources rich in vitamin D.

Hip Fractures

Hip fractures are becoming increasingly common, with around 70,000 to 75,000 occurring each year. According to the National Hip Fracture Database, the average age for hip fracture is 84 years in men and 83 in women, but they can occur at any age in people with osteoporosis (reduced bone density), and are therefore a type of fragility fracture.

Occasionally, the reasons for falling are purely accidental and can even occur after a simple slip or trip at home. However, the occurrence of a fall and the resulting hip fracture can often signify underlying ill health or a change in your mobility or ability to cope at home. As a result, approximately 10% of all patients with a hip fracture die within 1 month and about one-third within 1 year. Most deaths relating to associated medical conditions rather than the fracture itself. An emphasis on preventing falls and ensuring good bone health is therefore key to reducing the risk of hip fracture.

After falling over, the common signs and symptoms of a hip fracture include:

- Severe pain in the hip or groin
- Inability to move after the fall
- Inability to put weight through the injured leg
- Shorter leg on the injured side
- Leg or foot turning outwards on the injured side
- Severe bruising or swelling over the hip.

Any of the above signs warrant an assessment at your local Accident & Emergency department. Hip fractures can usually be seen on an X ray of the hip, but if the nature of the fall or the examination findings are suggestive of a hip fracture and it cannot be seen on an X ray, then an MRI or CT scan may be indicated.

The hip joint is a ball and socket joint (*Figure 17.1*). The ball refers to the round head of the thighbone (femur), which fits into its socket, the acetabulum, formed by the pelvis. A hip fracture refers to a break in the bone where the head is attached to the rest of the thighbone (*Figure 17.1*).

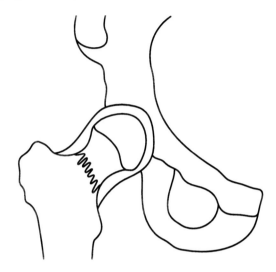

Figure 17.1 Fractured femur – the diagram of the hip joint has a fracture (irregular line) through the neck of the femur

Hip fractures almost always require surgery. Decisions made about what surgery you require are based on the location of your hip fracture and your general state of health.

The aim of surgery is to return you back to your baseline mobility. If you're already dependent on a walking stick or a Zimmer frame, then the aim of surgery will be to get you back to walking with a stick or Zimmer frame. If you were able to walk unaided before the fall, then the aim will be to restore your ability to walk unaided. The sooner you are able to mobilise after your operation, the lower the risk of infections, pressure sores and blood clots.

All of the above operations will be performed under either heavy sedation with a local anaesthetic injection in the spine to numb the hip region, or a general anaesthetic. This will depend on your general state of health as well as the preference of the anaesthetist.

National guidelines ensure that all NHS hospitals provide a high standard of multidisciplinary hip fracture care. Members of the team include, surgeons, specialised hip fracture physicians, physiotherapists, nurses, and occupational therapists. The aim is to ensure that patients are medically optimised for their operation and the immediate postoperative course. This helps patients to get back on their feet and mobilise after their operation, it also ensures there is a safe environment at home to return to.

The guidelines also focus on the prevention of further fragility fractures, treating conditions that are known to cause falls, giving medication such as calcium and vitamin D supplements to improve bone density, and providing walking aids at home designed to help them safely live an independent life. These are tailored to a patient's specific need.

Wrist Fractures

Wrist fractures account for around 18% of all fractures sustained in the elderly population. Risk factors are similar to hip fractures in that they result from a fall onto the affected side and often occur in patients with osteoporotic bone.

Common symptoms associated with wrist fracture include:

- A snapping or grinding at the fracture site
- Severe pain
- Bruising and swelling
- Difficulty in moving your hand
- Your wrist or arm may be an odd shape
- You may notice tingling and numbness in the hand
- There may also be bleeding if it is an open fracture and the bone is poking through the skin
- You may feel dizzy or sick following the shock and pain of breaking your arm.

If you think you have broken your arm or wrist, minor fractures can be treated at your local Minor Injuries Unit, but bad breaks need to be seen and treated by your local Accident & Emergency department. Avoid moving the affected arm as much as possible, stop any bleeding by applying pressure to the wound, and don't eat or drink anything in case you need emergency surgery to fix the bone once you get to hospital. Call 999 if you are unable to get to A&E or have multiple injuries.

On arrival to hospital, you will be given painkillers and a splint to help support your arm. Your arm and hand will then be examined and an X ray performed to confirm the diagnosis and determine the severity of the injury (*Figure 17.2*).

Treatment of your wrist fracture depends on the location on the bone and the type of fracture. In the emergency department, your doctor will often attempt to realign the broken bones with their hands. This is normally performed whilst you are awake, but with your arm numbed and medication given to relax you. Your arm will then be held in place with a plaster cast or splint and the position of your fracture rechecked with an X ray.

Provided your fracture is in a satisfactory position, you are given a sling to support your arm, painkillers to take home and a follow up appointment to monitor how your wrist is healing. Typically you spend 4 to 6 weeks in plaster to allow the bones to heal, although this may be longer if there are signs the fracture is not healing as expected.

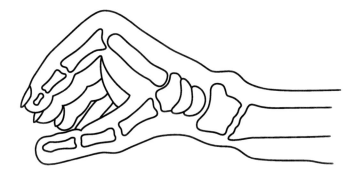

Figure 17.2 Fractured wrist – the diagram of the wrist joint has a fracture (irregular lines) through the radius, with deformity of the wrist

More serious fractures may require surgery to realign the bones and hold them in place with either wires, or a plate with screws. Occasionally the arm is held in place with an external frame.

Once out of plaster, your wrist will almost certainly be very stiff. You will be given some gentle exercises and stretches to improve the range of movement in your wrist, and if required a short course of physiotherapy. Decisions about when to return to lifting heavy weights and driving must be taken with your doctor.

Further reading

Falls in older people: assessing risk and prevention. Clinical Guideline: CG161. National Institute of Clinical Excellence (NICE). https://www.nice.org.uk/guidance/cg161

Falls – prevention. NHS Choices Website. http://www.nhs.uk/Conditions/Falls/Pages/Prevention.aspx

Vitamin D. Cambridge Nutritional Sciences Ltd. http://www.camnutri.com/vitamin-p-67.html?detail=7&cPath=22

Hip fracture: management. Clinical Guideline: CG124. National Institute of Clinical Excellence (NICE) https://www.nice.org.uk/guidance/cg124

Broken arm or wrist. NHS Choices Website http://www.nhs.uk/conditions/broken-arm/Pages/Introduction.aspx

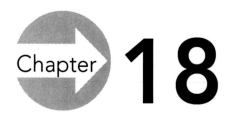

Chapter **18**

Putting your best foot, and leg, forward!

Nicola Bewes

Ageing affects many aspects of the leg and foot care.

Cold feet

Chilblains are the result of the microcirculation in the skin causing localised blood deprivation. A more severe reaction to the cold, than chilblains is **frostbite**, where the microcirculation does not recover, and tissue death results. By keeping the chilblain affected area at a similar temperature, or brought up to warm from cold slowly, tissue damage can be minimised. Smoking severely affects the microcirculation, exacerbating existing chilblains. *Penguins don't get chilblains, because they have short legs, plus the warm blood from their hearts, warms the cooler blood in the veins that wrap around the artery. This clever heat exchange cools blood in the feet, so not melting the ice, but warmer blood returning to the heart.* We humans have longer legs; so to keep the feet warm, the blood reaching the toes has to be warmer still. Wearing long johns and thicker warm tights, helps. When sitting still, the body becomes colder, as there are no additional movements to warm it. Just placing a blanket over the knees, does little, as the back of the legs is still getting cold. Sit on the blanket and wrap it around the legs, keeping both front and back warm. ***Please do not sit too close to a hot heat source.*** The heat from a fire will cook your skin, especially the thin skin of the shins. *Crispy skin is good on chicken legs, but not on yours!*

There are cold drafts at floor level, so if you don't like your feet up, place an old cushion in a box, and place the feet on the cushion. The walls of the box protect the legs from the draft. However, **do remember that your feet are in a box when you stand up!**

Exercise

Gentle exercise is beneficial for both the soul and the body. Just rotating the ankle while sitting, along with pointing the toes towards the ground and then up to the ceiling, helps the circulation.

It also keeps the joints supple and this aids with balance. Sitting for too long, increases the risk of suffering from **Deep Vein Thrombosis,** not only on aircraft, but also at home. Get up and walk about every hour, or at least once the movie on TV has finished. Walking up and down stairs is good exercise, and cheaper then joining a gym.

Swimming and gentle walking are excellent forms of low impact exercise. Bones become stronger with use, so walking not only helps to keep the body supple, but also strengthens the bones. Gentle walking with other like-minded people is not just good for the body, but also good for the soul. Many areas hold free, 'Health Walks' (see www.walkingforhealth.org.uk).

Footwear

Nature provides **cushioning pads** of fatty tissue under the heels and across the ball of both feet. These cushion the bones when walking, but with age, the pads become thinner. It feels as if you are walking on the bones! There is no way this natural protection can be replaced, but by wearing footwear with thick cushioning soles, the feet will be protected. This lack of cushioning also affects the knees and hips, so more cushioning footwear helps knees, hips, back and the neck (*de knee bones connected to de leg bone, is connected to de back bone etc.*).

Footwear ideally should tie on or buckle onto the feet, keeping the shoe firmly in place. Velcro is easy to use and is just as effective as laces and buckles, and it is kinder to the hands and fingers to use. When putting on footwear, sit down then, once the shoe or slipper is on the foot, tap the heel gently on the floor. This ensures the heel is in the correct place, and any space is up by the toes. Make sure you **fasten the footwear**. If the space is behind the heel, or if the footwear slips on easily, the foot slips backwards and forwards during walking, causing damage and pain to the toenails, as well as cramping the toes into the toe box. This can often be the cause of corns and hard skin or callous on the tops of toes; especially the littlest toe. If the toes are compressed into the narrower toe box, the toenails of one toe can dig into the flesh of the next. Not only causing discomfort, but also it can pierce the skin providing a route for infection.

The footwear that is most cushioning, and supportive, is the trainer. Not the most beautiful of shoe, but for comfort, trainers cannot be beaten. A reasonably priced pair of trainers is better for the feet than traditional slippers: keep smart shoes for smart occasions. Long handled shoehorns are a must!

Loose slippers can cause trips and falls, as to walk in a loose slipper the foot is shuffled along the floor. The back can also slip off the heel. *My great aunt was staying at friends, and walking up stairs to use the bathroom, the back of her slipper slipped of. She stopped on the stair and wriggled it back on, over balanced and fell down the stairs. Ending up in hospital with a fractured spine!* To be safe a slipper must grip the foot, and the soles must be intact and not worn through.

My grandmother's house shoe sole was flappy at the front, and walking back up the front steps, after paying the milkman, she tripped on the loose sole and fell holding the milk bottle. Bloody milk all over the place. The broken glass cut her hand, but luckily her wedding ring stopped the glass cutting her ring finger any deeper.

Rough, dry skin

As the skin becomes drier, any thickened skin around the heels can crack and become painful. If these cracks become deep enough, they can bleed. If this happens professional help should be sought. The dry hard skin, not deeply cracked around heels, can be gently removed by the use of an emery board, as used on fingernails. Rub against the dry skin, this smooth's the skin off as a fine dust, then apply the cream. Any slightly thickened areas of skin can be treated in the same way. Rub gently with an emery board, and keep softened with moisturising creams. These can be on prescription. Please do not use anything sharp on your feet. Do not dig with sharp objects, down the sides of the toenail, or into the skin, as any cut to the skin can be the entrance for infection. If there is dry or additional skin down the sides of nails, especially the big toe, use an old toothbrush to gently brush away any dry skin, from the base towards the free edge. If dry, apply cream.

Do not soak your feet, they only need gentle washing, with soap, water and a flannel, or a back brush can be used if bending is difficult. Place the wet feet upon a towel on the floor to dry, leaving the skin open to the air for a few minutes so the skin between the toes can dry naturally. If the toes are stiff, and cannot be dried in between with a towel, use **cotton buds** to dry. The addition of surgical spirit on the cotton bud will also dry the skin between the toes if it is soft and moist.

Skin

Due to changes in the circulation, especially within the skin all over the body, the skin becomes dry, and hair growth slows or stops. Leaving, especially the lower legs hairless. The skin sweats less, and with little hair, there are less natural oils secreted, both of which help moisturise the skin's surface. This leads to dry flaky skin that can become itchy due to the dryness. The skin also losses it's elasticity with age, combined with natural skin thinning makes the skin fragile and susceptible to damage. Even a gentle nudge will cause bruising, and this now delicate skin tears easily if damaged. Twice daily moisturising helps the skin become more resilient. Any **moisturising cream** will work, but **do not** cream in between the toes.

Stocking and sock aids

There are sock and stocking aids that can make putting socks on easier; these can be a flat flexible piece of plastic with long tapes. The plastic is used to open the sock aperture, holding the tapes, the opened sock is placed on the floor and the toes pushed into the open sock. The tapes are pulled up and the sock is pulled onto the foot, the plastic is then removed. There are 'soft top' socks widely available that do not cut into the leg; these are much kinder than tight digging in sock tops. The thick seams of socks can irritate the toes, and if you suffer with diminished feeling in the toes, these thick ridges of material can damage the skin without you knowing. Either wear the sock inside out, or move the seam out of the way. Clean hosiery should be worn daily.

Swollen legs and feet

Legs often become swollen, and this is often due to a reduced activity (resulting from arthritic changes in the back, knees and hips) and reduced return of the circulation via the veins and lymphatic system. **Varicose veins** severely hamper returning blood flow. This increased fluid retention within the lower leg tissue, causing swelling. This in turn compresses the nerves causing discomfort and pain, especially when moving the ankle. The stress on the tissues of the leg is such that small breaks in the skin can rapidly turn into considerably larger skin conditions. The **reduced blood supply**, means that healing takes considerably longer, and any resultant leg **ulcers** can take months to fully heal, often needing regular dressing from specialist nurses and bandageing regimes.

To help reduced swelling, when resting, sit with your **feet up** on a footrest or puffee. Compressive elastic stocking are often prescribed to provide support for swollen legs, it is vital that they are worn daily.

They have to be tight, to be effective. Putting them on before or immediately after getting out of bed helps, as the legs are at their slimmest, having been horizontal all night. If you sleep in a chair, try to sleep with your **legs up** as this helps to reduce swelling: if the chair reclines, even better.

The skin of your legs and feet should be checked daily for any changes in colour, such as new areas of redness or damage. This could be splits, cuts, or bleeding. To enable the sole of your feet and back of your legs to be seen, use a mirror resting or propped up, on the floor.

Toenails

As we get older, toenails like the skin, become drier. They become harder and more brittle. A lifetime of stubbing and injury causes the toenails to thicken, until they can be almost too thick to cut. Injury can be cumulative, or as a direct injury – dropping something heavy on the toes, causing the nail to blacken and sometimes fall off. The newly growing nail will invariably be thick and gnarled. By filing the nail with a good emery board or diamond dust file, this bulk can slowly be reduced, until the nail plate is thin enough to cut. By keeping the nail filed it will not become thick again.

Toenails should be cut following the line of the nail bed, at the free end. Filing the rough edges and any sharp corners. Once nails are short, they can be filed weekly, about three to five strokes per nail, when bone dry. This keeps them short and comfortable, and hosiery slips easily over the foot.

Verrucas

These are rare amongst mature people, usually caught in public changing areas, such as swimming pools and gyms. Upon investigation most *verrucas* on the feet of older people are actually corns. If concerned consult your local podiatrist.

If you are experiencing difficulties with your feet, there is help available:

For nail care, your local Age UK office may conduct a nail cutting service. They will have a list of local podiatrists.

Podiatrists (previously known as chiropodists), can advise and help with:

ingrowing toe nails, corns and callous, bunions and hammer toes, and 'policeman's heel – this feels like standing on a drawing pin, but there's nothing to see or feel except pain.

Your GP can refer those who have existing medical conditions that categorise them as high risk, to the local NHS Podiatry service.

The HPC (Health and care Professions Council) holds lists of registered practitioners that can be accessed via their website: www.hpc-uk.org

The Society of Chiropodists and Podiatrists have a useful web site that contains more information of common foot conditions: www.scpod.org

19

Your Brain, Nerves, Seeing and Hearing: the Nervous System

The nervous system is made up of the **brain** and **spinal cord** (the **central nervous system** – CNS), and all the nerves outside the CNS that form the **peripheral nervous system** (PNS). The PNS has two parts: a well defined set of nerves that supply your muscles, and bring sensation from the surface of your body and special sensory organs to the CNS – the **somatic nervous system**; and the **autonomic nervous system** (ANS), a fine network of nerves, that supplies the **heart**, the **smooth muscle** (in the walls of the gut and the blood vessels) and the **glands** throughout the body, and brings back sensory information from these deep structures to the CNS – the ANS is not under your conscious control.

In the somatic nervous system, you have twelve pairs of **cranial nerves** that pass directly to the brain, and 31 pairs of **spinal nerves** that pass to the spinal cord. When assessing this system, you have to consider the sensory and motor pathways. Sensory abnormalities include **altered sensations** of touch, pain and temperature (paraesthesia), and reduced vibration, position sense, recognition of shapes by touch and identification of numbers or letters written (with a blunt pointer) on your forearm. The cranial nerves carry these sensations from your face, and also the **special senses** of smell, vision, taste, hearing and balance.

On the **motor** side, damage to a peripheral nerve presents as **weakness** of the muscles that the nerve supplies. Weakness may be mild and only shown up by difficulties in dressing, or dropping and moving objects: there may be associated muscle wasting. If the problem is in the CNS, there may be muscle **spasticity**, as after a stroke. There may also be added movements, such as a tremor, and **incoordination of movement,** as with disorders of the cerebellum.

Disease of the brain interferes with your higher cortical (**cognitive**) function, i.e. your intellectual skills, with loss of knowledge and understanding, reducing your ability to recognise people or situations, or to understand and perform mental and physical tasks.

A doctor uses a mental state series of questions to identify whether your thinking capacity is diminished, your thought process is abnormal or whether both of these problems are present. You should ask yourself the same questions, and be ready to discuss them with your doctor. However, your assessment also depends on having sufficient insight to appreciate any abnormality should this be present.

Mental State Questions

Has there been alteration in your **behaviour**, such as lack of attention to your personal appearance and hygiene? How do you feel, is there a change in your **mood**, such as intolerance, irritability, disturbance of your sleep patterns, anxiety, depression or suicidal thoughts? Has your **speed of reaction** changed, such as your rate of thought, speech and deed; has your carrying out of mechanical tasks, such as dressing, feeding, typing and computing, changed?

What has happened to your **concentration**; have your attention span and task completion rate changed? How is your **memory**: short term, for tasks you had stood up to do, reliance on lists and losing your glasses and bus pass, and missing trains or planes; medium term memory of current world events; long term memory of your past experiences? Are you well **orientated** in time and space: time, day, month, year, train times; where are you now, can you visualise a frequently taken walk?

Cognitive and higher cortical function: can you read and write, recite a poem you know well and calculate sums to your expected ability, can you analyse problems and undertake critical and creative thinking in your field of interest?

Have you had any **abnormal** beliefs or experiences related to your environment, your body or your mind; were they in the form of hallucinations, phobias, compulsions or mania? It is likely you have ticked a few boxes in the above, but you probably also did in your, forties, when you were fully active! However, the abnormalities of this paragraph, when your **thought processes are abnormal**, and also **severe problems** with depression and progressive mental deterioration should be discussed with your doctor.

Headache

Pain is the most frequent neurological symptom, particularly headache and backache. You may have suffered from headaches throughout your life, particularly if you are subject to **migraine**. In this case you know how to recognise the symptoms, and the best way to reduce their effect. However, a new severe or persistent headache requires investigation.

Blood is particularly irritating to the brain, but the most severe bleeds, from rupture of a congenital aneurysm, usually occurs in your middle life. **Strokes** (page 44) are usually due to **blocking** of a brain artery, but diseased arteries may **bleed**, particularly if you are on anticoagulants.

Any disease expanding the contents of the skull gives rise to headaches. Specific examples are **cancers** and **infections**. Cancers may be **primary**, arising from part of the brain, or **secondary**, having spread through the blood stream from a cancer elsewhere in the body. Your doctor may see signs of the **raised pressure** inside your skull by looking into your eyes with an ophthalmoscope.

Other symptoms that may occur with raised intracranial pressure include: dizziness, vertigo (the world spinning around you, or you around the world), blackouts and drowsiness progressing to unconsciousness. **Epilepsy** (seizure) is a sudden discharge of energy through the brain producing convulsive movement of the body, accompanied by loss of consciousness, and often biting of your tongue and incontinence of urine. Although the late onset of these symptoms is often associated with a rise of intracranial pressure, it can be a congenital problem, be due to **drugs** or be residual effect of a stroke or trauma.

There may be abnormalities of the movement or sensation in parts of your body, due to generalised or to the localised effect of a brain cancer or other disease. Unsteadiness on your feet is termed **ataxia**, it can be related to damage in different parts of the motor system in the brain. If the damage is to the primary motor area of the brain, there is usually **paralysis** of the opposite side of the body, where movement is stiff (**spastic hemiplegia**).

Infection of the coverings of the brain (**meningitis**), the brain itself (**encephalitis**) or a cerebral abscess are relatively uncommon, but the aged are not immune, and the conditions can spread in institutions. Additional signs of meningitis are a generalised rash, drowsiness, a rigid neck and an aversion to bright light (**photophobia**). Meningitis is usually bacterial in origin, whereas encephalitis is usually caused by a virus: in tropical areas there are a number of worms, fungi and malaria that can affect the brain, but these are rare in the UK.

Other causes of headache include a high blood pressure, and problems of vision and hearing (pages 114 and 118).

Two specific problems can produce severe facial pain. **Trigeminal neuralgia** involves one of the three sensory divisions of the fifth cranial nerve (usually the middle and lower). It commonly starts late in life and produced excruciating, knife-like paroxysms of pain along the distribution of the nerve over your face and lower jaw. There may be a precipitating trigger point, such as when shaving. It does not occur at night and usually only affects one side of the face. The cause of the pain is ill understood, but the severity takes you rapidly to your doctor for advice.

If you have your first infection with **herpes zoster** (the chicken pox virus) in later life, it attacks a peripheral nerve, usually around the chest (**shingles**): the pain comes before a skin rash, along the line of the nerve, often leading to the misdiagnosis of a heart attack. The rash then erupts and scabs; these signs slowly disappear, but troublesome pain can persist.

Another variant (and why it is included at this point) is when the same virus attacks the seventh cranial nerve – a condition known as the **Ramsay–Hunt Syndrome**. Again the pain may precede a skin rash on the front of the ear and outside of the adjacent eye. In this case there may be other features related to the seventh nerve – it is the motor nerve to the facial muscles, and there may be weakness or paralysis of all or part of the same side of the face. Other features are vertigo, hearing loss and dizziness. You should see your doctor early on, as antiviral medicines can reduce the immediate and longterm persistence of symptoms.

The seventh nerve is also subject to a bout of paralysis, with usually minimal pain – a condition known as **Bell's palsy**. Although it is probably viral in origin, antiviral agents have not been so effective, steroids may help. Both these conditions usually recover fully in three to six months, but persistent pain and/or paralysis are very disturbing complications.

Backache

Backache is common in old age. The back is a complex collection of bones, ligaments and muscles, as well as housing the spinal cord; it thus provides a large number of possible causes for your pain. This presents a problem for your GP who has to identify possible curable causes and the few serious problems, from the majority that require long term symptomatic treatment.

Acute **muscle sprains** and **torn ligaments** are likely to be related to sudden twists or falls, although there may be no history of injury, or you may wake up with the pain, having slept in an unusual position. These injuries usually get better, but healing slows with age and it may take a number of months.

Arthritis of the joints between the vertebrae that make up your backbone is common. Inflammation around these joints is painful, and the enlargement and deformity of the joints can put pressure on the spinal nerves that pass nearby. Your bones also get softer and may start to **collapse**, adding to the problem. A general term often used for the pain is **lumbago**. Your neck is more mobile than the rest of your spine and is particularly susceptible to these changes, where they are called **cervical spondylitis**. Nerve pressure in your neck can give tingling, numbness and weakness down your arms.

So, what can be done to improve the symptoms? The initial treatment is pain relief with painkillers and possibly antiarthritic medicines; this is followed by graded exercises so that your back muscles are strong enough to prevent nerve pressure. Severe nerve compression gives pain and weakness related to the nerve involved; in the leg this is termed **sciatica**. These severe symptoms usually ease, but if they progress they require further investigation, to see if a procedure can be undertaken to remove the cause. Other forms of pain relief include injection of the plexuses of nerves supplying the limbs.

Cancers starting in the backbone are unusual, but it is a common site for **secondary spread** from other cancers, such as in the lung, breast and prostate. Symptoms are persistent and progressive backache is managed by your cancer specialist. Sudden collapse of an affected vertebra can produce paralysis of the limbs and requires emergency, usually surgical, decompression.

Pressure on nerves at other sites is uncommon; one example is from a **cervical rib**, an abnormality in your neck that may not trouble you until late in life, when pain and weakness of an arm take you to your GP. Other pressure sites are around the knee, elbow and wrist, the latter compressing the median nerve is the **carpal tunnel syndrome**. **Multiple sclerosis** is a disease of the nerve sheaths occurring in young adults, and **motor neurone disease**, a progressive destruction of the motor nerves in the spinal cord, occurs on middle life.

More common in later life is a generalised **peripheral neuropathy**. Here the problem is primarily reduced sensation of your fingers and toes, but this may be accompanied by disturbing tingling or other sensations. Burning toes at night is probably related, but is of an ill-defined cause and is usually treated with vitamin supplements.

A 'glove and stocking' peripheral neuropathy is common in diabetes. It also occurs in liver and renal failure, with certain drugs, with some cancers and in vitamin deficiencies, particularly when associated with alcohol abuse. Muscle weakness may also accompany some of these neuropathies, but **muscle diseases**, such as myasthenia gravis and the myotonias appear in early life.

Parkinson's Disease

Parkinson's disease is a disorder of movement, due to abnormalities of the motor pathways in the brain. The cause of these changes is unknown. The primary disease is one of old age, usually starting after 60; secondary causes include toxins, drugs, recurrent trauma and the late stage of many degenerative diseases. Whereas the diagnosis was traditionally on clinical grounds, modern scans have shown more diversity of the brain abnormalities than expected, and the term Parkinson's syndrome is more appropriate.

Clinically, there is muscle stiffness and **rigidity**, this giving rise to a paucity of movement (**akinesia**); the **tremor**, initially described by Parkinson, is a later feature. The initial mild rigidity slowly progresses: in your face there is a lack of expression, a mask-like rigidity and a serpentine stare. Chewing and swallowing are slow and speech is monotonous, weak and slurred. Rigidity and stiffness of the limbs and back produce a stoop and small forward steps; stopping is difficult once forward motion has started. The difficulty to control movement means that if you fall you go down like a pole.

Your writing is small and spidery, tone is increased and later there may be cogwheel rigidity; your muscles fatigue easily. The characteristic 'pill-rolling' sign is between your thumb, and the index and middle fingers. The mask-like face makes it difficult to assess your mood: the locked-in effect is accompanied by an emotional lability that may progress to depression. Intellect, memory and concentration are preserved until late in the disease.

The disease progresses unpredictably, over 10–15 years. Rigidity of your chest movement increases susceptibility to chest infections with subsequent slow resolution: this eventually can be a lethal complication.

Management is directed at preventing falls with rails, supports and other home improvements, exercise to maintain limb and chest mobility, and easy-to-manage clothing. Maintain a close liaison with your doctor, as specialist referral provides access to the latest medication in the field, and this may provide you with marked improvement.

Trauma

As you advance in age you probably have given up high contact sports, but you are still susceptible to road traffic accidents, and have an increased tendency to **fall**. With severe **head injuries** you are likely to end up in hospital and be fully assessed and monitored. However, there is one form of head injury that can occur in later life after relatively minor trauma.

The human brain shrinks with age and by so doing puts the vessels passing to it from the inside the skull on a stretch. The stretched veins are thin walled and can be torn with only mild trauma. The resultant blood clot (**subdural haematoma**) collects over the surface of the brain and may gradually expand. Unless the clot is over an area controlling a specific function, such as the motor area, the effects may be very gradual, and misinterpreted as 'ageing'. The deterioration may be missed or misinterpreted and your doctor has to be on the lookout for unexplained deterioration of this type, as the clot can be drained with minor surgery.

Severe head trauma can produce loss of consciousness, and it is worth considering other causes of **coma** when you encounter **unconsciousness** in the elderly. **Failure of many organs** and systems can result in coma, including kidney, liver, respiratory and endocrine, particularly too little thyroid, while **diabetics** may become unconscious on account of too little insulin or an overdose. The brain is sensitive to **hypothermia**, and the **toxic effects** of severe infection (such as malaria) and drugs, e.g. an overdose, alcohol or an anaesthetic. The causes of a **raised intracranial pressure** considered above (tumour, haemorrhage and an abscess) can all produce coma, and a period of unconsciousness follows a major epileptic attack.

A classification of the level of unconsciousness has been developed for trauma and is called the **Glasgow Coma Scale**. This determines your response to commands and verbal ability; results range from 3 to 15, the latter being fully conscious. If you come across an unconscious person, call for help and make sure there is nothing blocking the subject's airway.

Vision

Vision is one of your prized possessions, enabling you to read, write, watch TV and appreciate your surroundings: it markedly influences your quality of life. Conversely, loss of vision in later life is severely disabling, and may lead to loss of independence.

It is therefore essential you have annual visual checks to find any correctable defects at an early stage. These checks include the assessment of **visual acuity** (how small a print you can read); **perimetry** (are there any blotted out areas in your field of vision); **tonometry** (is the pressure in your eye too high); and **ophthalmoscopy** (on looking into the eye, are the nerve and blood vessels normal).

Some deterioration of vision occurs with ageing in everyone. This is not usually disabling, although diabetics suffer these changes at an earlier age, and they may be more severe; changes may also be increased if you are obese or hypertensive. *Figure 19.1* is a diagram of the anatomy of an eyeball, showing its layers. Light enters through the front and images are focused by the lens onto back of the eye, where sensors detect the image and pass this information to your brain for interpretation.

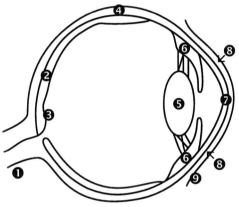

Figure 19.1 Eyeball

1. The nerve (optic) to the eye.
2. Retina: the inner sensitive layer that receives images focused on it by the lens.
3. Macula the most sensitive part of the retina, directly opposite the lens.
4. The outer firm covering of the eyeball.
5. Lens
6. Ring of muscle forming the coloured iris in front of the lens. It adjusts the size of the pupil, small to stop blinding light and large in the dark. The muscle also adjusts the shape of the lens to focus images onto the retina.
7. Transparent, bulging cornea: the front part of the eyeball.
8. Arrows indicate the only part of the eyeball that you can see.
9. Thin transparent conjunctiva covering the cornea: it extends over the inside of your eyelids to seal the eyeball from the outside world.

In your 40s, appreciation of small print in newspapers and on dress labels becomes difficult, and spectacles are the norm: although for some people, who were short sighted originally, these changes may make it easier to see!

Two severe problems occur predominantly in old age – cataract and macular degeneration.

A **cataract** is opacity of the lens of your eye, it is commoner in diabetics and may follow previous eye trauma. Cataracts reduce your appreciation of detail and of colour. Night vision is reduced and daytime images become foggy – just misty at first, but this becoming denser. Bright lights can dazzle, and occasionally you may see double.

A reliable operation is available to remove cataracts, in which the lens is emulsified and aspirated, and then replaced with an artificial one. Although the original results from cataract surgery were unpredictable, when bandages were removed after three weeks, current techniques make them remarkably good. The procedure is usually undertaken as a day case, return of colour vision is immediate, and recovery is complete within a few days.

Nevertheless, no surgery should be undertaken without careful consideration. The decision, made by you and your surgeon, is when a cataract, in one or both eyes, is markedly interfering with your normal lifestyle – preventing you reading, watching TV and undertaking desirable activities. When both eyes are affected, they are treated at separate operations, the worst eye first.

Macular degeneration is the most common cause of irreversible visual loss over the age of 65. The **central area** (macula) of the retina, where you appreciate the most precise visual information, degenerates, giving loss of central vision, with blurring, distortion and loss of colour. Wet and dry forms occur, the latter being less aggressive, but both show chronic progression. Vitamin supplements may help, as vitamins C and E influence pigment formation in the eye, and injection of certain drugs into the eye may slow progression of the disease (vitamins C and E are antioxidants and are present in fresh fruit [particularly tropical], and fresh green vegetables, tomatoes, oils and cereals). Other treatment measures are strict control of blood sugar levels and blood pressure, stopping smoking and avoidance of exposure to bright light and sunlight.

Glaucoma is increased pressure in the eyeball due to impeded drainage of the fluid from the front of the eyeball, Normal pressure is 10–20 mm Hg and pressures above this level can damage the visual nerve fibres, with potential blindness. The condition can occur at any age but is commoner in diabetics, has a familial tendency and is present in 1:100 of the population over 40.

Tests may detect increases in pressure before any symptoms, but when they occur presentation is with a sever headache above the affected eye. There is also blurring of vision, coloured halos around objects and loss of the outer aspect of the visual field. Eye drops can reduce the tension and are prescribed as an emergency. For recurrent attacks, surgery is needed to provide an alternative fluid drainage route.

Increased pressure within the eyeball occurs from other causes, such as hypertension and diabetes; these require management of their cause, but are not so serious, and do not require emergency attention as with glaucoma.

Diabetes and hypertension also produce changes in the vasculature of the eye, known as **retinopathy**. The arteries change and there may be small bleeds. In diabetics, the effects may be proliferative or nonproliferative: in the latter there are not only haemorrhages, but also fine new vessel formation that scars the retina, blocking its visual function. The effects are most marked when the changes are in the macular region. **Diabetic retinopathy** is the commonest form of blindness in diabetics.

Retinal detachment is a tear in the inner visual receptive layer of the eye, allowing fluid to get beneath it and lift it off. Such tears may be due to degenerative changes in the retina, but also occur after trauma and infection, and also in diabetics. The presentation is with a dark shadow across the visual field, and there may be accompanying specks and bright sparks.

Various surgical manoevers, applied to the outside of the eyeball to encourage reattachment, or inside, to remove fluid from beneath the retina, help recovery.

Floaters (black spots) and transparent films in the visual field are common in old age. These are often due to changes at the interface between the viscous fluid in the back chamber of the eye and the retina. Floaters may also be due to small bits of clot from arterial disease passing through retinal arteries. These may give rise to temporary (and very rarely permanent) visual loss (**amaurosis fujax**): the episodes require medical investigation and should be reported to your doctor.

The eyelids and the front of the eyeball are subject to infection (**conjunctivitis**) at every age, with abscesses of the eyelashes and glands along the edge of the lids. There may be a sticky discharge, redness of the eye and pain, all requiring attention, with possibly analgesics and antibiotics if they persist.

Tears are required to lubricate the front of the eye, to wash away debris and facilitate lid and eye movement. If tear production is reduces, drops of synthetic tears are an available substitute.

The multiplicity of potential problems that may affect your eyesight, some of which have serious effects on your vision, emphasise the importance of regular (at least annual) eye checks. Glasses should be of the right prescription for near and far vision. They must be up to date, well cleaned and looked after without scratches. Care must be taken not to loose them, but an old pair must always be available just in case. Look out for a large magnifying glass (possibly with an attached light source) to have available when you later need it, and learn tricks with your electronic equipment to greatly enlarge text and other items. Bright illumination facilitates all close visual tasks.

Fitness and a balanced diet are important, as in all health issues, and every effort must be taken to keep your blood pressure and blood glucose levels within normal limits. Smoking is harmful in many eye conditions and if possible this should be stopped.

Good lighting is needed for the partially sighted, to avoid bumping into things, and as sight further deteriorates, a white stick warns others of your disability, and they will ensure they are not in your way: they are also usually helpful. Bright lighting and bright sunlight should be avoided, and sunglasses can help. Subdued lighting allows the eyes to relax, and breaks should be taken from prolonged reading or staring, as in sewing or artwork. When medication, such as drops, are prescribed, they should be taken as directed.

When caring for others, the above rules apply equally: learn how to extend the subject's neck, pull the lower lid down and place a single drop in the gutter between the lid and the eyeball.

The Royal National Institute of Blind People (RNIB) provides extensive advice in their literature and website that should be accessed for further information.

Hearing

Good hearing brings to you the joys of music and theatre, and provides information from individuals, radio, TV and innumerable other sources. It enables you to communicate, to debate, to be aware of activity around you and alert you to unexpected danger.

This facility deteriorates with age, age-related-deafness having its own title of **presbycusis**: this is common after the age of 60, and affects 50% of people over the age of 70. The process, however, is slow, gradual and not inevitable.

The problem may be familial, and is accentuated by various factors, including prolonged exposure to noise (e.g. working in a quarry or mine), stress, and the usual health culprits of obesity, smoking, alcohol and high blood pressure. Other causes of deafness include local disease of the ear and its nerve supply, such as infection and trauma, together with diseases of the brain, such as strokes, trauma and tumours. **Toxins** affecting hearing include pesticides and solvents, and some drugs, such as antimalarial and gentamycin.

Whereas in many of the above conditions deafness will be looked for, the deafness of old age is **insidious in onset**, you may choose to deny or ignore it for a long time, and it can be quite advanced by the time of diagnosis. **Warning signs** include: turning up the volume of the TV set; having difficulty in following a conversation, particularly if there is a lot of background noise, or a number of people are talking at the same time; asking someone to repeat a question, to speak up or to stop mumbling; and having difficulty conversing on the telephone.

When you begin to notice deafness, you will also note many other **disadvantages**: the higher frequency voices, particularly women and children, are difficult to understand; there is reduction in your ability to communicate; it is socially inconvenient and frustrating, particularly if you like discussion; you can miss announcements, such as in an airport, and alarm bells; you start to be ignored, affecting your position in a community, with loss of personal esteem; as the condition progresses you miss information and stimulation, leading to loss of interest and giving up; the accumulation of these factors can lead to loneliness and depression.

The ear is concerned with both **hearing** and **balance**. Your hearing is from noise initiating **vibration** of your eardrums: each is a membrane (**tympanic membrane**) placed, out of sight, across the ear canal about three centimetres from the outside. These vibrations are transmitted through the ear and converted into **nerve impulses**, these in turn, are passed to the **brain** for interpretation.

Although vibrations can be transmitted to the same nerve through **bone**, they lack the definition of those from the eardrum. The problems of old age and their management relate primarily to the reduced appreciation of vibration from an intact eardrum. Very occasionally they can be accompanied by additional noises, generated within the ear, or the increased volume of certain tones.

Your **voice** also changes with age. There is reduction of power from your lungs; your vocal cords have a reduced ability to approximate and articulate; and reduced lubrication of your larynx combine to give a low volume, monotonal, uninteresting 'senile' voice. The male voice tends to become higher pitched and the female the reverse,

Hearing is **quantified** using audiology and is measured in units (decibels) of hearing loss (dB HL): mild loss is 20–40 dB HL: severe over 70 dB HL.

SO – what can be done to reverse this situation? The first thing is to **warn people** of your disability – they will usually appreciate, accommodate and adapt their approach. Initially it is important for them to attract your attention to let you know you are being talked to. Choose a **quiet**, non-public spot, without extraneous noise, such as background music or announcements.

When talking you should **face each other**, additional information being communicated through gesture and lip reading (although the latter takes time and training) – gesture can be particularly useful when wishing to change the topic of conversation. Ask the person to talk slowly, articulate precisely, talk a little louder (but not to shout), and not to have anything in their mouth, such as chewing gum. Difficulties may be overcome by the additional **written word**.

When communicating with a deaf person, show patience, and be positive, cheerful and courteous.

When you are **getting deaf**: look after your ears (do not blame them!); maintain good local hygiene – washing and drying the outside carefully; do not put anything, such as pencils, pens or keys, into them; water can be run out by leaning your neck to one side, if persistent, a cotton wool bud can be gently twisted around just inside the ear canal – removal of wax should be left to your doctor.

Avoid public swimming pools where ear infection can be caught and, if there is any suggestion of infection, with pain or discharge, consult your doctor; only use drops that have been prescribed specifically for you; in general avoid noisy places, such as open air music festivals and demonstrations, or situations where you could sustain a head injury.

Hearing Aids

There are many ways of improving your hearing: **earpieces** and **headphones** focus sound and remove extraneous noise, they can be plugged into music centres of all kinds, phones, both mobile and home, radios and TV sets.

You should consider some form of amplification when deafness is markedly interfering with your quality of life. The number of **hearing aids** is confusing. Some are **implanted** under the skin and send coded messages direct to the nerve. These are expensive, require personal programming and a lot of training – they are better suited to childhood and long standing deafness than an ageing problem: they are not considered further.

Hearing aids are usually placed behind the ear, within the ear or within the ear canal: there are also versions that attach to spectacles. The **cost** varies from under a hundred to a few thousand pounds, so you should seriously consider the free versions supplied by the NHS. They consist of **three parts**: a microphone that receives information; an amplifier than magnifies and modifies it; and a speaker that directs it at your eardrum. You can have one for each ear if needed, the combination also helping to determine the direction from which sound is coming.

Amplified sound is different from the sound you are used to and it takes a short while to adapt. Some adjustment may also be needed if the sound is too loud, if there is too much background noise, or there are various whistles or hisses. A great deal of research continues to address all these aspects, but if hearing is limiting your activities, an aid can revolutionise your life. Take good care of it, clean it with a damp cloth, do not immerse it in fluid or cover it with hair spray, switch it off when not needed, change spent batteries early and make sure none of the bits are left around for children and grandchildren to eat.

A valuable innovation has been the introduction of **loop systems**. These are defined encircled areas (transient listening environments) where an unlimited number of people with hearing aids can tune into a central transmitter to receive specific messages. Examples of their use are in airport lounges, railway stations and places of worship. Loop stations work to defined International Specifications. Not all hearing aids tune into the same frequencies, but all those supplied by the NHS do so. This form of focused communication is likely to increase.

Vertigo

When you move your head, treacle-like fluid flows around a system of three semicircular channels, set at right angles to each other and situated deeply in your ear. Fine sensory hairs within the channels note fluid movement and are able to tell your brain where your head has reached. Alteration of these sensations can confuse the brain producing the condition of **vertigo** – the world spinning round you, or you around the world.

The commonest form of vertigo is **benign paroxysmal postural vertigo** (BPPV) in which a crystal is formed in the treacle. When this lodges and gets stuck on a hair, it confuses the brain and results in vertigo, and this can precipitate a **fall**. You may feel sick and vomit, and your eyes may flick to one side (**nystagmus**).

BPPV can occur with head movements in bed and particularly on sudden looking upwards. Attacks my last a few seconds to a few minutes. They occur at any age, are twice as common in women and are commoner in the elderly. They may accompany other diseases or occur postoperatively, but there are often no precipitating factors. BPPV is usually self limiting over a few weeks, but tablets can help the nausea. If it persists or is recurrent, specific head manoevres move the crystal out of harms way. Once diagnosed, an Epley manoevre is usually successful in alleviating the problem. A trained individual can undertake the manoevre – and this includes you. It is written up on the Internet, but requires patients to learn and wait in the set positions long enough for the procedure to work.

Other forms of vertigo occur in motion sickness and disease of the inner ear, such as Meniere's.

Meniere's Disease

Meniere's disease can occur throughout life, but as it usually starts between the ages of 40 – 60, it is more common in the aged. The cause is much debated, but the symptoms are due to increased fluid in the organ of balance. Usually, but not invariably, the disease is confined to one ear. There are four principle symptoms that may occur singly or in any combination, and occur in episodes: a feeling of **fullness** in the ear; **deafness**; **vertigo**; and **tinnitus** (buzzing or other noises in the ear).

Attacks are unpredictable, without prodromal symptoms, and last for a few minutes to several hours: they may recur within weeks or years. In vertigo, everything seems to spin around you, and you loose your sense of balance. A severe episode of Meniere's disease may start with a **'drop attack'**, in which the sufferer can be injured, and this may be accompanied by marked sweating, nausea, vomiting and diarrhoea.

Tinnitus is the term given to buzzing, ringing and whistling in the ear, it is a common symptom in many ear diseases, and in chronic cases the sufferer has often to learn how to suppress the symptoms, as they are difficult to control. In Meniere's disease, the tinnitus and deafness only last for the duration of the attack.

A number of factors have been implicated in the initiation of an attack, and also as the possible cause of the disease. These include: exposure to severe noise, stress, viral infection, smoking, alcohol and various medications, including aspirin. Treatment has been directed at controlling these factors, together with salt restriction, diuretic and control of blood pressure: acupuncture, reflexology and relaxation techniques may also help.

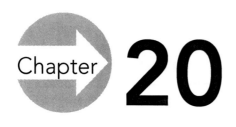

Dementia

Kris Warren

It is always important to remember that poor memory is a **symptom and not a disease.**

Dementia is one of the causes, but there are also many other conditions that can affect your memory.

As we get older, a mild degree of forgetfulness can be considered normal. However, dementia is **not a normal part of ageing**, and represents brain changes causing increasingly severe memory problems.

One of the reasons that many people view dementia as part of getting older is that it is a very common condition in old age. 1 in 3 people over the age of 65 years go on to die with a form of dementia.

Definition of dementia

Dementia is a clinical syndrome, characterised by a progressive impairment of multiple areas of your cognitive function that then interfere with your ability to function independently, in everyday situations, at home or at work.

If you have memory problems that are of recent onset (less than 3 months), that come and go or show signs of improvement, these are not dementia, and are caused by other conditions (e.g. physical illness, mood disturbance, stress)

Causes of dementia

Dementia is a common illness affecting older people living in the community, as well as in care homes. The prevalence and incidence increases exponentially with age.

The Alzheimer's Society estimates that there are 800,000 people in the UK living with dementia. With the ageing population, the numbers of people with dementia is set to increase, with double the number of cases within the next 30 years.

Dementia can also occur in younger age groups, and there are about 18,500 people with dementia aged under 65 years in the UK.

In terms of prevalence, dementia is one of the more common long term conditions. The prevalence of dementia is 5% in those aged above 65 years, rising to 20% in those aged above 80 years. The prevalence is much higher amongst residents living in care homes, with 80% affected.

Most people with dementia have yet to be diagnosed. The Alzheimer's Society estimates that currently only 44% of people with dementia in England, Wales and Northern Ireland have received a diagnosis.

The Government brought out a National Dementia Strategy in 2009 with the aim of improving the care for people with dementia and their carers, focusing on improved awareness, early diagnosis and "living well" with dementia, from diagnosis to death.

Types of Dementia

There are many different types of dementia, with different underlying causes and differing presentations.

Alzheimer's dementia

This is the most common dementia. It is a degenerative disease affecting the brain, starting in the hippocampus (memory area). It causes progressive structural damage and changes in neurotransmitter levels, with loss of cholinergic activity.

Onset is insidious. If you are a relative or carer of someone with Alzheimer's disease, you may not notice anything initially, but later when problems arise, you may be able to look back and retrospectively recognise that little memory problems had been going on for some time.

Short-term memory (memory for recent things) is affected early. But as things progress, other thinking abilities are also affected.

Progression is variable in speed, but generally there is a slow gradual deterioration over 5-15 years.

Vascular dementia

Vascular dementia is another common cause of dementia. There are differing subtypes of vascular dementia, with varying clinical features. Dementia occurs as a consequence of multiple strokes in the cortex of the brain or multiple subcortical (lacunar) strokes. It is now recognised that small vessel disease in the deep white matter and lacunar strokes are more important than strokes arising from larger vessel disease. High blood pressure in midlife and laterlife is a key cause of small vessel disease.

Onset is classically sudden, with stepwise deterioration following plateau periods, although some people experience a gradual decline as in Alzheimer's dementia. Cognitive impairment is patchy (due to preservation of function in nonaffected parts of the brain).

Progression is more variable than Alzheimer's dementia, and depends on if and when further strokes occur.

Mixed dementia

It is becoming increasingly accepted that the majority of people with dementia have mixed disease, with features of both Alzheimer's and vascular disease.

Other rarer types of dementia

Lewy Body Dementia

A person with this dementia characteristically has visual hallucinations, fluctuations in confusion and falls, associated with their progressive dementia.

Frontotemporal dementia

This condition causes a dementia at a younger age (typically under 65 years), with noticeable change in personality and behaviour early in the course.

Dementia of Parkinson's disease

This can occur when someone has had Parkinson's disease for many years. Their thinking slows down, just as their movements slow down.

Primary and secondary brain tumours

People with brain tumours may present with headaches and other symptoms relating to increased pressure in the head. But they can also present with a gradual decline in cognition, appearing to be a dementia. A brain scan will detect a tumour

In addition, there are numerous other causes of dementia, including Alcohol-related dementia, Posterior cortical atrophy, Creutzfeldt-Jakob disease, Huntington's disease and Multiple sclerosis – to name a few. Dementia associated with HIV and syphilis infections can improve with appropriate treatment.

Conditions that can masquerade as dementia

Delirium is acute confusion, and therefore has a recent onset. It presents with disturbed consciousness and fluctuations. It is associated with acute medical illness.

Older people (and children) have a lower confusion threshold than younger adults, because of reduced cerebral reserve. Therefore, minor illnesses (e.g. a urinary tract infection) can precipitate delirium, whereas a major insult (e.g. encephalitis) would be required to cause delirium in a younger adult

Delirium often occurs in patients with preexisting dementia, causing acute-on-chronic confusion. People with more advanced dementia have a particularly low confusion threshold. Hence, something as trivial as moving to a new environment may be sufficient to precipitate acute confusion in these patients (translocation effect).

Depression, anxiety and **stress** can cause memory problems, through causing distraction and poor attention and concentration. If information is not taken in properly in the first place, it is not recalled, and therefore the person can appear very forgetful.

Mild cognitive impairment is a similar condition but is not severe enough to represent dementia. A proportion of people with MCI go on to develop dementia in the coming years.

Learning difficulties can appear as dementia, but the key difference is that the problems are life-long.

Various medical conditions can also present as a dementia but can reverse with treatment. These include hypothyroidism, vitamin B_{12} and folate deficiencies, and epilepsy.

Drugs and alcohol (intoxication) can also cause confusion that might appear to be dementia. Common relevant drugs are sedatives, opiates (strong pain killers), corticosteroids and antiParkinson's drugs.

Sensory impairment, such as severe hearing or visual impairment can also cause problems misattributed as confusion.

Symptoms of Dementia

A person with dementia has variable insight into their condition. People with Alzheimer's disease, in particular, have limited awareness of their memory problem, do not recognise how severe it is and are generally unconcerned. It is much more noticeable to their family and friends. It is as if they forget that they are forgetful.

Accordingly, it is more likely for you to notice that someone else is developing dementia than it is for you to notice your own dementia. If you are very aware and very worried about memory problems, other causes may be responsible (such as anxiety and stress).

A key symptom is memory loss. This is predominantly difficulty recalling recent events or new information (short-term memory loss). You may notice that your relative or friend forgets conversations, appointments, and where they put things. They may become repetitive. The memories for things that happened many years ago are often very well established and remain intact, even in the later stages of the illness.

Short-term memory loss is the main feature of Alzheimer's dementia. Other dementias can also have prominent memory impairment, but it is not universal.

Dementia is defined by the presence of multiple areas of cognitive loss.

Other changes that you might notice include: difficulties finding words for things and problems with language (dysphasia); difficulties with planning, organising, completing tasks and problem solving (executive function); problems with attention and concentration; disorientation; impaired reasoning ability and judgement.

Often people describe these impairments in terms of forgetfulness ("I can't remember names and words" for dysphasia, "I can't remember what I was going to do" for executive dysfunction). But these are not true memory problems, and reflect damage in different parts of the brain.

Dementia can also cause subtle changes in personality. For example, the person may become more irritable or more mellow. Again, this is something you are more likely to notice happening with someone else, rather than yourself.

Dementia can also change someone's behaviour. For example, they may become aggressive, sexually disinhibited, or neglect themselves. However, many people with dementia retain good social skills, and in brief conversation may not appear to have any problems.

People with dementia can also occasionally develop symptoms of depression, delusions, paranoid ideas or hallucinations.

Over time, people with dementia have increasing difficulty managing their own affairs and carrying out normal day-to-day tasks. If you think that your memory is very poor but you continue to be able to manage all everyday living tasks with no change in your function or abilities, it is likely that problems other than dementia are responsible for your memory loss.

Making a Diagnosis of Dementia

Making a diagnosis of dementia is not a quick and easy thing. There is no simple test that confirms or excludes the diagnosis. Assessment involves a doctor talking to you or your loved one, gathering additional collateral information from relatives or friends, carrying out some memory tests, a physical examination and investigations (blood tests, heart trace and brain scan). All the results are then reviewed to consider the diagnosis. In rare cases, more extensive investigation is required.

Importance of making an early diagnosis of dementia

Historically, professional attitudes towards dementia have been negative, focusing on supportive and protective care in advanced stages. Management has been crisis-led, with intervention only occurring when behavioural problems make it unavoidable. It is still the case that many people with dementia present for the first time, to their GP or to A&E, at a time of crisis, e.g. when their carer can no longer cope.

There has been a considerable change in attitude with the arrival of the dementia medications, leading to demands for a proactive approach to detect people in earliest stage of dementia.

Early diagnosis allows you access to full assessment and investigation, with consideration of alternative diagnoses and on rare occasions treatment of reversible causes. It allows early treatment with drugs for Alzheimer's disease, delaying progression of the disease, and appropriate and timely referral to support services. Importantly, early diagnosis allows you the opportunity to discuss current and future healthcare plans, (e.g. advanced directives), and to make legal and financial plans (e.g. lasting power of attorney), before cognitive impairment is too severe. It can also allow access to various benefits and state allowances.

Early diagnosis is also beneficial for you if you are a carer for someone developing dementia. It leads to better understanding of behavioural and personality changes experienced by your loved one, and earlier assessment for carer stress, with timely referral to support services. (Carer stress can lead to you developing psychological or physical illness). It gives time to discuss future health and social care plans with your loved one, before cognition deteriorates too significantly. This results in shared decisions, reducing the burden of your responsibility. It may reduce the number of crises, and such situations can sometimes be irretrievable, and can lead to premature entry into a care home.

Reasons for why a diagnosis of dementia is often delayed relate to a counter-productive cycle of stigma, fear and misunderstanding, leading to lack of action. Stigma relating to the condition leads to a lack of open discussion. People have the false belief that it is a normal part of ageing or that nothing can be done. Healthcare professionals are also guilty, failing to seek or offer help.

The outcome is prevention or delay in referral for diagnostic assessment and onward referral for appropriate treatment and care.

Indicators for possible dementia

If you are worried about your memory or concerned about someone you know, the first point of contact is your GP. You or the GP may also notice other indicators that raise the possibility of dementia.

Possible indicators include:

- Symptoms suggestive of memory problems or other cognitive difficulties, e.g. difficulty carrying out tasks, disorientation, and/or a change in personality or behaviour, e.g. apathy, irritability, aggression
- A deterioration in function, such as difficulties at work, forgetting to pay bills, forgetting to take medication or accidental overdoses, neglecting appearance and hygiene
- A change in circumstances, such as neglecting the home, or becoming socially isolated or housebound, through no longer being able to use the phone or public transport
- Accidents such as falls, burns, road traffic accidents
- Frequent visits to the GP or A&E.

There may be many different things that can trigger a question of dementia. Diagnosis involves the GP carrying out a dementia screen and then, if appropriate, referral to a specialist memory service for assessment and investigation.

Management of Dementia

The aim is to maintain independence, and to manage and support the person within their own home for as long as possible. If this fails, appropriate alternative long term care is required.

Education about the diagnosis.

Understanding more about the condition can improve your ability to cope with it. Receiving a diagnosis may even be a relief, recognising that there is an actual medical illness causing the changes that you are aware of, legitimising your difficulties.

This can include appropriate treatment for the reversible medical conditions that can appear as dementia.

There are also drugs for Alzheimer's dementia (Acetylcholinesterase inhibitors) that slow the progression of the illness, and there are various treatments to modify the risk factors for vascular disease and to reduce to risk of further stroke.

Optimise function through maintaining health

This involves treating other medical conditions that might exacerbate confusion for a person with dementia.

Treatment of all concomitant illnesses – medical (physical illnesses, delirium) and psychiatric (e.g. depression, anxiety) – can improve confusion. Use of all medications needs to be monitored to ensure that they are appropriate and do not exacerbate confusion.

Lifestyle measures

Adopting lifestyle measure can help you cope with memory difficulties, and minimise the impact of cognitive problems on your day-to-day life. These include:

- developing memory management techniques
- establishing and maintaining familiar routines
- maintaining good nutrition and limiting alcohol intake
- maintaining physical and mental activity (e.g. hobbies, social engagements). Stimulating the mind is important for "use it or lose it".

Memory management techniques that you might find helpful include:

- memory aids (checklists, diaries, calendars)
- written prompts (e.g. a note on the fridge to remind you to take your medication)
- placement routines (e.g. a special place for your keys or glasses)
- rehearsal and repeated practice (e.g. repeating their name when you meet someone new)
- concentrating on important things to remember and ignoring minor things
- concentrating on doing one thing at a time and not rushing.

Provision of information

You as a person with dementia or as a carer need information about local support services that might be suitable now and in the future. This can include support from social services and from voluntary organisations and local groups. Local groups can provide peer support, and knowing that you are not alone and there are others in the same situation can be very comforting.

You may need information about legal and financial matters. This includes advice on claiming benefits, setting up direct debits, setting up an advanced directive or lasting power of attorney, making and changing wills.

A person with dementia may only grant lasting power of attorney if they are fully aware of the procedure and therefore it will need to be discussed in the early stages of the disease. Court Appointed Deputies are able to make decisions on welfare, healthcare and financial matters as determined by the Court, for those with mental incapacity but no LPA.

If you have dementia and still drive a car, you have a legal responsibility to inform the DVLA and your insurance company of your diagnosis of dementia. You should not drive until advised by the DVLA, who will review your individual case and state whether you can continue to drive. Sometimes they request a retest. Even if authorised to carry on driving, receiving a diagnosis of dementia is a suitable time to start thinking of alternatives to driving, as the issue will inevitably arise again as the condition progresses.

Provision of support and counselling

Specific counselling for the person (particularly in the early stages), the carer and/or family can help with feelings of distress.

Management of complications as they arise

Behavioural and noncognitive symptoms are very common, particularly (but not exclusively) in the more advanced stages of dementia. They include physical symptoms of weight loss, incontinence and falls, and mental symptoms of agitation and aggression, sexual disinhibition, wandering, sleep disturbances, delusions and hallucinations, depression and anxiety. They are often very distressing for the carers, as well as the person with dementia, and can result in admission to hospital or residential care.

Management of these symptoms should involve a person-centred approach to the problem. Drugs should be used with caution, because of side effects. Other management tools include modifying the environment, engaging with stimulating activity (e.g. reminiscing), developing communication strategies and advising/counselling carers.

Much of the use of tranquillisers called neuroleptics within care homes is inappropriate. Neuroleptics are used for treatment of schizophrenia and psychotic disorders, but are also often prescribed for nonspecific agitation, even though there is little evidence of benefit in this situation. However, neuroleptics may worsen cognitive abilities in dementia and may increase mortality. There are a few instances where neuroleptic are indicated (for psychotic or dangerously aggressive behaviour), but agitated behaviour can often be successfully managed by a holistic approach from dedicated, educated staff, without needing medication. Neuroleptics should never be prescribed as a substitute for good quality care.

Provision of continuing care and end of life care

Ultimately dementia is a terminal illness, although it can take many years to reach this point. Along the way, people with dementia need regular review, ongoing support for them and their families, and timely referral to appropriate services as needs arise.

This involves a personalised programme of support and monitoring, and recognition that your needs, as the person with dementia or as the carer, will change over time, and the management programme needs to adjust accordingly.

There is evidence that a programme of educational counselling, support, and advice given to family carers, together with timely referral to appropriate services, when need arises, can be effective in preventing or delaying time to nursing home placement.

In the final stages, people with dementia need access to palliative care measures, as for those dying with any other condition.

Risk Factors and Prevention of Dementia

Risk factors for Alzheimer's dementia:

The most important risk factor by far is age. Alzheimer's dementia simply becomes more likely to occur as we get older.

10–15% of cases are familial. These cases have young onset, typically before 60 years of age. Older age onset dementia is not inherited, and therefore you are not at any greater risk of developing the illness if you have relatives who became demented in old age.

Risk factors for blood circulation problems (hypertension, high cholesterol) are risk factors for Alzheimer's disease too.

Although at one time considered, there is no evidence that aluminium exposure increases risk of Alzheimer's disease.

Risk factors for vascular dementia:

Again, age is an important risk factor, as are risks factors for stroke – namely, hypertension, diabetes, high cholesterol, smoking, atrial fibrillation.

A previous stroke is a strong risk factor and about one third of stroke patients aged over 65 years develop vascular dementia.

Prevention of dementia

Prevention of dementia involves management of underlying risks factors in mid- and later-life.

Lifestyle measures recommended are:

- adopting a healthy diet (a Mediterranean diet has been recommended by many)
- maintaining regular physical exercise
- not smoking
- not drinking alcohol excessively.

Control of blood pressure and cholesterol are important for those over 40 years.
Where possible, you should avoid anything that causes a potential insult or injury to your brain. This includes head injuries, and anything that causes loss of consciousness (e.g. severe low blood sugar or low blood pressure, but also self inflicted causes such as binge drinking). If these events occur repeatedly, they can lead to cognitive decline.

Further reading

The Alzheimer's Society (www.alzheimers.org.uk) provides a whole range of information for people with dementia and their carers on all types of dementia and all aspects of care.

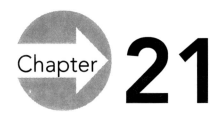

Chapter **21**

Geriatric Psychological Issues of Mental Health

Richard Sherry

Ageing well, and therefore living well, requires you to look at the emotional perspective that you hold of life. If you are negative or pessimistic in this respect, it dramatically reduces your appreciation of how extraordinarily rich this point in your life can be. Although this is a deceptively simple idea, psychologically, it is fundamental to every aspect of your life. Being mindful, open and connected provides you with a wise presence that enables you to evolve and reach your maximum capability.

Issues in and around mental health at any age are all too frequently overlooked, and this can be especially true within the area of geriatric psychological health. Examining the spectrum of your lifetime experience captures the accumulation of some of your worst and best qualities. For example, issues related to loss of control, impaired body and mind, and feeling like a burden can become the primary resonating factors during later life. Also, psychological trauma, loss and material factors can markedly affect your perception of circumstances. It is not that negative factors should be ignored, but to focus on them to the exclusion of positive aspects, unnecessarily increases anxiety, depression, vulnerability and a pessimistic outlook.

One of the key aspects that can challenge how you relate to ageing is how you judge your own accomplishments and whether you feel that you have achieved your lifetime goals. The psychological opinion you hold of yourself, regardless of what society thinks, has a profound effect on how you judge whether you have had a good life or not.

Your vulnerability and resiliency are linked to the relative emphasis and focus you give to life events: negative and positive patterns of responses have predictive power in many diverse areas. Vulnerability is a hallmark of, and reinforces, negative cycles and social processes. Conversely, positive indicators hold a protective factor in your management of psychological trauma, and your interpretation of life events. A positive mindset is protective, it helps you better manage stress, it increases the enjoyment of relationships with others and it improves your health. The more positive your input, the more you will get out, in terms of the quality of your life and in loving and compassionate relationships with yourself and others.

As an individual, you probably show a bias toward a positive or negative, more pessimistic, reaction. This usually becomes more pronounced as you get older. Rate yourself for levels along a scale with negativity at one end and positivity at the other: zero being completely negative and one hundred completely positive. On this scale, how negative or positive do you think you are; what do you think about those around you; and what about the world in general?

Your earlier experience informs your psychological mindset, which in turn influences your subsequent beliefs. These patterns of thinking and acting change with the support and care you experience. It is possible to make changes within these areas toward a more mindful and positive direction at ANY point in your development or at any age. Thinking more about the later stages of life and development help you to live better throughout the entire course of your life.

You can help to create a more thoughtful environment to think and talk about ageing: this removes the avoidance, and all too frequent shame about the subject, to something that can positively focus on the socioeconomic environment, available resources, and family and community support. These factors all play a part in and around your experience of compassion and care and whether you can meaningfully connect with support structures and the complex relationships that are a part of longer lived experiences. The approach can be improved by having a more positive psychological framework available: you can work both individually, and collectively to share a healthier view of ageing. In this way it may be possible to improve the higher level developments of consciousness and wisdom that ideally should be present during this life stage.

Mental health for the elderly population needs to be understood as a two-way contract and commitment from the younger as well as the older members of society. Both sides have to work together to improve this time of life. The younger generations have to be more supportive and the older population needs to help take a more proactive responsibility of not attacking themselves or others with an overly pessimistic mindset.

Another key issue that you should help address with the whole of your community, is to ensure that old age is not treated as an illness or something shameful and to be avoided if not downright feared. This is one of the greatest disservices to yourself or others: it can have a profound impact on society, and is a measure of how enlightened we are in our communal responsibility.

In looking at these issues of the end-of-life stages it can help you see how crucial the psychological framework is in guiding your life. These psychological organising functions of your personality structure can be seen to work comparatively, like highlighting health concerns. Taking a more mindful preventive health approach significantly reduces problems and increases your wellbeing. Awareness of issues around preventative care, enable you to experience this very rich emotional and creative period that has literally taken your lifetime to create.

Huppert et al's (2005) book, The Science of Well-being, is like a cookbook for preventative health and positive psychology. Applying these principles, from having the right nutrition, cultivating a positive philosophy of life, promoting/encourageing the application of exercise, as well as having meaningful relationships, all of these aspects take the interface of your body and personality to highlight your relationship to yourself, other people and to the world at large. These interconnecting relationship spheres unfold throughout your lifespan. Ideally, later life can provide you with a space to sum up and appreciate the positive nature of your lifetime experiences. Earlier times can be overwhelmed by the tasks and challenges that you face during different developmental stages, such as schooling, family or work. Your psychological perspective fundamentally shapes the core of experience throughout your life span. This emotional filter can radically change how you interpret, experience, and frequently how you react to people as well as the world around you.

In this chapter you have seen how your psychological disposition can have a profound impact upon your emotional experience of older age. Central to this is correctly benchmarking your levels of negativity versus positivity. Having a clear idea of this perspective provides you with strategies and interventions that can help you during this dynamic, complex and potentially creative period of your life, and to enjoy it to the full.

Further reading

Huppert, F.A., Baylis, N., and Keverne, B., (2005) *The Science of Well-being*. Oxford: Oxford University Press.

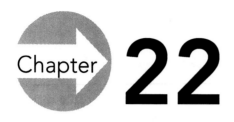

Chapter 22

Cancer

Tim Oliver

Cancer treatment in the Older Generation and relevance of the Sanatorium Movement (1850–1950) to cancer prevention

In 1850 Dr Penny Brookes, in creating the Much Wenlock annual community Olympian contests which survives to this day (http://www.wenlock-olympian-society.org.uk/history/william-penny-brookes/), did not have in mind the gladiatorial contest of the modern Olympics that Coubertin started in 1894. Rather he saw "… *the encouragement of out-door recreation, and by the award of Prizes annually at public meetings for skill in Athletic exercise….*" as an antidote to the illnesses Victorian society was witnessing from the dark satanic mills and increased urbanisation. Brookes' legacy was an annual local competition that continues to this day but it also led to increasing sports in schools across the UK and the birth of the Sanatorium movement. This built on his observations and also the increasing knowledge at the beginning of the 20th Century about the health benefits of the sun and the invention of personalised sunlamps, which followed the award of the Nobel Prize to Niels Finsen in 1903 (https://www.nobelprize.org/nobel_prizes/medicine/laureates/1903/) for demonstrating healing of Tuberculosis in the skin. By the 1930s the Sanatorium movement had demonstrated that the key to gaining the best health benefit was a combination of Exercise and sunshine and advocated this in the UK through organisations such as the Peckham and Finsbury Health Centres Rickets disappeared and TB deaths fell between 1900 and 1948 by 67% long before the advent of antibiotics.

Over the next 30 years the health benefits of sunshine and exercise were forgotten, in part because the successes of the previous 50 years were attributed solely to other public health measures, such as improved housing, nutrition and judicious use of cod liver oil and sun lamps. Sports in schools diminished as antibiotics "conquered" infectious disease. As increasing obesity ensued in the years 1996-2005, low-fat diets were wrongly seen as the solution, diminishing the absorption of fat-soluble Vitamins such as Vitamin D. There followed the shame of reemergence Rickets and TB in our inner cities. At the same time sunshine was blamed for the mounting skin cancer epidemic from sunshine holidays. Even worse, sun lamps were being vilified because of linkage of sunbeds to melanoma in "tanorexic" inner city children in poor areas of our cities unable to afford summer weekends in the country or winter "easyjet" weekends in the sun as treatment for their undiagnosed "nonseasonal seasonal affective disorder". This was in part because fashion magazines promoted tanning but also because the kids recognised that sunlamps cured their depression ("nonseasonal seasonal affective disorder") due to their 24/7 lifestyle being better than their GP's drugs. In response to the skin cancer risk, the scientific community has classified UVB part of sunshine as a "Class 1" carcinogen as bad as cigarette smoking and Lawyers ensure that no doctor or Government agency can advise outdoor activity in case they are sued for causing a melanoma. The 21st Century has seen the emergence of antibiotic resistance due to inappropriate use, both in General Practice but more so in our indoor farming industry. Even more troubling has been the emergence of "morbid" obesity starting in Childhood and its associated increased risk of deaths from Diabetes, Heart disease and Cancer as well as Dementia. Since 2014 the NHS Public Health England has at last begun to recognise the importance of exercise, though only promoted without emphasis on outdoor activity, let alone the fact that all data on the health benefits of exercise are confounded by the health benefits of sunshine (https://www.gov.uk/government/publications/health-matters-getting-every-adult-active-every-day/health-matters-getting-every-adult-active-every-day#contents).

How is exercise and increased sun exposure relevant for Cancer prevention in the over 60s

By the time one gets to the ripe old age of 68 about 50% of all cancers have manifested themselves and even killed more than 50% of the sufferers. However for those who live beyond that age, cancer will undoubtedly be an increasing proportion of illnesses that present in their later years. It is the aim of this chapter to firstly present a thumbnail sketch of how it is thought cancers develop, then discuss how they present and are treated, and finally consider how one can maximise symptom free living if the disease spreads beyond the limits of conventional treatment. It then ends with a brief explanation of the principals of palliative care and how non-healthcare persons can make the life of end stage cancer sufferers happier by helping them to travel hopefully and not arrive at their destination too quickly.

Cancer Causes and How a Cancer Develops and May Be Prevented

One of the problems with getting a true perspective on preventing cancer, is that if one listens to the media one is overwhelmed by the fact that there are too many, not too few, suspected causes of cancer. Despite this, when one actually meets someone who has cancer it is rarely clear what has caused it to develop at the time it does occur. However, what science has now proved beyond all doubt is that all of the known causes of cancer act by leading to damage to DNA and/or a reduction of the body's ability to repair DNA damage. Furthermore, as illustrated by the increased susceptibility of people with ginger hair to skin cancer from sun exposure, the risks of any given carcinogenic influence are modified by the genetic inheritance of the individual and the multiplicity of hits.

The consequence of this is that, even for the most closely examined cancer cause, i.e. smoking, this risk factor is associated with less than 20% of regular users developing cancer after more than 40 years' use. This is one of the facts that contribute to why many youngsters fail to heed the message. However, the most telling message about smoking is not being emphasised. This message is that it is the number of cigarettes smoked per year during the body's pubertal growth phase before the age of 18 that are most important in predicting the later risk of getting cancer by the age of 50–60. Getting the growing brain exposed to the addictive substance by the age of 18 while growth is actively taking place is as relevant in inducing addiction to nicotine as it is to alcohol and other addictive drugs such as heroin and cannabis. However, even though for smokers it is the first few years that are the most important individually, it is the total number of years that ends up making the real difference, and so any time spent off smoking helps reduce the risk, though the longer the better. Even today stopping people smoking remains the single most productive population based step to reducing cancer deaths, though were it to return to its original use in American Indian communities as the occasional Pipe of Peace, it is unlikely to be a health hazard.

With the exception of stomach and bowel cancer there are few other cancers with simple messages that help with prevention. However, because they act throughout a lifetime, it is worth reiterating these two exceptions now, because they will help to understand how safe sun, safe sex and regular exercise may help to reduce the occurrence of cancers.

For stomach cancer, it has now been established that the lifetime equivalent of one orange's worth of vitamin C taken daily is sufficient to virtually eliminate the risk of stomach cancer. This is because the chemical action of vitamin C acts to block the action of DNA damageing cancer causing chemicals and bacteria in the stomach. For bowel cancer, it has taken more than twenty years to prove that regular high fibre diet with vegetables reduces the risk of deaths from cancer of the large intestine by stimulating the passage of food residues, though paradoxically it does not seem to affect the risk of the early polyp stage developing.

Safe sun and men's cancers

The Chinese philosophy of Ying and Yang recognises that there is good and bad in everything and nowhere is this clearer than in the effects of the sun on development of cancer. The sun keeps us warm but burns the skin if the dose is excessive and you have low skin pigment. If you burn your skin excessively, and particularly as a child, and get blisters, you increase your risk of getting a skin cancer called Melanoma which can kill people as young as 20–30 years of age. If you have 50–60 years of chronic sunburn you end up with a different type of skin cancer called squamous cancer. Though this is less malignant it can keep recurring all over the sunburnt areas and be quite disfiguring.

However, there is now new evidence emerging that sun can have important lifetime benefits as well. It has long been known that sunlight reduces the risk of tuberculosis and helps it heal. This is now known to be due to the sun stimulating the body to make vitamin D which helps the body's scavenging phagocytes to resist the tuberculosis infection (decreased outdoor sports, low fat diets, as vitamin D is a fat soluble vitamin, and more indoor computer games and clubbing, could be unsuspected factors adding to the resurgence of tuberculosis and rickets in this country). It is now emerging that a regular but intermittent lifetime sun exposure (for average white skin about 30–40 mins 2–3 x a week, while Asians and Africans require more frequent up to 60–80 mins 3x a week) may be helping to reduce the risk of bowel, breast and prostate cancer, possibly by the same mechanism. In the UK and particularly in Scotland where most people are Vitamin D deficient in winter months, it is advisable to take supplements or increase food rich in Vitamin D such as oily fish and livers of sea and land animals. As currently there are some conditions associated with Vitamin D deficiency that have not responded to supplements, the question arises as to whether there are some additional benefits from sunshine. However it may be also a question of dose, something which will be resolved when follow up of large trials currently in progress is complete.

The Vitamin D induced scavenging phagocytes are equally effective at eliminating early stages of cancer. Recent research is suggesting that this effect may be indirect. This research has provided evidence that Vitamin D's role may be more important in controlling a group of bacteria that can grow without access to normal levels of Oxygen and so colonise scar tissue anywhere in the body. The best known example of this is Helicobacter pylori. This has now been proven as a cause of stomach cancer and the combination of Vitamin C and Vitamin D deficiency over a long period as much as 30–40 years enables this bacteria to cause low grade damage to cells lining the stomach, such that DNA mutations accumulate in the stem cells and the early stages of cancer develop. Five to ten more years of low Vitamin C & D enables the early silent stages to progress to inoperable cancer as more DNA mutations occur.

Recently scientists have begun applying the DNA technology developed to study the Human genome to study the bacterial content of the human body. The most exciting but still preliminary results of this work has been the suggestion that there are examples of these low oxygen dependent bacteria present in colonic, pancreatic, prostatic and possibly also breast cancer, all of which are cancers reduced by exercise

What is not known is, what is the safe dose of sunshine and exercise to maximise the benefit against most cancers, but not increase risk of skin cancers?

Safe sex and good diet in prostate and testicular cancer

For testicular cancer, there is increasing evidence that an early onset of puberty increases the risk, though the exact mechanism is not clear. As discussed below, under the effects of exercise, it is thought to be mediated in part via an effect of the body's sex hormones, although there is evidence that sexually acquired infection can contribute to increase this risk. There is also evidence emerging in respect of prostate cancer, that early onset of puberty is increasing risk, and here there is beginning to be a more clear cut explanation. Recent work has suggested that it is because at a younger age men are more prone to damage their prostates by developing an asymptomatic form of "honeymoon prostatitis", (which is the male equivalent of the honeymoon cystitis women often experience when they first begin sexual activity with a new partner). In contrast to women this is usually without causing any or only minor symptoms: 40% of men get at least one attack before the age of 50. In some people, who are more susceptible, this may lead to a lifetime's hidden persistence of mild infection which is amplified by repeat exposures. Inadequate dietary Vitamin A and D, by reducing function of immune cells and phagocytes, may facilitate this persistent infection. This chronic damage to the prostate seems to encourage DNA mutations to accumulate and prostate cancer ultimately develops 25-50 years later.

These observations have led to the hypothesis that a possible late effect of the anti-AIDS safe sex campaign of the early 80s, may explain the unexplained decline of prostate cancer deaths in the UK in the late 90s before the availability of PSA screening. Reports that 6 month condom use can lead to regression of the early stages of cervix cancer and limited evidence that condom use can also reduce prostate cancer is encourageing greater focus on education in puberty about these risks, in an attempt to reinforce the 1980's safe sex message that is being forgotten by today's youth. This is a message that is equally relevant to later generations as there is increasing recognition of rising incidence of STDs in these age groups. Recently there have been reports that the sun-sensitive low oxygen dependent acne bacterium has been detected in prostate cancers of 60–70 year old men. If this becomes lodged in the prostate when the individual is low in Vitamin D it could be acting like Helicobacter in the stomach to accelerate the development of prostate cancer

How can regular exercise prevent testis and prostate cancer?

While it has long been known that exercise reduces risks of heart disease, the message that exercise is good for prevention of several types of cancer, such as breast, bowel, testis and prostate cancer, is less well known, as is the fact that it may also contribute to increase survival after diagnosis in all cancer sufferers.

For testis cancer there are thought to be two mechanisms that may be acting together. Firstly, lack of exercise leads to a greater sedentary existence. Sitting down, particularly in tight underpants, heats up the testicle and this is known to damage the sperm stem cells from which testis cancers develop. The second mechanism is that regular exercise has a beneficial effect on regulation of sex hormones that control puberty and this leads to a more gradual development of puberty, thus reducing the deleterious effects of an early puberty. It is a similar mechanism that is thought to be a factor in why exercise, particularly in schools, is beneficial in reducing later risks of prostate cancer, though it may also be that those who take more exercise have more sun exposure and better vitamin D levels. As with heart disease prevention, it is by no means certain that exercise has to be excessive. The critical thing is developing a regular pattern and maintaining it over a lifetime.

How could we demonstrate the benefit of education on these issues in schools and the workplace?

Today more than 95% of men developing testis cancer can be cured. With such a high cure rate why are we worried? What good are we going to do by creating worried teenagers when the risk of testis cancer is only 1 in 500 during the years between 12 and 50? Despite the last decade of increasing recognition of the benefits of early diagnosis, the average size of testis cancers has only reduced from 5 to 4 cms. Still today, more than half the men diagnosed with testicular cancer are taking 4-8 months to be diagnosed. Even today this delay is much more frequent in teenagers who are understandably shyer and less aware about these issues. While this delay no longer affects the cure, because treatment is so effective, treatment is far more complicated and can leave lasting consequences. Today, if diagnosed early, it may only be necessary to give one day's chemotherapy treatment after diagnosis. However, at present all patients need to lose a testicle for diagnostic purposes. If we could reduce delay so that the tumours were less than 2cms it might then be possible to avoid the routine loss of a testicle. It is for this reason that all men by the age of 12 need to know of the importance of selfexamination and early investigation if there are any changes.

However, it is clear from the preceding discussion on safe sun, safe sex, diet and exercising, that there are several equally important messages that are relevant for both sexes and may reduce their lifetime risk of cancer, that need to be learned at the time of puberty and maintained throughout life.

An equally important lifetime lesson to learn at this age, like selfexamination of the testis, is to learn the importance of foreskin hygiene. Despite the relative rarity of penile cancer, attention to foreskin hygiene is also important for other areas of genital health in both men and women, such as HIV infection, cervix and also prostate cancer.

If one limits the campaign to teenagers, it may take 40–50 years before one can expect to see a reduction in deaths from all cancers. However, there is some evidence suggesting that population based PSA blood testing may give an early indication by the age of 25–30. Extending these messages into the workplace, to family planning and vasectomy as well as sexually transmitted disease clinics will ensure that the benefit of the message is also reinforced at later stages.

However, long before the impact on all cancer deaths can be fully evaluated, there are other interim check points that could highlight the progress being made. The first of these would be a further reduction in the incidence of teenage pregnancies, one of the more embarrassing statistics on which the UK used to lead the rest of Europe. Secondly, there could be a reduction in sexually transmitted diseases and even the early stages of cervix cancer. Thirdly, there might even be a reduction in the occurrence of depression and suicide in young men, as exercise and sunlight have both been shown to reduce risks of depression

Relevance of these messages to older readers

It is clear that even after diagnosis of cancer, regular exercise outside is a simple precaution that can be implemented. What is more controversial is the issue of what should be the advice about sun exposure and use of sun blockade. For the last 20 years the primary message of cancer research organisations is to use sunblock whenever out in the sun, because of the risk of skin cancer and particularly melanoma. The authorities even went further and the World Health Organisation has classified UVB as a class 1 carcinogen and banned use of sun beds to people of under 18 years of age because of the behaviour of "Tannorectics", teenagers in low level sunshine areas of the UK becoming addicted because they found it was effective in dealing with minor depression. Recent research has demonstrated that pollution and particularly heavy metals such as chromium from traffic fumes acted as a cocarcinogen with UV in causing melanoma. As all data on health benefits of exercise are confounded by the fact that the historic epidemiology data didn't take into account that it was mainly outdoor exercise, and modern research has shown that outdoor exercise is the best way to raise serum vitamin D level, attitudes are changing.

As a consequence until such time that there is further research to resolve these issues, what is the best advice? The first issue is that until it is resolved it would be wise that not all personal exercise is done in gyms with reliance on Vitamin D supplementation to make up for lack of sunshine, given that to date the results from trials in cancer patients have been very inconclusive. Trials in treatment of blood pressure have led to the discovery that there are other factors produced by sun exposure such as nitric oxide. Given these observations and the inconclusive trials in cancer patients it would be advisable that 20–30 minutes mild exercise in the midday sun is taken as a routine whenever possible. Judicious use of sun beds and or "Easyjet" long weekends during winter months should be considered. This aspiration is even relevant for terminal patients as will be discussed in the later section, which have a greater focus on the curative treatment. After a brief discussion of screening, the final three sections explore these issues in detail and what is needed to resolve the uncertainty.

Screening of the aged population

While screening for cervical cancer has been credited with reducing cervical cancer in the West, it is unaffordable in the areas of the world where there is most cervical cancer. This is because of the cost of a large amount of "over-diagnosis" needing expensive intervention. It has avoided education until recently that it is a sexually transmitted disease involving both men and women. Even now that the focus is on HPV vaccination, this is only given to girls but not boys despite increasing evidence of the HPV virus being involved in oral cancers arising in both sexes from the increase in oral sex. Progress in simplifying HPV testing and second generation vaccines is leading to hope that this approach may make it more affordable in the countries where it is most needed.

Breast screening is undoubtedly the most successful in terms of the numbers of women who have apparently benefitted and in terms of reductions of breast cancer deaths. However confounding factors such as decline in organo-chloride pesticide use and lead-time bias are leading to a re-examination of the early premise of these programmes, which are even more unaffordable in low income countries than cervical screening. Lead-time bias is due to early diagnosis increasing detection of early latent breast cancer that would not have presented during that individuals lifetime, causing increased worried well suffering over treatment.

PSA screening for early prostate cancer detection has been even more controversial. While it has been associated with a reduction of prostate cancer patient with metastases and some reduction of prostate cancer deaths, it has been at the expense of vast amount of over-diagnosis and suffering of side effects of treatment. This is due to exaggeration of the benefits of screening and underestimating the lead-time bias in early diagnosis which is more than 10 years. Furthermore the trial data shows that it takes 8 to 10 years after the first screening before the 7-10% benefit begins to appear. In individuals starting screening over the age of 70 this minor benefit virtually disappears. As a consequence, most authorities even now are not advising routine screening. Because PSA does predict people with an increased risk of death from prostate cancer even at the age of 40, it's use is being focused more on patients under 65 with prostate symptoms and populations with increased risk, such as those with multiple cases in the same family and those with African ancestry.

As a consequence in the aged population, the focus should be more on prevention and early diagnosis if symptoms arise

Conventional Cancer Treatments

Local recurrence is one of the worst things that can happen to a cancer patient. Because of this careful and complete excision of any mass where there is a strong suspicion of cancer without preliminary biopsy with clear margin is the standard of best care. However this must be safe without risk of damageing vital neighbouring structures. For more difficult locations such as head and neck, central nervous and pelvic tumours, such a policy can often produce disfigurement and loss of function. In such situations a preliminary biopsy is considered a safer option, so that provided cancer is confirmed by pathological examination, radiation with or without chemotherapy can be used either as a preoperative procedure to minimise the amount of tissue damage from surgery or, in some instances if complete destruction of the tumour can be proven by post treatment biopsy, avoid surgery completely.

For the patient diagnosed with cancer, the sometimes prolonged series of treatments necessary can lead to a considerable loss of fitness and a tendency to withdraw from normal day-to-day activity. Giving increasing evidence that sun-deficiency and inactivity leads to depression, an unrecognised component of cancer recovery is to try, however hard it is, to get as much daily physical exercise outdoor (though keeping any areas treated with radiation protected from sunlight). In addition to the long term survival benefit this has, there is more immediate benefit in terms of recovery from side effects of chemotherapy and hormone ablation treatments of sex-hormone dependant cancers, such as breast and prostate cancer.

Clinical trials and recent advances due to discoveries from genetic research in cancer

Medical practitioners are so called because from the day they start to the day they stop they are learning from the individuality of each patient and accumulating experience that can be of benefit to the next patient that is treated. In the past this was all doctors had to go on, and depended on their teachers passing on this knowledge during their apprenticeship. The science of clinical trials has evolved on the back of progress in statistics and increasing numbers of patients are required in trials to make true progress, as most new treatments show only 5-7% improvement. This has led to increasing cost and complexity of trials so much so that even in America until the Obama healthcare act only about 50% of the patients on the highest band of insurance could get access to all new drugs as they become available. In many of the emerging economies only the very richest citizens actually get any access at all. As a result of the AIDS epidemic being centred in Africa and ingenuity of start-up Pharmaceutical companies in India, newer approaches are being tried out in this setting that are also helping to develop simpler trial processes that could benefit the richer Western countries.

This progress could not have come at a better time, as the Pharmaceutical companies are getting increasing numbers of genetically designed drugs, because of progress in understanding the genetic changes that accumulate in the development of cancer. These drugs have somewhat different side effects and are less toxic than conventional chemotherapy; though to date there have been few patients totally cleared of cancer and able to come off treatment. None the less this progress, particularly in breast and prostate cancer, which get a disproportionate access to these agents, has led some specialists to suggest that cancer is becoming a chronic disease, which like diabetes though not curable can be stabilised for prolong periods.

Palliative care, Immunotherapy and "Complementary" Medicine

Most of conventional postsurgery therapy with both radiation and chemotherapy is "palliative" in the sense that they don't offer long term cure but shrink the tumour enabling symptom control for a measurable period time: it is only after this has failed that the specialist palliative care comes into its own. It is often that death comes to cancer patients at unexpected times, in one patient coming when there is only a small amount of cancer while others survive for prolonged periods with large volumes of metastases all over the body. Examples of the former are cancers causing a large amount of "metabolic" mayhem disturbing vital organ function from generation of "poisons" that disrupt a specific organ function in the patient. One example of this is calcium poisoning from the cancer producing too much of a calcium controlling hormone causing absorption and mobilising of calcium into the blood from bones. Another cancer cell product is the cellular signalling molecule called Tumour Necrosis Factor or Cachexin. Over-production of this molecule by the cancer leads to loss of appetite and severe weight loss. A final example is a small tumour growing at a location where surgery would destroy vital structures such as in the brainstem.

Palliative care developed as a speciality whose role was to look after those cancer patients whose disease had failed all conventional treatment and, through trained nurse support in the community, aimed to keep patients living with symptoms controlled in their own home, but provide a link to deal with any of the multiple different problems that can develop as the cancer progresses. Though well known for their prowess in dealing with pain control and in particular regulating morphine dosage, it is often manageing patients with the metabolic mayhem who prove the more difficult, of which constipation and anaemia are the most frequent. As well as being a troublesome side effect of patients on morphine and those with abnormal calcium control, constipation is also more troublesome when cancer involves nerves controlling motility of the large bowel.

The most troubling part of palliative care is in the large group of patient that have relatively few symptoms but growing metastases, often small at first but visible on scans, so that the patient is left with the Sword of Damocles fear, without any specific therapy to grasp. Such patients are open to any snake oil salesman of alternative therapy with a good story to tell, most of which have an element of truth or based on extrapolation from previous research. In the past these products were not studied in properly controlled randomised trials. However recently this has changed. This is with publication of a positive placebo controlled trial of tablets of purified food extracts as they are not as tightly regulated as pharmaceutical trials and so require less funds to undertake. It was "immunotherapy" trials in the 1990s which first showed why placebo based trials are necessary. In trials of Gamma Interferon the placebo response occurred in up to 10% of such end stage cancer patients.

Today it is more than 60 years since the MacFarlane Burnet thesis that it is an intact immune system that is constantly rejecting cancers. In both melanoma and lung cancer there have been encourageing durable cancer complete remissions and long term control achieved from a new series of immune regulatory molecules tested against placebos in randomised trials. Evidence that part of the reason that cancer control is more prolonged in patients who exercise, is via an immune mechanisms due to higher Vitamin D levels, gives hope that the next decade will witness considerable improvement in cancer survival even in late stage patients from knowing how best to exploit this new understanding.

Conclusion

The concept of U4U is that individuals should be in control of their own destiny. Nowhere is it more important than in relation to prevention and in those individuals who develop and are living with cancer. This chapter has reviewed the evidence that most cancers are caused by a slowly developing process which is amenable to slowing or even reversal by self help in some individuals. This requires education that needs to take place throughout life, though at no age is it too late to learn the message. More importantly U4U individuals are in a unique position to have the time and the increasing access to Grandchildren to encourage their education about the life long benefit of exercise.

Chapter 23

Your Doctor

Although we are all going to die at sometime, the timing of this event remains difficult to predict, and it is important not to sit around waiting. You can prepare personal affairs related to finance, property and possessions, and aim to lead a full, interesting, enjoyable, contented life, in a comfortable environment, keeping your mind and body as active as possible.

Nevertheless, illness can interfere with these ideals, and previous chapters have suggested when you should discuss abnormal symptoms and signs with your doctor. This chapter brings together these features and considers when various treatments, such as medicines and sometimes surgery, can improve the quality of your life.

All your organs gradually wear out. You have probably noticed that your **joints** are getting a bit stiff, and mild exercise and tablets can help retain mobility and improve discomfort. Joint replacement might seem a good idea, and it certainly relieves severe pain and deformity, but no operation is without risk, and you have to be fit and motivated enough to rehabilitate to gain maximum benefit.

Your **faculties** can deteriorate faster than the rest of you, and dealing with poor **vision** and **deafness** are considered in the relevant chapters. **Mental deterioration** and **dementia** are one of the greatest horrors of ageing, and recognition and monitoring of change need professional help and understanding, Ongoing deterioration requires advanced planning while you are still able to do so: this includes deciding where you are going to live and be looked after, and the preparation of advanced directives and an advocate of your choice.

It is your heart and lungs, the furring up of your arteries and the uncontrolled growth of parts of your body as a cancer that usually lead to death, but the problems they produce can be markedly alleviated with medical help.

Furring of your **arteries** makes them more rigid leading to a raised blood pressure, that damages delicate organs such as the kidneys and the brain, where a haemorrhagic **stroke** can have a devastating effect on you and those close to you. Furring also blocks arteries not only affecting the brain, but also your legs, producing pain on exercise and eventually at rest. In the **heart**, it not only causes the acute heart attacks more common at a younger age, but also gradually leads to heart failure. Failure of the pump in any fluid system produces backpressure and in your body **heart failure** produces swelling of your legs and fluid in your lungs. The latter gives breathlessness, and the heart may show its displeasure with loss of a regular rhythm, producing palpitations and chest discomfort.

Your doctor can help many of these problems, such as controlling your **blood pressure** with tablets and, if blocks in your arteries have been identified, referring you to a specialist to see if they can be unblocked. **Strokes** and **heart attacks** need emergency hospital care, as may acute breathlessness, but your doctor can prescribe tablets to support a failing heart and help your symptoms. **Irregular rhythms** may need to be controlled with tablets and anticoagulants prescribed to reduce the chances of blood clotting in your arteries, due to the turbulence of the irregularity. Other measures are controlling obesity, and any related secondary diabetes, with dietary advice and an exercise programme.

Chest problems of breathlessness are not only linked to heart failure, but also primary **lung** disease, such as the infection of bronchitis and pneumonia, particularly seen in smokers. Appropriate antibiotics are needed in these and for infection elsewhere, such as in the urine. Failure of other organs, such as the kidneys and liver, may only be picked up on routine blood testing, and vague feelings of being unwell, particularly if recent, are worthy of a visit to your doctor.

Cancer

The term cancer can strike fear into you, raising thoughts of an immanent and painful death. As this is rarely so, some facts are worthy of consideration.

You develop from a single cell from each of your parents, these join and then divide many billions of times to produce your adult form. When you have reaches a genetically predetermined size, your cells stop dividing. Although some cells retain the ability to divide, such as the skin to repair injury and bone to repair fractures, most cells do not do so for the rest of your life.

If any cells usurp this normal process and keep dividing, they can produce a lump – also termed a swelling, a new growth, a neoplasm (or a tumour). If this swelling is small, well defined, not pressing on anything vital or producing harmful products, it is said to be a **benign** tumour. Problems arise when a swelling starts to grow into (**invade**) and destroy the surrounding parts of the body: this abnormal uncontrolled growth is termed a **malignant** tumour or a cancer (malignant tumours of some deeper structures are termed sarcomas, but it is easier to think of them collectively as cancers).

Another problem with cancers is that they can grow into blood vessels, and bits can break off, get carried around the body in the blood stream and start growing elsewhere. These are termed secondary tumours (secondaries or **metastases**): the term **primary** tumour is applied to the initial site. Every type of cell can undertake this uncontrolled division, but common ones relate to the skin, the lining of the gut and lungs, and the glandular tissues of the breast and prostate: blood cells can also become involved. Much research is being undertaken to work out why cells should suddenly change and how to prevent this division.

Most cancers produce symptoms before they produce secondaries, and any unexplained indigestion or alteration of your bowel habit, weight loss or the appearance of blood in your vomit, stool, sputum or urine, must be investigated. Early cancers can usually be cut out and cured by **surgery**, or destroyed by various forms of **radiotherapy**. It is thus important to be aware of any **changes in your health** and to discuss them with your doctor. In the UK particular emphasis is given to population screening and early diagnosis of cancer.

Drugs are used to control cancer once it has spread (and sometimes after other treatments, just in case bits got away). They have to be carefully controlled so that they only attack the cancer and not the rest of the body. A number of drugs and drug **combinations** are used, and they are continually being refined. In view of the importance of stageing the size and invasiveness of a cancer, and the amount it has spread, a **multidisciplinary team** of clinicians usually manages cancer, tailoring treatment to the needs of each individual to obtain optimal care.

These developments have turned much cancer management into chronic rather than terminal care, and long term **monitoring** of the disease is the norm. Nevertheless we all die of something and **many treatments** are available to manage pain, breathlessness or any other disturbing symptoms of the disease. In view of the reputation of the disease, many seek second opinions and probably half of those afflicted consider complementary medicine. The unpredictability of outcome of an individual cancer makes it difficult to judge the effects of any treatment outside a controlled environment, but measures that manage your general wellbeing, both mental and physical, have considerable beneficial effect.

Cancer of the **skin** presents as a lump that may break through and bleed: show this to your doctor if it is progressing. You cannot usually see deeper cancers so be on the lookout for symptoms – with **lung** cancer these are a cough (the sputum may be bloodstained, and different from any long standing problem) and breathlessness. With cancers of the **gut** look out for changes of apatite, indigestion and weight loss from the **stomach**, and change in your bowel habit with the **lower bowel**. The latter may also have blood in the stool and if the cancer blocks the bowel you may become distended, have abdominal pain and constipation.

Female cancers are of the **breast, ovary** and **womb** (**uterus, cervix**). Breast lumps: changes in the feel the breast or nipple discharge, should be checked by your doctor. Postmenopausal vaginal bleeding or discharge must be checked, but other symptoms, from the womb, like those of ovarian cancer, are usually vague abdominal discomfort and distension – report anything unusual to your doctor – it is better to be safe than sorry. **Men** are subject to cancers of the lung and bowel, but **prostate** cancer is a specific male problem. This is very variable in its severity, and it is probable that every man over 90 has some cancerous change in the prostate – emphasising its benign course that you can live with. However, other forms need specialist care.

Your doctor may well refer you for a **specialist opinion** if they confirm or suspect something is wrong, as a specialist has more experience in a particular area and also access to more sophisticated forms of investigation. Ask your doctor how long the waiting time of your referral is likely to be so you can check an appointment and ensure you do not get lost in the system.

Occasionally your journey to the hospital may be as an **emergency**, you are probably not in control of this situation and should accept the advice of the professionals around you. Such occasions may be due to an accident, a major bleed, acute pain or collapse. These incidents are best left to the experts and you can get more involved when you get there – if someone considers you need emergency attention you probably do.

Consent

By visiting your doctor you in effect agree to talk to them and they will ask your permission to examine you – it is sufficient to respond in words or a nod of acceptance. Similarly procedures such as taking your blood or receiving an injection are consented verbally.

For more elaborate interventions and any form of anaesthesia or sedation, a doctor has a legal requirement to obtain your written consent. Usually the consultant concerned discusses any potential procedure with you, and you will get a chance to ask questions then, and if you think of anything else, at a later date. You will be told of the benefits and common small and all major risks of the operation, including their likely occurrence, and any available alternative treatments. It is worth having someone with you so you can discuss the procedure later: there may well be a printed handout to provide further information. You can refuse a procedure, even if there is no rational reason and it is considered by others to be in your best interest.

When you go into hospital for the operation you have to sign a consent form after another full explanation. This must be before any sedation, it is not necessarily by the consultant, but must be by an appropriately trained and qualified doctor, who fully understands the procedure, can answer all your questions and knows the rules of consent: both of you sign the form, as it is a legal joint agreement on a mutual partnership.

The consent form confirms that you understand the procedure and are mentally competent to make the decision to proceed; you are fully informed of the risks (common small and all major complications); that all your questions have been answered; that you have signed voluntarily without coercion; that there is no guarantee that the procedure will be undertaken by a named surgeon (although this is usually the consultant you have discussed it with); and any additional procedure would only be undertaken if it were lifesaving and dangerous to delay (e.g. if your heart stopped and the surgical team had to take measures to resuscitate you – but they are not legally able to add a bit of 'cosmetic' surgery, even if it seemed to the surgeon a useful addition).

When anaesthesia is being administered, a similar visit takes place to explain and for you to consent to the anaesthetic procedure – the type of anaesthetic will have been discussed with you by your consultant, but you may wish to ask further questions of the anaesthetist.

If you are not mentally competent, you may have appointed an advocate with lasting power of attorney, as discussed with advanced directives, but if this is not so, there is extensive case law on how the court can appoint a deputy – this is usually a member of your family, as it will also involve them in your aftercare.

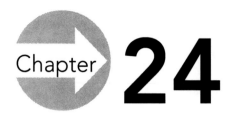

Chapter **24**

The Role of the Pharmacist in the Care of the Elderly

Sumaira Malik

The role of pharmacists has changed over the years, where currently, not only do they help manage your medicines, but they now offer a wide variety of health related services, most of which are free of charge and readily available.

What services can pharmacies provide?

Ideally you will need to visit to your local pharmacies to see exactly what services they provide as some services are locally commissioned based on the needs of the population.

What to look out for?

Pharmacists expanding role has led to the introduction of Healthy Living Pharmacies (HLP). A HLP is a pharmacy that follows an approved framework that ensures the delivery of high-quality services to meet the health needs of individuals. Not every pharmacy is a HLP but it is a status that more and more pharmacies are looking to achieve.

Qualities of a Healthy Living Pharmacy:

- A skilled team that is fully aware of national and local **strategies to improve health**

- A pharmacy team that full understand principles of **health and well being**

- A team that is proactive in tending to the health-related needs of the community via effective **community engagement**

- An engagement in **health promoting activity** and the provision of easily accessible **information** on topics such as smoking, cancer, managing long term conditions and flu

- A pharmacy that is fully equipped for purpose; i.e. promoting and maintaining health and well being.

Example of a Healthy Living Pharmacy: Green Light Pharmacy (London, Euston, NW1 2NU)

Founded in 1999, this bright and welcoming pharmacy has specifically been designed to help patients navigate through the pharmacy, offering lots of space for patients to have one-to-one contact with pharmacy staff members. The pharmacy provides lots of services such as Medicines Use Reviews, health checks, smoking cessation and travel vaccinations and there are private consultation room to facilitate this. The pharmacy also supports lots of Public Health Campaigns throughout the year.

The pharmacy has been heavily involved in bringing the local community together and empowering people on health topics and health related issues. Green Light organises a weekly walk for both men and women of all ages around Regent's Park; a chance for fresh air and light exercise as well as providing an all-important social gathering. They also run health talks for the older population, where common health issues are explained and discussed with the opportunity for healthy refreshments after.

Over-the-counter medicines

Pharmacies stock a wide variety of over-the-counter (OTC) medicines aimed for conditions that can easily be treated. Sometimes it is easy to misdiagnose ourselves and believe that we are suffering from a more serious condition than in reality. Speaking to a pharmacist can help clarify when you need to see your doctor or whether you require prescription medication. Pharmacists do not require appointments to speak to, making it easier to address your symptoms sooner. You can describe your symptoms to the pharmacist; and it may well be the case that it is a condition that is easily treated over-the-counter, in which case the pharmacist will make sure the treatment is safe for you to use and explain exactly how to use it.

Minor Ailment Scheme

The minor ailments scheme gives you free access to medicines without having to visit your GP. In the scheme, you are offered a consultation with a community pharmacist without the need for an appointment and depending on the symptoms you present with, may provide you with treatment.

The scheme covers treatment for common and uncomplicated health conditions, some of which are listed below:

- Athlete's foot
- Colds
- Constipation

- Cough
- Dry skin conditions
- Earache
- Haemorrhoids
- Hay fever
- Pain.

Three prerequisites are essential in order to be able to access the free service. The first is that you have a prescription exemption (note prescriptions are free for all who are over the age of 60). The second is the locality of your GP practice. The minor ailment service is based on local access; pharmacies will only be able to accept patients who are registered with approved local GP surgeries. Lastly, you will need a voucher, which can be provided by your GP practice upon request, and will contain some of your personal details on it. The voucher is what you will need to present to the pharmacy, and it allows the pharmacist to record any medication that is given out.

Medicines management

Pharmacists don't just dispense your medications. They are there to try and make taking medicines easier for you. There are lots of ways pharmacists can help to accommodate your needs. If you are experiencing any issues with your medicines, no matter how small of an issue, speak to your pharmacist about it; it is highly likely that many others have discussed the same issues with their pharmacists and so solutions have been made readily available.

> **Important note:** If you stop taking your medicines that your doctor has prescribed, or are thinking of stopping taking your medicines for whatever reason – perhaps you are suffering from side-effects that are affecting your daily activities, remember that pharmacists are not there to judge you! Manageing an illness and medicines isn't always easy, and it is important to realise there are lots of ways to receive support; one of which is through your pharmacist.

Examples of ways to better manage medicines:

Sometimes it is difficult to read the name of the medication on the box, as well as the dosing instructions. Pharmacists can create larger labels for you that have a larger text size, making it easier for you to read the all-important instructions of your medicines.

Taking different medicines at different times of the day and at different quantities can be addressed in a way which means you don't even have to worry about these issues at all! Monitored Dosage Systems (MDS) is a very simple type of medicines storage device aimed to simplify the routine of taking medicines, especially if you know you are one to accidently miss taking doses. The system has individual pockets to store your medicines for each day of the week and the time of day you are required to take the medicines (i.e. morning, lunch, dinner and bedtime). It also contains information about each medication such as its strength appearance. Once the pharmacist has sealed your medicines in place, all that is required from you is to pop out the contents of the pocket at specific time intervals. Your pharmacist can arrange for your medications to be packaged in this way and your GP will also need to be notified about this.

To be aware, not all medicines are able to be stored via MDS due to special storage requirements that affect the integrity of the drug, or medicines that come in the form of liquids – in which case, these medicines can be given separately.

The following is the basic structure of a Monitored Dosage System.

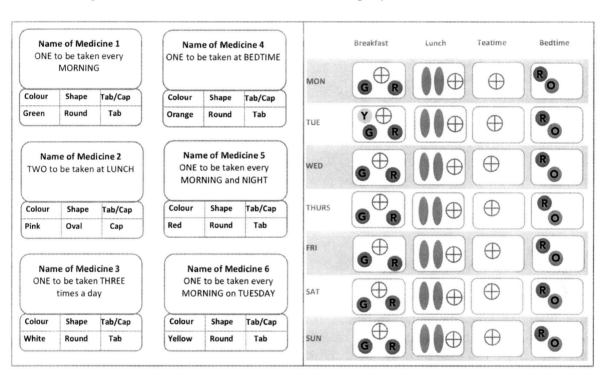

Letters have been added to show real-life colours: R - red; G - green; O - orange; Y, yellow; the oval shapes are pink and the crosses white.

Another way pharmacists can help you make better use of your medicines is by assessing the suitability of medical devices. An example of this is with inhalers. There are various types of inhalers available; one particular style may be more suited to you depending on your level of dexterity and preference. The correct inhaler technique is critical for its effectiveness and a specific inhaler device may mean the correct technique is easier to achieve. Pharmacists can check and demonstrate inhaler technique, discuss inhaler options, show you what is available to you and suggest possible alterations to your GP.

Medicines Use Reviews

Polypharmacy is a term that relates to the use of multiple medicines. As you get older you are more likely to suffer from chronic illnesses and inevitably this can mean there is a need to be taking more medicines, often more than four of five. Sometimes this can make manageing your medicines more difficult, for example ensuring your medicines are being taken at the correct times, and it can be difficult to identify which medicines are responsible for certain side effects.

Pharmacists can conduct free, yearly and confidential Medicines Use Reviews, which are specifically aimed to help you manage and understand your medicines better, to identify any side effects or problems and offer appropriate solutions. Either your pharmacist will offer you a review, or you can request for one yourself.

If you suffer from asthma or COPD, or are on heart-protective medication for example, you are *more likely* to be selected for a review, as you are considered most likely to benefit from a thorough discussion of your medicines.

Your pharmacist will go through each of your medicines, recapping on how and when to take them, and can give you more information on each medication so that you are fully aware of why you have been prescribed them. It is a chance to discuss any concerns that you have about your medicines, whether you are suffering any side effects, or if you are unsure about whether they are working. Your pharmacist will discuss possible solutions with you, and work together with your GP to create the most effective treatment plan for you.

New Medicine Service

This service involves a series of consultations which aim to support those with long term conditions *and* who have been prescribed new medicines. When taking new medicines, people often encounter problems with them. For example, it is easy to forget new information about your medicines, you may experience side effects or you may have difficulties taking your new medicines. The New Medicine service is split into 3 stages and aims to address these issues and help you use the medicine in the safest way possible.

Although it is a free service, it is only available for people who are on *new* medicines for certain conditions:

- Asthma/ COPD (chronic obstructive pulmonary disease)
- Type 2 diabetes
- Hypertension
- People suffering from conditions that require blood thinning medicines.

Stage 1 of the service begins when you first receive your medicine(s) from the pharmacist. Here the pharmacist will give you information about your medicine and how best to take it. The pharmacist will obtain your contact details in order to check in with you over the next few weeks.

Stage 2 of the service usually happens 1–2 weeks after first receiving your new medicine. Your pharmacist will contact you (can either be a face-to-face consultation or over the phone) and it is a chance to discuss how you are getting on with your medicine and whether you have encountered any side effects or problems. The pharmacist at this point can offer advice and solutions.

Stage 3 is the final follow up and usually happens about 3–4 weeks after receiving your new medicine. It is a chance to discuss whether any issues that you encountered have now been resolved.

Electronic Prescription Service (EPS)

This service is now very widely available, and if you agree to the service, it means that after seeing your GP, your prescription will be sent electronically to a pharmacy of your choice instead of the GP handing you a paper prescription to take to the pharmacy. It holds the advantages that the pharmacy can start preparing your medicines as soon as you have finished your appointment with the GP at the very earliest and your medicines will be ready to collect sooner (of course this also depends on how busy the pharmacy is on the day). It is usually advised to call the pharmacy before you want to collect your medications to ensure they have prepared it and will save you an otherwise wasted trip. It also eliminates the chances of your prescription being misplaced or lost. With every appointment with your GP, you have the chance to opt to change the pharmacy of where you want your electronic prescription to go.

The EPS system has been developed so that it is completely secure and confidential. Your prescription will only be seen by people in the GP practices, pharmacies and NHS prescription agencies.

Repeat Prescription Service

If you are on medicines that you take regularly then the Repeat Prescription Service is the simplest way to receive your medicines. Usually when you want another supply of your regular medicines, you would have to select the medicines you want on your repeat prescription slip and hand this in to your GP surgery or pharmacy, It will then get sent to your GP who will approve the repeat request and your prescription will be made available for you.

The repeat prescription service is a way of accessing your medicines regularly without having the need of handing in your request to the pharmacy or GP surgery. Once you sign up to the service at your chosen pharmacy, they can request your medication from your GP surgery on your behalf, they will then receive the prescriptions from your surgery directly (usually electronically) and the pharmacy will then prepare your medicines and notify you (via text or phone call) when your medicines are ready to collect. Once you have selected your pharmacy, your prescriptions will always be sent there unless you choose to cancel the service or opt to change pharmacy. It is a good way to ensure you have a continuous medicines supply, without the hassle of requesting the same medications again and again. You can have medication supplies of various time frames (e.g. 1-month supply, 2-month supply or 3-month supply), and this would have been previously agreed by, with your GP.

It is a good idea to keep in contact with your designated pharmacy as you can select which medicines you require in any given time. For example, you may find that you have a large excess stock on one medicine, and you can notify the pharmacist to withhold requesting it from the GP until further notice. It reduces the wastage of medicines and allows your medicine regime to be specific to your needs.

With most medications, a review with the GP (possibly including a blood test) may be necessary from time to time as medication requirements can change. It is important to attend your reviews regularly in order to avoid disruptions in your supply of medicines.

Home Delivery

Even though visiting your pharmacy gives you a chance to speak to your pharmacist, sometimes collecting your medicines from the pharmacy can be a burden. There are many reasons why personally collecting your medicines may not be the best option. Getting your medicines delivered is great for people who live far from their nearest pharmacy, have a lot of medicines to carry, do not have someone at home to collect on their behalf or struggle to get out especially in the cold winter months.

Your medicines will be packaged and delivered in a confidential manner and usually, as long as the address is local, you are able to change the delivery address depending on where you are staying. This is a service that not all pharmacies offer, but it is a service that more and more pharmacies are starting to introduce. Contacting your local pharmacies will allow you to identify which pharmacies offer this service.

Emergency Supply

Sometimes you may find yourself in a situation where you have run out of medicines and are unable to obtain a prescription on the same day. Running out of medication will mean that you miss one or several doses, which can compromise your current health status. Through an emergency supply it is possible to receive a limited supply of your medicines until a prescription can be made for you. Any pharmacist can offer you an emergency supply and if you do not pay for your prescriptions, it is free of charge. The pharmacist will usually need to speak to you or a carer (ideally face-to-face) and will assess the need for the emergency supply on a case-to-case basis. It is essential that you have taken the medicine before (preferably on a regular basis), and the pharmacist needs to be satisfied with the strength and dose. Therefore, the more information you can provide about your medicines, the more likely the pharmacist will be able to approve an emergency supply. You do not have to visit your regular pharmacy, however the pharmacy that provides the supply will eventually require a prescription and they will usually make a request on your behalf to your GP.

Depending on the situation, and the next available chance to obtain a prescription, your pharmacist can supply you with up to 30 days of medication. Some medicines have strict regulations like certain pain killers and for this, an emergency supply will not be possible. For some items, like creams and inhalers, the pharmacist will provide one full, unopened pack.

Health Checks

Many pharmacies now offer health checks, both privately and via the NHS. A health check is a quick way to get a general idea of your risk of conditions such as heart disease, diabetes and stroke.

NHS health checks are available for people between the ages of 40 and 74, and who do not have a preexisting condition. If you fall under this category, it means you will have access to a free health check every five years and usually you will receive a letter, reminding you of this. If you do not fall within this category, there may be other ways to access free health checks, depending on the available commissioned services in your local area.

You can arrange for a health check by simply speaking to the pharmacist; it may even be possible to get your health check done there and then depending on how busy the pharmacy is. The health check will take around 20–30 minutes and will involve the following tests:

- Weight
- Height
- Blood pressure
- Blood sugar
- Cholesterol.

The results of the health check are quick to process and your pharmacist will discuss them with you at the end of the consultation. Your pharmacist will also ask you a series of questions relating to your diet, activity levels, and general health, and all the information you provide (as well as the health check results) will contribute towards a *risk score*. Your risk score will tell you the percentage risk of developing a heart-related problem over the next 10 years. Generally, the risk will increase with age, and unfortunately genetics may also play a part in the likelihood of developing heart disease. However, your pharmacist will explain the individual test results to you and give you tailored lifestyle advice in order to minimise the risk as much as possible.

Note about Diet:

We all want to live longer, but we need to make sure that we look after ourselves in a way that means the *quality* of life we have is not compromised. Controlling what we eat and drink can play a huge part in our overall heath, and by eating the right foods, we can *prevent or delay* the onset of diseases such as diabetes and even cancer. Adding or increasing plant-based food into your diet is one of the best ways to decrease the risk of getting diseases, improve your body on the outside and inside and to help boost energy levels.

It can be difficult to change longstanding eating habits, but it is important to remember the most successful eating habits can be created by making realistic and gradual changes. Not only is this less likely to overwhelm you, but it is more likely that these changes are sustainable. There is little benefit from abruptly and completely neglecting certain foods (which you used to enjoy) that may have been harmful to your health, only to revert back to these foods a few months, weeks or even days down the line.

During your health check, your pharmacist can help you create achievable, healthy eating goals, as well as discussing healthier substitutions to foods you usually enjoy but aren't so good for you.

Smoking Cessation

Smoking is a notoriously difficult addiction to stop, even though most of us are aware of the impact it can have on your health (as well as those around you), and not to mention, your wallet. This is why many pharmacies offer an NHS stop smoking service to provide you with as much support as necessary in order to help you quit. Statistics show that you are *four times* more likely to quit with support, than attempting to quit smoking on your own.

The NHS offers a free 12-week programme, that combines one-to-one support along with nicotine replacement therapy products, such as nicotine patches or nicotine gum. The products are free if you do not pay for your prescriptions. There are now many different products and combinations available, which means that you are likely to find a treatment plan that is most suited to your needs.

Even if you've had unsuccessful attempts at stopping smoking in the past – this is an issue that your pharmacist will address with you, and will discuss the reasons why you think your attempts were unsuccessful and how to make sure you don't face the same obstacles.

Remember, it is **NEVER** too late to stop smoking. The effects of giving up smoking can start to show merely within the first 20 minutes and the following timeline shows how your health will only continue to improve.

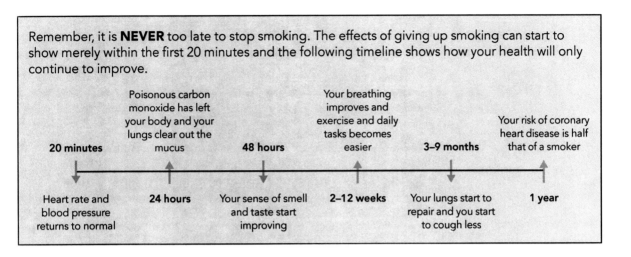

20 minutes	Poisonous carbon monoxide has left your body and your lungs clear out the mucus	**48 hours**	Your breathing improves and exercise and daily tasks becomes easier	**3–9 months**	Your risk of coronary heart disease is half that of a smoker
Heart rate and blood pressure returns to normal	**24 hours**	Your sense of smell and taste start improving	**2–12 weeks**	Your lungs start to repair and you start to cough less	**1 year**

Winter Health

The cold weather sees a rise in conditions such as colds and flu, coughs, sore throats, painful joints, dry skin and worsening of asthma. There are no quick fixes for colds and flus and it is mostly unavoidable, but there are many selfhelp measures you can take to help your body deal with these ailments. Colds and flu are caused by viruses, which means that antibiotics are usually unnecessary, as they are only effective in bacterial infections.

Pharmacies can offer advice, over-the-counter products, and can advise you on whether you need to see your GP.

The following are common measures to take when suffering the symptoms of a cold, or when feeling run down. It is important to discuss which products are suitable for you to take with your pharmacist as some over-the-counter products can interact with medications and may not be suitable to take with certain conditions. For example, diabetic patients should not use cough medicines containing sugar and some ingredients may exacerbate conditions such as high blood pressure. On top of this, it is important to eat well, get plenty of rest and to keep hydrated.

Ailment	Treatment and selfhelp measures
Cough* *Coughs are usually of two types; a chesty cough is when mucus or phlegm is brought up when coughing, and a dry cough usually feel tickly and without the presence of mucus.* *Coughs can either be bacterial or viral; a thick coloured mucus (yellowish, green) is a sign on a possible bacterial infection, in which case, you should see your GP where antibiotics may be required.* Note: for a cough that has lasted longer than 3 weeks -you must tell your doctor. It could just be a persistent cough, or it could be something more serious that requires investigations.	• Simple Linctus for a soothing effect • Cough drops or boiled sweets (to soothe and moisten a dry throat) • Expectorants e.g. guafenesin for chesty coughs • Cough suppressants e.g. pholcodine for dry coughs • Antihistamines (to aid sleep) e.g. diphenhydramine
Sore throat *Sore throats can also be viral (most common) or bacterial. A viral infection is treated with selfcare and a bacterial infection will require medical treatment.*	• Gargle with warm salty water • Warm honey and lemon drinks • Lozenges and Pastilles • Local anaesthetic-containing-products (mouth sprays)
Headache *Headaches are often a symptom in coughs and colds, and is usually due to sinus pressure from inflamed sinuses. These headaches often present as a constant dull, throbbing pain in the upper face, typically on one side (but can be both)*	• Paracetamol • Ibuprofen • Decongestant nasal sprays e.g. oxymetazoline
Aches and Pains *Aches and pains are commonly associated with the flu, but they can also appear in a severe cold. Sometimes you may feel achy all over, or the pain may be restricted to specific joints*	• Paracetamol • Ibuprofen (oral or topical) • Heat therapy (patches, gel) • Rubefacients (cause warmth)
Fever *A fever is generally classed as a temperature above 37.5C (99.5F) Our body usually raises in temperature when we are ill, as it is our body's natural defence to fight pathogens. Usually a fever will subside over a few hours or a couple of days at most, however, if your fever is no going away or you are concerned about the severity, medical attention should be sought.*	• Paracetamol

| Blocked nose

Blocked noses are the result of inflamed blood vessels in the sinuses and usually makes it difficult to get a good night's rest.	• Steam inhalation • Humidifier • Mentholated products e.g. Menthol, Eucalyptus • Vapour Rubs • Saline nasal drops/ spray • Decongestants e.g. Pseudoephedrine
Runny Nose

Caused from an excess of mucus production. Sometimes this excess mucus can run down the back of the nose to the throat, which is referred to as post-nasal drip. | • Antihistamines e.g. diphenhydramine- can dry up nasal secretions
• Saline nasal drops/spray
• Steam inhalation |

*There is limited scientific evidence to suggest that cough products are an effective treatment. On the whole, there is no real evidence for or against over-the-counter medicines for acute coughs. For this reason, selfcare measures are strongly advised, and can be very helpful in providing symptomatic relief.

There are lots of herbal products which are used to boost the immune system, prevent colds and shorten the duration of illnesses. Some come in the form of teas (e.g. peppermint tea). The evidence for the effectiveness of herbal products is unclear; some people swear by it and others claim it to offer no relief. It is safer to purchase herbal products from pharmacies or other shops, as opposed to online, where the quality and safety of the products cannot be guaranteed.

Erectile Dysfunction

Erectile dysfunction (the inability to get and maintain an erection) can be a sensitive subject, but it is not uncommon and there are things that can be done about it. It is important to speak to a health professional as there are many different causes, and in order to treat it, we must first understand the reason behind it.

Some pharmacies have the authorisation to supply medication to help treat erectile dysfunction without the need to see the doctor or obtain a prescription. This service is available to men who are 75 years of age and younger. It is a discrete and confidential service, usually advertised within pharmacies, or you can speak to staff members about it.

It will require a consultation with the pharmacist, which will be held in a private consultation room. Here, you will be asked a series of questions about your symptoms, medical history, medication and general health. Your blood pressure will also need to be monitored. There are strict criteria regarding who is eligible for this service and the decision to supply medication will depend on the assessment results. If you are not eligible, it is a matter that will need to be seen by your doctor.

Travel Vaccinations and Malaria Prevention

Lots of pharmacies provide a private travel clinic service, depending on the pharmacy it may be possible to receive vaccinations via a walkin appointment, or you may have to book for specific days of the week. Your GP practice may also offer travel vaccines free of charge, however, some vaccines can only be attained privately through pharmacies and clinics. The prices vary between pharmacies, but usually the consultations are free of charge. Once you have received your vaccination, you pharmacist will also provide you with a certificate

As long as you provide the details of where you are travelling, and are able to provide a history of your previous vaccinations, your pharmacist can tell you what vaccines you will need and whether any booster shots are necessary. Your pharmacist will also be able to tell you whether malaria prevention is necessary and some pharmacies will also be able to provide you with medication on the same day. There are various different antimalarial medicines available, with different formulations, prices and side effects, and your pharmacist will advise you on which one is most suitable for you.

Further reading

Information on minor ailment service, including a link to locate local pharmacies

http://www.nhs.uk/Livewell/Pharmacy/Pages/Commonconditions.aspx

Coping with colds and flu

http://www.nhs.uk/livewell/coldsandflu/Pages/Coldcomfort.aspx

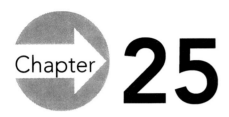

Chapter 25

Having an Operation

Andrew Rogerson

Coming into hospital for an operation can be daunting. However for many people having an operation can be a definitive treatment for a health problem and therefore of huge benefit. It can also be an excellent opportunity to reflect on your health and lifestyle, and if necessary to make changes for the better.

There are many ways to take control of some of the process, improve your experience of the hospital stay, speed up your recovery after an operation, and improve your long term health and quality of life. This chapter explains some of these at various stages of the surgical pathway: before surgery, during the hospital stay, and after your return home.

Before an operation

This is a time for gaining an understanding of what the operation and the recovery process will involve, as well as preparing for the practical aspects of the hospital stay.

Information gathering/shared decision-making

The decision to have an operation, and which operation to have, is one that requires close communication between you and the surgeon. The surgeon will advise on the most appropriate treatment option, but your opinion and values are crucial to this decision-making process. It is important that you ask the right questions and understand the answers before you decide. This process may take more than one visit or consultation: you may need to go away, reflect, and come back to the clinic with further questions before arriving at a shared decision. You must have all the information you need before you give your consent to surgery.

Some key questions to ask your surgeon (there may be many more specific questions):

1   What are we trying to achieve by doing this operation?

2 What will happen if we don't do the operation?

3 Are there nonsurgical options?

4 How is the operation performed?

5 What complications should I be aware of? e.g.:

- infection
- bleeding
- delirium
- failure of the procedure
- long period of rehabilitation
- surgical complications specific to the procedure
- death

6 Are there any other pieces of information that may change my mind?

7 How long should I expect to be in hospital?

8 How long will it take until I feel back to normal?

Lifestyle changes before an operation

Smoking

If you smoke, stopping smoking is the single most important step you can take to both improving your chances of a successful recovery after surgery and improving your long term health. The earlier you stop, the more benefit you will gain. It will reduce the risk of postoperative pneumonia, improve wound healing, reduce the surgical recovery time, and reduce your risk of emphysema/chronic bronchitis (smoker's lung), cancer and cardiovascular disease.

Alcohol

People who drink more than 14 units of alcohol per week are at increased risk of surgical complications and long term health problems including liver disease, cardiovascular problems, dementia and cancer. You should aim to keep your alcohol intake within government guideline limits during the period before an operation (and long term):

- Maximum 14 units/week (equivalent of 6 standard glasses of wine or pints of regular strength beer/lager)

- Spread your drinking over 3 or more days per week if you drink up to 14 units/week.

Exercise

Your muscle strength and aerobic fitness influence your recovery from an operation. These functions are very trainable. The longer you work on improving your fitness the better (5–6 months is optimal) but you can make significant improvements within a period of 3-4 weeks. It could be any aerobic activity that makes you sweat a little and increases your breathing rate. This could be walking, cycling, swimming or any activity you enjoy doing. Aim for 30–60 min, at least 3 times per week. The addition of range of motion resistance training adds additional benefit. You can obtain such a plan form your GP, a physiotherapist or a personal trainer.

Nutrition/weight loss

You should aim to eat at least 1g protein/kg body weight/day in the period before an operation. Good sources include meat, fish, eggs, pulses, soya and dairy products. Aim to keep your intake of carbohydrate and fat within recommended proportions (page 70).

If you are overweight (i.e. have a body mass index of greater than 25 kg/m^2), losing some weight prior to the operation may reduce your risk of postoperative complications and improve your recovery from surgery. This is not universally the case: for example patients with cancer are unlikely to benefit from restricting calories. Ask your surgeon/doctor first.

BMI calculation: body weight (kg)/ (height in metres)^2

Losing weight can be difficult, but the principles are simple:

- take regular exercise as above

- eat smaller portions (aim for 1/3 less on your plate at each meal)

- increase the proportion of fruit and vegetable in your diet

- Minimise cakes, biscuits, chocolates, crisps and sugary drinks from your diet.

If you can do this for a sustained period of time, you will almost certainly lose weight, feel healthier and have more energy. You should aim to keep this lifestyle going for long term health benefits: if you can maintain a BMI in the 20–25 range long term, it will improve your life expectancy and risk of cardiovascular disease in the future.

Medications

Before you come into hospital, you may need to withhold or change some of your medications. The list below is a guide to some common medication changes preoperatively, but should not replace the advice of your surgical/preoperative assessment team.

- Aspirin – in most cases this can be continued up until, and after, the operation

- Clopidogrel – this will usually be stopped 7 days before the operation

- ACE inhibitors (drugs ending in –pril) or angiotensin receptor blockers (ending in –artan) will usually be withheld on the morning of the operation

- Warfarin and other anticoagulants (drugs that reduce the risk of clots) – are usually be stopped 4 days before the operation. In some instances you will need to take an alternative (usually an under-the-skin injection) during these 4 days. Check this with your surgical/preoperative assessment team

- Diabetes medications (tablets or insulin) – you will need a tailored plan for what to do with these medications in the days preceding and after the operation. Check this with your surgical/preoperative assessment team.

Environmental/social considerations

Before you come in for an operation it is important to plan for the event in advance, to minimise challenges in the postoperative period.

An occupational therapist may be available in the preoperative period, but not all hospitals have this service. If available, their advice and support can be very helpful. Occupational therapists provides practical support to people who have long term conditions, disability, or those experiencing the effects of ageing, to do the things they need or want to do. They aim to help you to adapt to the changes that you may have in your day-to-day activities before, during and after your surgery. For example:

- Assess you in clinic or at home before surgery to see how safely and easily you manage, and suggest equipment (like bath seat, hoist or raised toilet) or adaptations (hand rails for example or ramp) you may essentially need to be more safe and independent

- Give you advice on how to conserve your energy or simplify tasks to get the most out of your day and manage any fatigue or breathlessness

- Coordinate with other organisations /services /professionals in your local community to offer you continued support in view of your upcoming surgery

- Assess and refer you to local services to provide you with suitable equipment, adaptations and even refer you for a wheelchair if needed for long term use or advise you on where to hire wheelchairs for short-term use

- Give information, education and support to you and your carers /family on managing your everyday activities at present or after surgery.

Since not all hospitals have a preoperative occupational therapy service, it is worth asking yourself questions as to how you're managing at present, and what difficulties you might have following your operation. Things you might want to consider:

- Am I /will I be having difficulty with personal care – washing, dressing, toileting, taking or remembering when to take my medications?

- Am I/will I be having difficulty with walking, getting in and out of bed, bath, on/off chair and toilet? Will I still be able to manage the stairs or do I need to have an extra stair rail or be on one level?

- Am I falling at home or felt that my balance has reduced and is fearful of falling?

- Am I/will I be having difficulty cooking, shopping, cleaning and doing most of my household chores?

- Is my memory compromising my safety at home?

- Am I socially isolated?

- If I am looking after a partner or dependant, will they manage on their own when I come in to hospital? and am I still manageing as the sole carer?

The answers to these questions may prompt you to plan in advance for the period after you return home from hospital. This may mean for example moving a bed downstairs, cooking and shopping in bulk, and arranging with family/friends to stay and support you and/or your partner/dependant for a period of time.

It is also helpful to familiarise yourself with the available services in your community. You can do this by visiting your local council's website if you have access to the Internet or by speaking to your GP. If you think that the help you will require is only with domestic tasks, it might be worth contacting your local Age UK or Red Cross charities to know what help they can provide as Social Services may not be able to offer help solely for domestic support.

It is always best to make anticipatory plans and cancel services if no longer required than to have no help planned and then struggle.

Your stay in hospital

You will usually come in to hospital on the day of surgery to a surgical admissions lounge. In some circumstances you will need to come into hospital the day before the operation. You will need to stop eating from 6 hours before the operation and stop drinking (apart from small sips of water) from 2 hours before the operation. You should take your morning medications as usual unless directed otherwise. The anaesthetist will meet you on the morning of the operation and explain the anaesthesia process to you. After this you will be taken into the anaesthetic room for the anaesthetic to be administered before you are wheeled into the operating theatre.

After the operation, you will stay in the theatre recovery room until you are ready to go to the ward. If you have had an anaesthetic, you may feel very sleepy or confused for a period of time after you wake up. This is normal.

Once you arrive on the ward, you will usually be able to eat and drink straight away. It is important to start eating and drinking as soon as you feel able to do so, but do so with small amounts on a "little and often" basis, as your gut may not be ready to absorb large amounts of food and fluids. The sooner your get your body back into a normal routine, the quicker you will recover, and the more likely you are to make a full recovery.

Simple measures you can take to speed up the recovery process are:

- Sitting in a chair rather than lying in bed
- Choosing day clothes to wear during the day and night clothes at night
- Walking to the toilet (with assistance if needed)
- Washing yourself in the bathroom if possible
- Feeding yourself if possible (asking for assistance if you need it)
- Having a rest on the bed after lunch
- Working with the physiotherapists on the ward to improve your strength and balance
- Dinking plenty of fluids throughout the day
- Walking to the dining table if there is one
- Getting out to the garden, café or day room with any visitors
- Walking to the bathroom to brush your teeth before bed
- Recruiting the help of family or friends to help you do your recommended exercises
- Making sure you ask the nurses for pain relief if you need it as pain can hamper your recovery
- Getting a good night's sleep if possible. If you are not sleeping well, inform the nursing staff who may be able to obtain ear plugs/eye shades if these help
- If you need to use the toilet at night, try to get out of bed to use a commode or the toilet.

Some common postoperative complications

Delirium

Delirium is a state of confusion and disordered thinking that can occur during illness or after an operation. Having dementia, cognitive impairment, other health problems, or drinking alcohol increases the risk of developing delirium. Surgery can trigger delirium on its own, but there are many other triggers such as sedating drugs, dehydration, salt imbalances, pain, infection, low oxygen levels, constipation and disruptions in bladder function.

It is characterised by poor concentration (inattention), muddled thoughts, hallucinations/ delusions, and drowsiness. Not all of these features are necessarily present. It usually has a fluctuating course, with lucid and relatively normal periods alternating with drowsy, confused periods. These fluctuations can happen several times over the course of the day. Often patients with delirium are very sleepy during the day and very awake and sometimes agitated at night. They may see or hear things that are not there. Personality changes are often seen, with swearing and shouting being common. Delirium is often a very distressing experience for patients as well as their families and friends, and some people feel ashamed of their behaviour and have unpleasant memories of the experience after it has resolved.

The recovery from delirium can be improved by:

- treating the underlying cause

- maintaining adequate nutrition and hydration

- ensuring pain is treated

- regularly reminding the delirious patient of the date, time, and where they are

- engageing in calm and reassuring conversation

- visitors bringing in some things from home such as a clock/bedside lamp/ pictures of friends and family

- getting a good sleep at night and avoiding sleeping during the day

- ensuring usual spectacles and hearing aids are brought in to hospital and worn

- engageing in physical activity

- avoiding drugs that cause drowsiness.

It is important to be aware that, in most cases, delirium will resolve completely. The recovery time varies between a few days and several weeks. In some cases it can take months to fully resolve, and occasionally some people do not fully recover, but this is less common.

Constipation

This is a very common occurrence in the period after an operation. There are several causes, including the use of painkillers in the morphine drug class, reduced activity levels, reduced intake of food, eating low-fibre hospital food, and the "bowel-stunning" effect of abdominal surgery. Constipation can worsen the effects of delirium, cause pain, reduce appetite, make urination impossible, and cause incontinence, diarrhoea, nausea, vomiting and lethargy. It is important to tell the nurses if you have not opened your bowels for more than a day, as prevention is better than cure. In almost all cases it can be prevented by taking an appropriate laxative. When constipation becomes established, it takes longer to treat and may necessitate suppositories or enemas.

Ileus

Ileus is a phenomenon that occurs frequently after abdominal surgery, when the bowel is handled or manipulated. After such an operation, the bowel can become "stunned", which often leads to reduced/absent bowel activity, constipation, severe bloating, nausea and vomiting, and griping abdominal pain. It usually resolves after 2-3 days but can last a week or more. The recovery process can be helped by avoiding the use of morphine class painkillers; taking small amounts of fluids only and avoiding large amounts of food; keeping moving; and taking medications that stimulate the movement of the gut. Sometimes the surgical team may insert a tube through the nose into the stomach to release the pressure in the gut and reduce vomiting secondary to ileus.

Pain

Pain occurs after almost all operations and is a normal response to surgery. It will be managed during the procedure itself by general or local anaesthesia. After the operation you will require painkillers to manage the pain. Some people require large amounts of painkillers while others require very little. It is important to admit when you are in pain and ask for painkillers to help manage it. Untreated pain can cause delirium and pneumonia, and make it very difficult for you mobilise, which will slow down your recovery after surgery. Pain can also be greatly improved by talking to others, keeping your mind and body active, and making sure you stay relaxed and in a positive frame of mind.

After discharge from hospital

The recovery process continues long after you leave hospital. You can expect to feel more tired than normal, for weeks of even months after the operation. You may also experience low mood and lethargy. This is because the body is working hard to heal itself and adapt to the changes that the operation has brought about. During this period it is important that you continue to work hard to regain your independence, mobility and general health.

Depending on the type of surgery and your health needs afterwards you may require a period of rehabilitation following discharge from hospital. This may occur in a rehabilitation unit or in your own home. Not everyone requires this and your individual needs will be assessed by a specialist team who will give you advice and support during this process. The choices you make during this rehabilitation phase will have a huge impact on how quickly you recover and the completeness of your recovery.

As discussed above, you may not be able to do some basic activities of daily living at the beginning, such as cooking, cleaning or even going to the toilet independently. While you should not do things that are unsafe, it important that you work towards regaining your ability to perform these tasks by doing a little more each day. The practical support and understanding of your family and friends are very important in this process. Their help will often be very valuable and necessary. However they may sometimes want to help you with things that you can manage yourself, in which case ask them to let you try it on your own as this will speed up your return to independence and give you a sense of achievement.

Your physiotherapist in hospital should have provided you with a list of exercises to perform while in hospital and after discharge. Working on these diligently will help you recover and get back to normal functioning, so keep working at this.

While recovering from an operation you will need more protein than usual. You should aim for 1.5g protein/kg body weight/day for the first 2 months after the operation. If you have diabetes, good control of your blood sugars (aiming for glucose readings in the 4-11 range) aids the healing process.

Although for many people having surgery is a frightening prospect, it can bring very positive, lasting changes to your health and lifestyle. The above steps will allow you to take control and optimise both your surgical recovery and long term health. Embrace it!

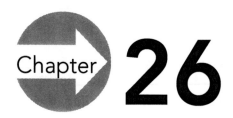

Chapter **26**

Post Hospital Nursing Care

Carol Forde-Johnston

Your nurse is a highly trained professional and, like your doctor and pharmacist, is able to provide support and advice on a wide range of health issues. This chapter focuses on post-hospital nursing care that is particularly pertinent to the elderly.

Hospital discharges and readmissions

Although there is good nursing and medical practice delivered across UK health services, many of us will know a person who has experienced a rushed hospital discharge and the negative effects that this had on the individual and their family. In 2011, the Parliamentary and Health Service Ombudsman reported on older peoples' hospital discharges. Findings indicated that there was evidence of poor communication on discharge, older people being moved home too quickly and a lack of sufficient care being in place at home. A positive view of community staff was reported, as they were able to spend more time on the delivery of care than hospital staff.

Over the past decade, emergency hospital readmission rates have risen, especially in the over 75's. Readmission is defined as an unplanned readmission within 28 days of you leaving hospital. The readmission rate is 50% higher for those over 65 years, in comparison to 18-64 year olds (Laurie and Battye 2012). Nursing care that is not adequately planned for can lead to a difficult time at home following your hospital discharge, which increases your risk of readmission. The better equipped you are to anticipate your care needs before you leave hospital, the more chance you will have of receiving the correct support at home.

Prepare before you leave hospital

Professionals in hospital are responsible for clearly explaining what is happening to you and answering any of your questions. Do not be afraid to write a list of questions down for the doctors or nurses who can answer them during their bedside rounds.

This chapter aims to enable you to understand what is happening to you, and how you can manage your care on discharge. Asking key questions about your care will help guide you. See some example questions below:

- What investigations, procedures or surgery are taking place in hospital and how will it affect me?
- What are the usual timescales for recovery?
- What are the potential complications?
- What can I do to prevent complications when I am discharged home?
- Will I need a new medication? If so, what is it for? How will it affect my body? Are there any side effects?
- Will I be able to move, walk, eat, drink, go to the toilet, wash/dress myself, see and hear normally? (Questions will depend on why you are admitted to hospital)
- If I am restricted in anyway when I am discharged how long will this last?
- What extra support do you think I will need when I am discharged?
- How long will I need this extra support for?
- Do I need to pay for extra support or is it provided free?
- Who do I need to contact when I am at home to ensure I receive the correct support and/ or follow up?
- Will I need to come back to hospital follow up clinics or outpatient treatments? If so how often and where will they take place?

If you are warned that you may be immobile for a few weeks when you are discharged it is unrealistic to plan to run a half marathon in a month. People make the mistake of planning for the minimum amount of time to recover following their discharge, when their body may need a little extra time to heal.

It is helpful for staff planning your discharge to know about your normal routines and daily life at home before discharge, and any hobbies you have. This information will help professionals when they are advising you to plan for your future life at home. If you live alone, nursing staff will discuss what you may need to put in place at home and advise about the community support available to you. They should liaise with your GP and local District Nurses to ensure you have a safe discharge.

The different health care professional roles

During your hospital stay a Medical Consultant will lead your medical care and many professionals may visit you in a short space of time. It is helpful to know the roles of each health care professional and how they can support you at home. An overview of health care professionals' roles is provided in the table below.

Health care professionals and their roles linked to your discharge and post hospital care

Roles	Key responsibilities
Registered Nurse	• Initiates discharge planning procedures and responsible for a safe discharge home • The key link person between hospital and community care and will liaise between you and other health care providers in the hospital and community, e.g. the GP, district nurse team, community physiotherapist • Ensures all nursing care plans are in order at the time of your discharge and at home • Teaches the patient and family, e.g. how to take a blood sugar, how to care for their wounds/sutures and prevent discharge complications
Physiotherapist	• Aims to improve your range of movement and flexibility when you have injuries that limit physical activities in hospital or at home • Assists you with carefully planned, regular exercise routines to build up your strength and independence • Educates and promotes healthy methods to improve your movements • Helps manage pain or disease using good posture and techniques • Identifies equipment and aids to promote mobility and your safety
Speech & Language Therapist	• Finds out what is causing your speech or swallowing difficulties • Conducts a swallow assessment to assess whether it is working properly • Decides whether you are safe to eat and that you do not choke • Identifies the best treatment to enable you to speak, or swallow, to the best of your ability • Educates using swallowing and speech exercises to improve your condition and symptoms • Finds the right equipment and communication aids to promote communication between you and others
Occupational Therapist	• Aims to improve or regain everyday life skills, e.g. washing, dressing, eating, painting, sewing and reading • Works with people who have disabilities, trauma injuries or impairments from long term conditions • Assesses you in your home, or in areas made to look like a home environment in hospital, e.g. kitchen • Assesses your capability and helps you find the right equipment or adaptations to promote meaningful activities • Advises on methods to help you achieve your goals living at home, e.g. reorganising rooms and placing objects differently to help you use them more easily

Roles	Key responsibilities
Social Worker	• Understands social issues within the community • Advises you when you have social problems linked to housing, disability, benefits, poverty and abuse • Supports communities, families and individuals with social challenges in life using a holistic approach
Dietician	• Expert in human nutrition and diet • Assesses nutritional health by finding out your weight, favourite foods, and eating and exercise habits • Assesses your risk of malnutrition using a risk assessment tool. • Sets dietary goals to meet your nutritional daily requirements • Prescribes additional, nutritious meals and drink supplements • Prescribes bottles of feed if you need to be fed with a tube. This is called nasogastric feeding

Practical support during your first few days at home

It is essential that you plan your first few days at home with the nursing and medical staff responsible for your discharge. You may lack mobility, or have a wound or new treatment. If you have restricted access to local services due to immobility, pain or the need to rest, you will need to plan how you will manage as independently as possible at home. Plan to have enough grocery shopping at home by contacting friends or family. The day you are discharged from hospital, your immediate care needs are transferred over to your GP and a community team of professionals.

Post hospital nursing care

Within this section practical nursing advice is provided, however, please note that only general guidance is offered. Your care will differ according to the severity of your symptoms and medical condition. If you have a specific condition that requires specialist treatment you must check with your Consultant or GP first. If you have any sudden deterioration, such as difficult breathing, sudden severe pain or loss of consciousness, you **should always dial 999 and contact the emergency services**.

Breathing

The guidance below may help a person who has a long term condition that affects their breathing or wants to know how to promote good breathing, e.g. after surgery when movement is restricted. **If someone is having breathing difficulty or has an airway obstruction, call 999 right away.**

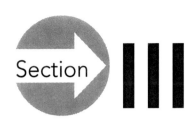

Section III

ADDRESSING CHANGE

Chapter 27

Retirement

By the age of 50 many individuals have reached the height of their career and are looking for new challenges. Like the rest of the community, they feel 10 years younger than their chronological age and are expecting another 25 years of sustained activity. Yet 50% of the same individuals approach retirement totally unprepared: half would like to carry on for financial reasons, another quarter for enjoyment or personal job satisfaction, and a smaller number wish to continue for health reasons or to retain a group of friends.

Retirement, redundancy and job loss affect your life style, rather than your physical or mental health. They can have a marked affect on your self esteem and your position in the community:

- Status change from a leader to a has-been

- Reduced support from secretaries and staff

- Reduced mental (and possibly) physical demands

- Increased personal time and responsibility

- Fear and uncertainty of what is expected of you, both by yourself and others

- Resultant insecurity and slowing of mental and physical activity.

Other examples of life changing events include: taking on new paid or voluntary employment; changes in your financial status (affecting payment of facilities, home improvements, a car, holidays and pensions); change in housing (changes in location leading to loss of friends and long standing community support); and loss of a partner, resulting in bereavement, loneliness and boredom.

The **stress of life changing events** can be a major factor in producing disenchantment, confusion, insecurity and instability, leading to bitterness and depression, with loss of interest, apathy and general inactivity.

These effects can result in diminution of the rate and accuracy of your thoughts, activities and responses, these symptoms and signs being noted by both you and others around you. It is important to understand these changes, and thence consider how best to adapt, reinvent yourself, and ensure you are appropriately prepared for your future.

These situations require a **relook at your personal life**. They often require taking on new responsibilities for yourself and others, such as looking after medication, cooking, shopping, cleaning and repairs. Although some events may have rendered a severe blow to your morale, and a realisation that you are not indispensible, you are not unique, and most people have come out the other side strengthened in their resolve. Your aim must be do the same, and become fitter, stronger and happier.

If these events are happening later in life other factors enter the equation. The wear and tear of life eventually gets to various bits of you. Your movements are slower and stiffer; you may be short of breath after minimal exertion; your bowel and waterworks may be playing up; and you may be thinking more slowly.

However, these changes do not occur all together, or at the same rate, and they do not mean that you have lost it. Frailty of body is not synonymous with frailty of mind (with perhaps the sad exception of sufferers from dementia). Not all oldies are oldies – some feel like this in their forties, while others deny it in their nineties – remember **you are an individual**. This text advises you as an individual on how to maintain your wellbeing, and by so doing, aims to **extend your independence and autonomy**.

You may think a bit more slowly, but your brain usually serves you well to the end of your days, and it is essential that you fill it with **meaningful activity.**

You may have to address the stigmata of retirement (at whatever age!). It is worth remembering that when pensions were introduced in the early twentieth century, less than half of the male population passed the retirement age – it is perhaps not surprising that the sums no longer add up.

There is the possibility of your being perceived as a noncontributor, a nonperson who has had his or her day and should slide into oblivion. You may be branded as a burden on your family and society, and a social appendage that is likely to need constant supervision and care. Terms such as golden oldie, over the hill and pensioner abound. The scenario may be played out through loss of respect, being ignored and left out of decision-making, rejection and relegation (perhaps physically as well as mentally).

This lack of respect, and perhaps worse the patronisation, make you feel unwanted, unheeded, unneeded and a failure. When you encounter poor decisions that you are unable to influence, you are likely to lose interest, switch off and enter into **social isolation**.

In fact – as you know well – **the above is a false conception**.

You are a valuable knowledge resource, loaded with distilled information and pearls of wisdom. You have unique skills, experience, expertise and an unparalleled institutional memory; you have been there, and handled and coped with change. You have accumulated social skills that take a lifetime to develop, in leadership, critical thinking, cooperation and collaboration.

You have the soft skills so necessary in networking – far more important than a list of qualifications (that you probably have as well) – and knowledge of how to listen, negotiate and deliver, calmly and successfully. You may not think these all relates you, but it is worth a little reflection to realise your true value.

SO – **how are you going to make use of these attributes**?

Do you need to take up a **job**, does it need to be reimbursed and does it complement your intended lifestyle?

This text is not intended to prepare you for a job interview, but it is heavily weighted towards reinventing your outlook, image and attitude, by exploring new activities and ensuring you are **occupied**.

It is important that you set this pattern when you are still relatively young and fit: it should be **something you really want to do,** and is sustainable for the foreseeable future. This section does not attempt to provide answers, but provides the questions that you should be asking yourself. It is suggested in the chapter on finance, that you should be considering these matters a decade before you retire, but whatever your status, this means now!

What would you like to do? It is hoped that your life's work has given you much satisfaction, and you feel that you have contributed to whatever your area of employment. If you are still fit and active in your mind and body, it is important to undertake something that satisfies your potential. Retirement provides time, freedom and the opportunity to reexamine your outlook on the world, none more so than in **work satisfaction**. Although this is of particular importance in voluntary work, it also applies to any reemployment you are considering.

Paid Employment

Linked to the question of reemployment, is whether you want full of part-time work. The former requires commitment and responsibility, and a fixed working pattern. Part-time allows you more time to relax and may also include **flexibility** to accommodate future change. You may never have experienced part-time employment, but the responsibility is likely to be less, and you may have to be the recipient of orders that you used to deliver.

Do you wish to: continue in the same job; continue in a similar job; continue with the same employer; consult in your field; consider a new field; develop new skills; or undertake unskilled work?

You need to find out whether any such **opportunities** are available and the chances of getting one if you applied. You may have to do a lot of searching, and make some hard decisions on what job you would be willing to do if offered, and how this meets your financial aspirations?

Salary may be a key factor, and whether it enables you to maintain your accustomed lifestyle. You may have already decided to downsize your home, and the **location** of a new residence may be a deciding factor in your future place of employment.

Unpaid Activity

Unpaid work includes both voluntary and leisure activity – it allows you more emphasis on enjoyment and satisfaction; consider whether these factors equate to the energies that you intend to put in. Take time to explore these opportunities.

Everyone needs help and advice, and finding an area for long term interest is an example of where you need to take **multiple opinions**. As with all jobs, however, if you are taking advise from a potential employer, have some idea of the advice you would and would not accept and bring these factors into the conversation, otherwise you may have the embarrassment of refusing, or being obliged to take an unwanted offer.

In your **networking**, searching on the **Internet**, and exploring local institutions and **charities**, consider whether your expertise and core skills match the interests and needs of a targeted position, and whether you may be able to transfer them to mutual advantage. Taking such a position may be at a lesser level of responsibility than you are used to. It is essential to know that you would be able to **contribute** and be **wanted** (a reward far more desirable than financial remuneration). You need to be involved, integrated and part of the decision making process, and not just a token presence – you would be wise not to consider the latter.

In your field there should be opportunities to consult, advise and mentor individuals in training. Outcomes relate to the initial decision-making, and in many fields are a balance between benefits and risks. If you are working in these areas, ensure you are working in a true partnership, and failures cannot be attributed to or blamed on age-related criteria. Part-time voluntary work is usually more appropriate, but you still need to consider the time given, and the **location** and accessibility of the workplace, or whether this could be managed electronically from home.

You may have to learn new skills, and undertake **training** on appropriate courses. A new field of interest can give you lots of enjoyment and ensure that you are enthusiastic and motivated to go forward. Nevertheless, decide whether this is at your own expense, and whether it is worth it.

Does the training provide you with a saleable commodity, with or without a certificate; is it from a respected institution, is it an area you are going to enjoy and does it match your desired employment? In a new field, it is important that you are competent, fit for purpose, able to pass external and self assessments, and you are comfortable with what is expected of you.

Specific areas that you should consider for personal development, and in which you may be lacking, include IT and all aspects of management. Aim to become independent on electronic media and understand their advantages, particularly as a means of communication.

Remember that charity begins **at home**, and there may be a number of previously neglected areas that deserve your attention; examples include, decorating, gardening, cooking and caring for others, possibly your partner or a family member. Do not neglect home comforts and social engagements.

In **leisure activities**, classes are likely to bring you into contact with new social groups, and plenty of advice is given elsewhere in the text, such as in the arts, health care and more vigorous endeavours, such as walking, bird watching, swimming and exercise programmes. Other hobbies include: clubs; cards; photography; painting; visits to galleries, museums and sporting events; concert and theatre visits; reading; lectures (giving or attending); writing; and consider whether your travelling days are over or whether you would consider a cruise.

As everyone is different, both mentally and physically, this chapter has avoided being prescriptive, however, the one message that is universal, and much repeated is that you must be **occupied**.

Note that while retirement is a key life-changing and challenging event, it is also a time to put in place long term disease-control measures. Learn what symptoms to look out for, when to consult a doctor, and what medication you may require. Consider how you can learn through education and other sources, how you can become a skilled contented elder, and also by applying this knowledge, how you can help others.

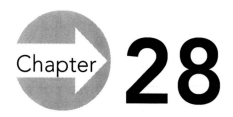

Chapter 28

Family and Friends

Family

Throughout the animal kingdom parents nurture their offsprings, and the human Family Unit is based on love, sex and the birth of children: within this powerful bond, parents are responsible for the care of their young. The Unit provides companionship for like-minded individuals with shared interests, and develops mutual respect and a framework to support financial, housing and home needs, together with child education and holidays. The rules for the Unit are established for all to work together: likes and dislikes, and habits, good and bad, are known and accepted or tolerated within the umbrella of dependency.

Although many of these features may be put to the test, the Family Unit is usually inviolate during the upbringing of the children. Children start to leave home in their late teens, although dependency may extend into their midtwenties (and much longer in some parent's view). At this time parents are usually in their fifth and sixth decades and it is a time for reappraisal of the Family Unit.

With the release of immediate parental responsibility, it is a time for reexamination of parental compatibility. Differences that may have been tolerated, perhaps with minor arguments, for many years, are freed for vigorous assessment. Differences are most apparent when there is a marked age gap between parents, as this can have a substantial impact on the relationship.

The younger member of a couple may be keen to follow an active life, filled with entertainment and friends, with youthful ideas and interests. In contrast the older member may have reached retirement age, and have started to look for a quieter, less active life and home comforts. Unfortunately the acceptance of 'getting old' is a state of mind that promotes and becomes a self fulfilling prophecy: lack of exercise is accompanied by weight gain, and lack of attention to grooming and clothing; all shortening longevity as well as partner acceptance.

The impact of a mismatch and diverging interests may be substantial. Agreement may be reached to live separate lives, with freedom to follow independent lifestyles and possibly changes of sleeping arrangements – continuing a marriage of convenience. This may prove an effective living arrangement, as complete loneliness is diverted and mutual support can still be given in an emergency. If the situation is intolerable, external advice should be sought, such as from a marriage councilor. The problem is just between the parents and not for family friends or the community to be involved in, or to give judgment.

If a solution is not found, some form of separation is desirable. Ideally this is by mutual agreement without residual hatred, or a messy divorce that can incur expensive legal fees. When both parents are earning, this allows considerably more leeway and independence, and previous prejudices against divorce have reduced in recent years. It is of interest that, whereas the UK incidence of divorce has fallen over the last 15 years, it has risen in the over 65-year-olds.

Although the last few paragraphs have unfolded the problems encountered when children leave the Family Unit, in most cases it is a time of celebration and rekindling a loving relationship for the parents. Financial responsibility is reduced and disposable income increased: this may be accentuated by downsizing of the family home. Possibly for the first time in their lives they can consider enjoying themselves with added luxury in holidays, clothing, entertainment, house decoration and a car upgrade.

You can expect to be targeted by financial advisors, life insurers, travel agents and other sales personnel: enjoy reading their literature (especially the travel brochures), but beware, there is no such thing as a free lunch, if it's too good to be true, it is, and it's better to make initial enquiries from close friends and relatives whom you trust.

The responsibility to children and potential grandchildren never goes away. Your children may have moved away, even gone abroad: although this may be distressing, communication can be maintained through electronic media and visits in either direction can be looked forward to. Nearby offspring's can be a mixed blessing. If the relationship with the child is a loving one and this extends to their partner, the arrangement is very convenient and enjoyable, and allows monitoring of the health and wellbeing of the parents. Parents must ensure that the arrangement does not impose any detriment to the social life of the child or their partner. This must be particularly guarded against when living under the same roof, such as in an annex.

Parents may have moved to a rural area, as this trend has increased markedly in over 65-year-olds over the last 15 years. They may still be in easy access to at least one of the children, and when both parents are alive and active, this is an excellent arrangement. It can, however, raise problems in making new friends, if one of the parents dies or if they stop using a car and public transport is limited.

When grandchildren arrive it is natural that grandparents will be asked to babysit. However, this must not become a burden or interfere with their own social life – for them this is the priority, and rules must be in place to ensure this does not happen. With this understanding the arrangement is a common interest, looking after the baby being a reward in its own right.

When grandchildren grow older they can be fun for grandparents, as witnessed by the t-shirt slogan – 'if I'd known grandchildren were such fun, I'd have had them first'. Again rules must be in place as to the time and lengths of visits, and the parents' rules must be adhered to – it is not for grandparents to dictate or interfere with the parenting techniques of their children. Old traditions such as family get-togethers on holidays and festivals must be discussed, so that they do not become an unwanted ritual, and can be abandoned or modified when needed.

Gifts, of any size, to children and grandchildren give pleasure to both the donor and the recipient; a pleasure lost to the parents if only passed on through an inheritance. However, such gifts should be proportionate to the future needs of the parents, such as for care, must be fair to all the family and should not be looked on as a bribe. Also check with the current laws concerning inheritance tax – gifts over a set limit are taxable if the donor dies before seven years have elapsed.

These various arrangements can be made to work well until the inevitable death of one of the parents. This can be a life-shattering event, particularly if the dead parent was the carer for the second. Immediate support from family and friends is usually present in abundance, with everyone rallying round; but when the funeral is over and everyone has gone home, problems of care can arise.

The health of the remaining parent is a key factor, and whether they are fit and able to live on their own. A member of the family may be designated to move in and look after the parent; but this can be severely detrimental for the chosen one. Moving in with one of the children is another option, but the success of this move is dependent on the previous relationship between the parent and child, and other members of the child's family.

The parent may well find the relationship untenable. The hierarchical order is changed; their opinion may be ignored or overruled, leading to frustration and anger that cannot openly be expressed. With good planning these issues should have been subjects of discussion between parents and children in advance, as well as the possibility of moving into a care home. As considered in many chapters of this text, the aim is to grow old with dignity and grace, retaining enthusiasm and independence, and living what you, the parent, considers a quality lifestyle.

Friends

Your circle of friends varies throughout your life, with changes of residence, changing interests and activities, such as team and other sports, and your places of education. When you are actively progressing through life, friendship opportunities also change, and you are probably not noticing the gradual transition. Work and family life take over, and friends become linked through your employment and children.

Retirement brings a new element into your life, and may also bring a change to your circle of friends. It may be that you do not need new friends outside your family circle, and you are self-sufficient, with enough personal activities to fill your time: a positive decision that may serve you well for many years.

Nevertheless, humans are by nature sociable creatures and need someone to talk to, rather than sink into a world of loneliness – a contented life as a recluse is unusual.

Some friends with whom you have a particular affinity are retained, even when separated, communication being maintained by electronic means, or at least by Christmas cards. However, later life can be accompanied by loss of close friends, as well as relatives, and some you may consider irreplaceable.

It is difficult to replace someone with whom you have shared life's secrets and events. Yet it is important to retain a network of friends to avoid loneliness and social isolation in your latter years. This can be more difficult if you are living on your own, with few external contacts. If you are not used to socialising it requires a great deal of effort and courage to start.

The first step is literally the step that takes you out of your home. You probably have a local newspaper; look through it to see if there are local events advertised, such as sporting activities or local theatre productions that could motivate you to step outside. Once you get to one of these events you are likely to be surrounded by like-minded individuals of all ages. If someone smiles at you, smile back and have a chat; once you've done this once you will find it easier and may even initiate the sequence.

Getting used to communicating has to be remembered or relearned. In other spheres, religious leaders and community centres welcome new members. If you are a dog owner you wont have to relearn, as the dog does it all for you. Internet dating is a growing trend for all ages, and the elderly should not be excluded. Take advice on how to become involved from someone who has been there (usually a younger associate). Ensure that the first meeting is in a public space, such as a public house. If you are intending to enter into this arena, you must be confident enough to tell someone that you do not wish to see him or her again when the occasion arises.

If you want to know what is happening in the community, the local library is the place to start. The skills of the staff are directed at information gathering and distribution, and this encompasses information on all local activities. Here you can find out about community activities and classes that could interest you, as considered in chapter 31. If your specific interest is missing, discuss with the library staff the logistics of setting up the relevant group – they have the skills and possibly the space to help.

Voluntary work may interest you and this will introduce you to a large and diverse collection of enthusiasts from across society. Remember that if you intend to work with children or the disabled, you need a Disclosure and Barring Service (DBS formerly CRB) Certificate issued by the police – ask the library for details.

Don't expect new friends to suddenly replace ones that had an understanding built in over many decades. Friendship encompasses many levels, starting with a casual acquaintance leading to mutual agreement to meet again. These meetings in coffee shops, pubs and restaurants define commonality of interest and lead to joining groups and building up a network of like-minded individuals that address problems of loneliness; dispelling any doubts you may have had about your social skills.

Deeper friendship is based on mutual interest, understanding and trust, giving much pleasure and enjoyment. Such friends are there when needed, giving mutual support, sharing many aspects of your life, including regular meetings, outings and possibly holidays: such friendship has been shown to increase longevity.

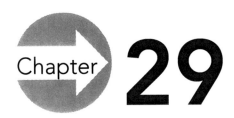

Chapter **29**

Homes for the Third Age

Ed Green

"We don't stop being ourselves as we get older, we don't suddenly become a different kind of human being, prepared to accept just anything…"

Hugh Pearman, RIBA Journal July/Aug 2011

Over the next twenty years, the number of people over sixty is predicted to rise by 43% from 2013[1], and a third of the UK population will fall into the 'older person' category. Improvements in quality of life mean that we can now expect to live twenty years past retirement age, for half of which we are likely to be active and healthy. This concept of an active third age represents a significant change in the social fabric of Britain that our homes, town and cities were not designed to accommodate.

The UK housing crisis is well documented. We have a shortage of quality, affordable homes that rises year on year, affecting all types of resident, because demand for new homes continues to outstrip supply by around 200%. Much of the response thus far has focussed on new homes for first time buyers. However, studies have identified a clear shortage of housing suited to older people. Part of the issue is the British penchant for home-owning. Only 18% of people in the UK rent privately, compared with 51% in Switzerland or 40% in Germany.[2] Combined with a shortage of good housing and inflated prices, this makes us less inclined to relocate. As people grow older and their needs change – either gradually, or suddenly with an illness or a fall – many become trapped, stranded in large family homes they no longer need, but unwilling to downsize (or 'right-size') to accommodation they consider to be substandard. By building age-appropriate housing, we would be unlocking family homes, with a clear opportunity to impact on the housing crisis.

---

1   Silver Linings p.8
2   Office of National Statistics, Census data 2013

The UK is also saddled with the oldest housing stock in the developed world; more than eight million of the twenty five million UK properties are more than sixty years old. Interestingly, while this does not make our homes eminently suitable for older people[1], neither does it make them less suitable... A hundred years of reuse and adaptation testify to the flexibility of Victorian bricks and mortar, in comparison to many more recently built homes. Older people currently have three options – mainstream housing (including adaptation), specialised housing (homes designed for older people) or residential care homes (HAPPI, 2009). As a generation, they spend 70–90% of each day in their home (a statistic that increases with age), so housing design has a huge impact on quality of life. To further complicate things, dementia is predicted to increase by 44% among over 65's by 2025[2]. Frailty, immobility, dependence and deterioration of the senses lead many older people to a paradoxical plight that has been described as 'needing help, but wanting independence'.[3] This chapter discusses homes for the third age, under the following sections:

From here to where?	a look at mainstream housing and the alternatives
Moving house	what makes a good home?
Staying put	adapting your home to changing needs
Forward thinking	designing for dementia and the future of homes for the third age
From here to where?	A look at mainstream housing and the alternatives

"Older people consistently say they want to stay in their own home. It's where they have lots of experiences and memories and home is a key part of their identity; it is about having familiar surroundings, their own things and space, and a sense of belonging with their friends and neighbours. It's also about maintaining privacy and independence and not losing control over their own lives." *Stephen Burke, chief executive, Counsel and Care*

Most people living in the UK do not intend to live anywhere other than general needs (mainstream) housing as they grow older. More than 60% would choose to stay in their family home with support from friends and family, while 56% would remain in their own home with professional care. Just over one third would be prepared to downsize to a smaller home of their own, while less than a third would move into sheltered housing with a warden[4]. However, for those willing to relocate, a number of different housing 'options' exist, some of which are specialist, i.e. designed for older people. These alternatives are designed to cater for differing 'needs' in terms of physical and/or mental impairment, with higher levels of care typically offered by more institutional settings. Some alternatives are embedded in mainstream communities, while others create communities of 'elders'.

In their recent publication 'Designing with Downsizers', the University of Sheffield / DWELL

---

1 Part M of the Building Regulations relating to 'accessibilty' was not published until 1995
2 ILC UK, 2008
3 Centre for Housing Policy, 2008
4 Derek Wanless, *Securing Good Care for Older People*, report 2006

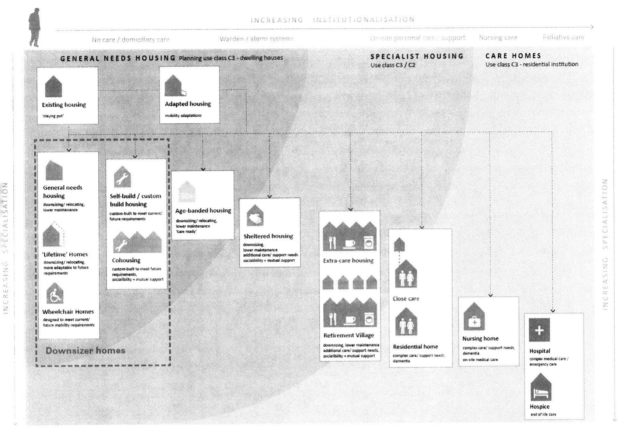

Adam Park, Friederike Ziegler and Sarah Wigglesworth, *Designing for Downsizers*, report 2017

team distinguished between housing options by degree of institutionalisation, and by degree of specialisation, to map out the housing types and tenures that might be considered age-appropriate:

Lifetime Homes

The Lifetime Homes concept was developed in the 1990s by a group including the Joseph Rowntree Foundation and Habinteg Housing Association, prompted by concerns that many modern homes are inaccessible and inconvenient, to ensure that new homes are accessible and inclusive. Lifetime Homes are often mainstream, and are designed to sixteen criteria that add to the flexibility and adaptability of the home, supporting the changing needs of households at different stages of life. For many years, social housing and some private homes have been designed to meet Lifetime Homes.

Self build and custom build housing

In many European countries, large housebuilders are only responsible for a modest proportion of housebuilding. Instead, between thirty and fifty percent of all new homes are built (self build) or directly organised (custom build) by individuals or by communities[1]. This means employing an architect or choosing a house design from a catalogue, and then hiring a contractor or fabricator to build it. In Berlin around a sixth of all new homes completed in recent years were directly delivered by local building groups (baugruppen), saving around 25% of total cost. In the USA more than 50,000 homes have been delivered by charitable organisations that help people on lower incomes to do some of the construction work, to keep costs down.

In Britain less than 10% of homes are currently built this way. However, a recent IPSOS Mori survey (NaCSBA, 2014) suggested that 14% of the UK population is currently researching how they might build their own home. The end result can be innovative, tailor-made housing that meets the occupants' needs. Working together to procure their own homes creates cohesive communities that are proud of their neighbourhoods, look after their localities and support each other.

Cohousing and Intentional Communities

Cohousing provides intentional communities, created and run by residents. Each household has a private home, but residents come together to manage their community, share activities, and often to eat. Cohousing is a way of combating the alienation and isolation that many people experience today, by recreating a community spirit. The first purpose-built cohousing community, Sættedammen in Denmark, was established in the 1960s. A group of fifty families, inspired by the article 'Children should have one hundred parents' by Bodil Graae, built a different type of neighbourhood, with a strong community spirit. The concept of community-led housing is now beginning to catch on in the UK, and over the last few years, hundreds of small-scale pioneering projects have been built. In 2013, there were 14 cohousing communities in the UK, with many more at various stages of development. Some are aimed specifically at older people.

The neighbourly relationships of cohousing are particularly important to older people. Becoming part of such a community, whether intergenerational or of a narrower age-range, offers continued active involvement in the life of a group of people, and a mutually supportive environment. Residents are usually encouraged to bring their particular skills and experience to bear for the benefit of the wider community. The rise of cohousing provides an opportunity to find a new place for the third generation, in communities that are actively looking for the support, experience, and enrichment that 'elders' can provide.

---

1   Ed Green and Wayne Forster, *More/better* report, 2017

Intergenerational living and homesharing

As the housing crisis has deepened, home ownership has slipped beyond the grasp of many young adults living in the UK, and there is pressure on families to live together for longer. As a result, extended families are increasingly found living under one roof. While intergenerational living is a source of frustration and resentment for some, it can also be liberating; building stronger communities and allowing family members to recognise mutual benefit (such as childcare provision within the home). Different housing models are now emerging that provide sufficient long term flexibility to cater for intergenerational living, with scope for a balance between community and privacy.

Homesharing typically involves two people, one of whom has a home that they are willing to share but needs some support. The other person needs accommodation, and is willing to give some help in return. Homeshare is a specific way of going about sharing a home, and is promoted by the charity Shared Lives (which used to be called NAAPS / Adult Placement). Both the householder and the homesharer can feel valued and respected for what they are contributing to the situation, allowing them to enter into the arrangement with dignity and enthusiasm.

Sheltered housing

Sheltered housing, sometimes referred to as retirement housing, offers individual homes – usually self contained apartments – along with limited communal facilities and services. Accommodation is usually provided under one roof and is commonly accessible, via a central lift. Most schemes comprise flats, but bungalow estates also exist. Most newer schemes offer one and two bedroom properties. Units can be designed with the particular needs of older people in mind, although many are not. Communal facilities might include a lounge, visitors' room, communal garden and laundry, and may be used to provide social events. Schemes typically have a full-time or part-time manager, paid for by a service charge, whose role is to provide support and advice to residents. Properties may typically be bought or rented.

Extra care / assisted living

The primary aims of Extra Care are to foster "independence, enablement and choice" in older people[1]. Extra Care schemes were conceived as an alternative to residential care environments

---

1   Extra Care guidance, Welsh Assembly Government, 2005

that, historically, have been institutional in character and have eroded independence, rather than reinforcing it. The intent is to provide 'homes for life', with a flexible support network that can offer care and assistance to suit the needs of the individual resident. Typically, schemes are comprised of at least forty flats (smaller than this, facilities such as on-site catering are not financially viable), and provide a range of communal facilities.

As a result, Extra Care schemes are inevitably large buildings. However, in spite of the 'under-one-roof' approach, it is crucial that they are embedded in a wider community, not stranded in isolation. They aim to be domestic, rather than institutional, in character, and to strike a balance between privacy, comfort and support. In more successful cases, they can also provide a resource for the surrounding community, by offering day care facilities and the like. A range of tenures are available, with a complex mixture of care and support packages to respond to differing needs.

Retirement villages

The first retirement community was Sun City in Arizona, built in 1960 and now home to more than forty thousand people. Retirement villages are common in the United States, New Zealand, Australia and South Africa, and are emerging in the UK as the baby boomer generation moves towards retirement. In a typical retirement village, houses are grouped around country-club-style facilities, with care and support available on site. Facilities often include restaurants, fitness and treatment centres, a library, classes and lectures.

Some villages include extra care schemes and even care homes. Residents buy their own home and retain their independence, a key difference to conventional care homes, safe in the knowledge that if their needs change, they have a range of options available 'on site'. A study by the International Longevity Centre (in partnership with Audley, the Extra Care Charitable Trust and sheltered housing managers Retirement Security People) suggested that residents of care villages are less than half as likely to move to an institutional care home after five years than those in conventional housing.

Residential care homes

A care home is a residential setting for older people to live, usually in single rooms, with access to on-site care services. Homes range in size from small family businesses for a handful of residents up to expansive complexes, many of which have in excess of a hundred bed spaces. All meals are provided, either in residents' own rooms or in a dining room, and communal facilities usually include lounges, activity rooms and a garden. All inclusive costs range from around £300 to £1,000 a week. Hairdressing, chiropody and other services are generally available but charged for separately.

For some older people, moving to a care home is a positive choice. Daily chores become a thing of the past, and care is always at hand. Many care homes offer a wide range of excellent services. A philosophy that supports frailer older people to maintain, and in some cases regain, independence is gaining ground. This shift, in turn, can reduce the institutional nature of residential care facilities. Many care homes specialise in caring for older people with dementia, and do so with great professionalism, skill and sensitivity.

On the other hand, most care homes provide only limited private space – usually a single room, though increasingly with an *en-suite* bathroom. Their focus is on the provision of personal care, including assistance with moving, toileting, bathing and dining. Some homes also provide nursing care. In the main, care homes are for older people who need a higher level of care than can be provided by a professional carer visiting the home.

In summary

A range of housing types are available to suit different needs and budgets. However, while a minority of asset-rich elders have plenty of options to choose from, most of the UK's elderly population is relatively poor. This impacts on their ability to afford alternatives, and generates a lack of choice in the marketplace. It also has implications for the funding of alternatives: entities such as mixed tenure extra care schemes do not even exist in Wales, where too few prospective residents have sufficient assets to afford modern, purpose-built accommodation. Even asset-rich individuals may aspire to retain any wealth for their family (especially given that the cost of housing now excludes many younger families from home ownership) or for the provision of care in the future. For homeowners throughout the UK, it is likely that housing will become an increasingly important contributor to income (through equity release), as pension provisions diminish over time.

Finally, it is also worth noting that the facilities on offer in many such settings are often not all that they could be, particularly when one considers the varied needs and aspirations of older people, many of whom are independent, active and able-bodied. The majority of people in need of care are over the age of 75, and therefore children of the 1940's. As Nial McLaughlin notes, "they belong to a generation who valued state provision of care and are often touchingly grateful for it. The next generation of postwar babies have very different attitudes. They have a far stronger sense of their rights and individual entitlements."[1] If this is indeed the case, then we can expect a significant shakeup in the types and the quality of accommodation available for older people, as the next generation of more demanding, more discerning residents insist on better design, higher performance standards, greater innovation and more sensitivity in the delivery of places that must serve as both home and community.

---

1   'Why not ask the old folks?" Niall McLaughlin, RIBA Journal July/Aug 2011

Moving house: what makes a good home?

Buying a house is a complex business, and decisions are made based on a wide variety of factors, which vary considerably from person to person. However, there are consistent underlying issues which become increasingly pertinent with older age. Key issues have been prioritised, as follows:

Primary issues: Location, Access, Energy efficiency
Secondary issues: Flexibility and adaptability, Security, Potential for expansion
Tertiary issues: Outside space, Natural light and legibility, Lower maintenance

Primary issue A   Location

The importance of location cannot be overstated. For all of us, where we live defines us to a certain extent. It says something about who we are and what we feel is important, whether this is convenience, culture or conformity. However, location becomes even more important for a sector of the population who are likely to develop mobility issues, and may well cease to be able to drive. As we get older, the prospect of driving becomes more intimidating and, for many, physical impairment or medication may make it impossible. Proximity to amenities – and to public transport – is extremely valuable. For the same reason, finding a home that is close to family, to community, to recreation and to healthcare, is likely to be of considerable benefit.

Primary issue B   Access

"Accessibility and the creation of accessible environments is absolutely central to good design and architecture; it is not something that is separate or added on. For too long, accessibility was all about ramps and handrails, but it is much more than that. It is actually about providing environments that are fit for people with a range of abilities."[1]

Accessibility is unique, in that it is of little relevance to the majority, but of critical importance to people with mobility issues. Access can be broken up into two categories; access *into* the property, and access *around* the property. Level changes from outside to inside are commonplace. Very often, they are a product of geography, and cannot be avoided. In many cases, they can be overcome, so long as they are not too significant and/or there is plenty of space between the dwelling and surrounding public realm.

Internally, level changes are inevitable in all but single storey dwellings. Careful thought should be given to the ways in which accessibility could be improved within the dwelling (see following section). Where this is not possible, an assessment should be made of the facilities that can

---

1   RIBA News, RIBA launches new guidance for inclusive design, www.architecture.com/NewsAndPress/News/
    RIBANews/News/2009/RIBALaunchesNew
    InclusiveGuidance.aspx

be provided at entry level. Bungalows and larger houses may be sufficiently generous that all 'essentials' are provided for on the ground floor. House types have been developed (by the Extra Care Charitable Trust among others) with a ground floor that can be converted into a flatlet, future-proofing for periods of reduced mobility. In general, a footprint of 45-50sqm makes this feasible.

Primary issue C   Energy efficiency

The average UK household's energy bills are now well over £1000 each year, with a thirty percent rise in real terms predicted by 2020. More than five million households suffer from fuel poverty, which means that more than ten percent of their income is needed to maintain comfort in the home. For this reason alone, energy efficiency has an increasingly important part to play in the selection of homes in the future.

Energy Performance Certificates (EPCs) are required whenever a property is built, sold or rented. An EPC contains information about a property's energy use, and includes recommendations for reducing energy use and saving money. The certificate gives a property a rating from A (most efficient) to G (least efficient). Other things to look out for include double glazing (in addition to being energy hungry, single glazing reduces the perceived comfort in a warm home, and raises the risk of condensation which can lead to health issues), whether or not the roofspace and walls have been insulated, and the age of the boiler or central heating system.

Secondary issue A   Flexibility and adaptability

Because of the many and varied challenges facing older people, it can be difficult to anticipate how a person's needs will change in the future. Certainly, as we age, it is likely that modifications will need to be made at various points, if we are to enjoy living in the same home for a long time. Generosity of space is beneficial in providing flexibility – a 'spare' room that can double as a downstairs bathroom or a bedroom for a carer, or sufficient space in the kitchen for a wheelchair.

Perhaps surprisingly, homes built of bricks and mortar are relatively adaptable. Masonry takes additions such as handrails and chasing out for wiring well, and new openings can be formed in a convenient – if messy – manner. In contrast, timber frame homes are often highly engineered, making it more difficult to form new openings or remove walls without specialist knowledge. Whatever the construction, giving some thought to the different ways that a home could be adapted is likely to be time well spent.

Secondary issue B   Security

Security is a point of concern for most people, but is particularly relevant for older people, who may feel vulnerable. Many publicly funded schemes designed with older people in mind are Secured by Design accredited, a national programme administered by the police with a focus on security and community safety. However, older schemes and private properties are unlikely to have any specific accreditation in this regard. In the absence of formal accreditation, key criteria to consider include:

Overlooking of outside spaces – natural surveillance plays a big part in both perceived and real safety. Ideally, a property will have windows overlooking all surrounding external areas.

Boundary treatments – clearly defined boundaries establish defensible space between private properties and the public realm. Boundaries should not be so high as to create hidden areas.

CCTV and external lighting – both provide deterrents for crime and criminal behaviour, although the impact of CCTV on reducing crime is less clear than its benefit in prosecuting perpetrators. Well lit, open, overlooked spaces reduce the likelihood of burglary, vandalism and antisocial behaviour.

Secondary issue C   Potential for expansion

Mobility aids and home improvements that are designed to make life easier for older people tend to consume more space, and lack of space is a common shortcoming of housing in the UK. The longer term solution to many mobility impairments is to expand part of a home, to provide more facilities on one level, or to accommodate increases in space required as a result of changes in mobility, intergenerational living or the integration of care in the home. Relaxations in planning legislation mean that it is now easier to expand dwellings with single storey extensions, but to do so requires some capacity on site. Generous, level gardens, without complex party wall arrangements, provide the best possible chance of a simple extension to provide valuable additional internal space.

Tertiary issue A   Outside space

Over 700,000 over 65's don't leave the house more than once per week[1], and 80% of 65-74 year olds are not getting recommended levels of exercise[2]. It may be no surprise to learn therefore that two thirds of NHS clients are over 65[3]. One reason for this lack of exercise is the numerous barriers that may exist between an older person's home and the outside world. Modest gardens combined with terraces and balconies at each level of a property provide easy access to the outdoors, encourageing mobility and a more varied lifestyle, even when moving about becomes more difficult.

1   Help the Aged (2007) Spotlight Report
2   Silver Linings, RIBA (2013)
3   Later Life fact sheet, Age UK (2013)

Tertiary issue B   Natural light and legibility

There are approximately one million blind and partially sighted adults in the UK, about 5% of whom have no sight at all. The nature of sight loss varies considerably, but is rife among older people and increases with age[1], placing elders at increased risk of falling, one of the leading causes of death for the over 75's. An abundance of natural light is a clear asset in reducing the risk of falls, and assisting residents who suffer from visual impairments. Tall, generous windows throw light deep into spaces, and windows facing more than one direction provide a more even quality of light, and reduce glare and shadow. Sunlight also provides other benefits, in psychological and medical terms (as a source of vitamin D_3). An appropriately oriented, well-lit home will absorb sunlight throughout the day – lighting its rooms, heating its spaces, and enriching its character.

Tertiary issue C   Lower maintenance

Maintaining a home is something that many people find challenging, and for the frail, the infirm or those with mobility issues it can be a very daunting prospect indeed. Complex roofs that catch leaves, extensive gardens that must be managed, and surface finishes that require regular treatment all present different challenges. Internally, surfaces that become slippery, rooms that suffer from mould growth, windows that require regular cleaning; all pose additional, and in some cases considerable, risks – even to more able-bodied older people. A healthy, sustainable home for an older resident is one that requires little or no maintenance, and for which the majority of these challenges and risks have been considered and then carefully designed out.

Staying put: adapting your home to changing needs

There are many ways to improve the quality of life for an older person who is finding it difficult to manage at home. A variety of organisations provide advice on the range of options, depending on personal needs and circumstances. Social services will also advise regarding the receipt of care in the home, but if the main issue is the unsuitability of the home itself, a range of 'physical' options exist that may be of more direct assistance. These modifications are the subject of this section:

---

1   One in five over 75's have a recognised eye condition, while one in four will have sight loss by the age of 80.

Adaptation	Price	Disruption	Impact
Stair lift	££	low, short term	mobility
Platform lift	£££	medium, medium term	mobility
Handrails and grab rails	£	low, short term	mobility functionality
Ceiling mounted hoist	£££	medium	mobility functionality
Accessible bathroom	£££	high, medium term	functionality
Accessible kitchen	££	medium, short term	functionality
Telecare and assistive technology	££	low, short term	comfort, safety, function
Security and door entry	££	low, short term	mobility, comfort, safety
Improved heating	£££	high, medium term	comfort, affordability

Price guide:			
	£	modest	£50–£500
	££	medium	£500–£5000
	£££	expensive	£3000–15,000

Stair lifts are mechanical devices for lifting people up and down staircases. For sufficiently wide stairs, a rail is mounted to the stair treads or wall, and a chair or platform is attached to the rail. Different models suit straight and curved staircases and different seat sizes are available, although all require a continuous run – preferably on the outside of the staircase, with sufficient space at one end to safely store the folded stair lift. Some are sufficiently large to take a wheelchair. Different control mechanisms, safety features and finishes are also available.

Platform lifts are designed to raise a wheelchair and its occupant in order to overcome a step or level change. They can be installed internally or externally, and are available in a wide range of sizes, and to suit different changes in level. Domestic models are compact, and will usually fit into a 'shaft' of around 0.8metres by 1.2metres. Many are self supporting, which means that they do not need a structural wall from which to be hung. When an appropriate location can be found, these lifts can function discretely and quietly, and open up areas of a home that would otherwise be inaccessible.

Handrails and grab rails are commonly used to address a range of mobility impairments. Both are fixed to a wall via brackets, or mounted on balusters, typically between 0.9metres and 1.0metre above floor level. They are available in a range of materials and finishes. Handrails are generally used for movement, whereas grab rails usually assist with stability while performing other tasks, such as standing at a wash basin. The issue most likely to be encountered when installing a handrail or grab rail is finding a robust fixing. In timber frame, a patress may be required – a plate or board that acts as intermediary between the brackets and the studwork behind. Bracket centres are usually no more than a few feet apart, but wider centres – for example spanning across a broad window – can be overcome by reinforcing the handrail from bracket to bracket. In external applications, specialist handrail coatings are available that remain warm to the touch regardless of external temperature.

A **hoist** is a device used for lifting or lowering a person. Manually or electrically driven, they are designed to reduce the physical strain on a family member or carer who is moving the hoist user from one part of the home to another. Hoists can be freestanding, or hung from the ceiling where supporting structure permits.

Accessible bathrooms afford users with mobility issues access to one of the most personal domestic areas. Bathing can be one of the more challenging daily rituals, one that many older people are forced to carry out much less frequently when the task becomes increasingly difficult. Walkin bathtubs provide a partial solution to the problem of getting in and out of the bath, but the process of waiting for the bath to fill and to drain is time consuming and can be demeaning. A shower is a better solution for most people, although many users require the assistance of a shower seat. Level access showers do not have the step up of a conventional shower, reducing the trip/fall hazard, and permitting access in a wheelchair. Level access trays are available in a wide range of sizes, and some are large enough to accommodate a wheelchair. Moveable shower screens – either half height or full height – assist greatly in limiting water egress from the shower area. Flooring should be carefully chosen for its nonslip properties (with a slip resistance designed to suit bare feet, not shoes). Adjustable height basins are available, and can be manually or electronically operated, although they are not cheap. Accessible WC's are usually a few inches higher than conventional WC's to make them easier to use, and a limited range of WC seats are available with spacers that raise the sitting height. Some cisterns are designed to offer back support, and paddle flushes suit arthritic fingers. Well located grab rails make the process of going about these various tasks considerably easier, maintaining dignity and independence for people who would otherwise lose it.

An accessible kitchen ensures that a resident who would struggle to use a conventional kitchen has access to basic functions as a minimum. Mid height ovens reduce the need for bending over, and maximise visibility of this high risk area. Side opening oven doors are more convenient for wheelchair users than conventional bottom-hung doors. Most kitchen manufacturers provide base units that are height adjustable. The main downside is a reduction in storage capacity. Accessible kitchens often provide only core areas such as the sink and hob on adjustable height brackets, to ensure that storage capacity remains sufficient. The general consensus is that electric appliances are better than gas, as people with sensory impairment are less likely to notice gas in the air, and more likely to be burnt. Modern ceramic hobs have high heat conductivity. Models should be chosen that have legible controls located along one side, where they will not cause pans to catch, and clear 'hot hob' indicators. Artificial lighting in kitchens should be bright and well spaced, and should ensure an even spread of light.

Telecare and assistive technology are relatively recent innovations, although much that is good about assistive technology draws from well established principles of good design. **Telecare** offers remote support, providing users with the care and reassurance needed to allow them to remain independent in their own homes, by providing person-centred technologies that support the individual. Some technologies mitigate harm by reacting to defined events such as a fall, and raising assistance. Others, such as lifestyle monitoring, have a preventive function that identifies deterioration or behavioural issues at an early stage. **Assistive Technology** includes adaptive and rehabilitative devices that promote greater independence in older people, by enabling them to perform tasks that they would otherwise struggle to accomplish. The advent of personal mobile technology has transformed the remit of assistive technology. A huge range of personal and environmental sensors and alarms can be integrated into the home, including telecare, remote monitoring, occupancy sensors, fall sensors, flood sensors and CO_2 detectors. There are now more than ten thousand health-related apps on the market, capturing physical and environmental data such as pulse, blood pressure and body temperature, providing related services such as navigation, and supporting vulnerable people to remain independent for longer.

Security and door entry systems are a key concern for many older people, whose feelings of isolation can easily turn to vulnerability. Security must be increased carefully, as too much security can be counterproductive – increasing isolation and even trapping residents in their homes. Door entry systems, on the other hand, can be useful in combatting feelings of vulnerability. An audio video door entry system provides the resident with as much information as possible, and empowers them to accept or refuse guests safely and securely from the comfort of their home.

Improved heating cannot be ignored, given the number of households struggling with fuel poverty, and the impact, which adverse changes in temperature can have on older people. Many people on a low income or in receipt of benefits are entitled to assistance with home improvements like new boilers and additional roof and wall insulation, which together have the potential to significantly reduce heating bills. For those who are eligible, improvements are completely free. For those who are not eligible, grant aid is still available, and many of the improvements remain worthwhile, with modest payback periods that result in significant financial and energy savings – and much greater comfort – in the medium and long term. Anyone interested can find out more, and apply online, at www.affordablewarmthgrants.co.uk

Hopefully, this section of the chapter demonstrates that there are many tools at the disposal of homeowners to make their living environments as suitable as possible, and to improve quality of life even when a home does not ideally suit the needs of the resident.

Forward thinking: designing for dementia and the future of homes for the third age

"The time has come for a national effort to build the homes that will meet our needs and aspirations as we all grow older. We should all plan ahead positively, creating demand for better choice through

a greater range of housing opportunities. Housing for older people should become an exemplar for mainstream housing, and meet higher design standards for space and quality. Local Planning Authorities should play a key role to ensure delivery of desirable housing in great places, tuned to local need and demand." Manifesto, HAPPI report, 2009

A lack of housing specifically designed for older people means that most currently choose to stay in their 'family' home for as long as possible – houses that may be bigger than needed, difficult to maintain, expensive to heat, and in some cases challenging to live in. Meanwhile, initiatives such as Lifetime Homes – which attempts to improve accessibility and adaptability for all – increases the cost of 'conventional' family housing by making it bigger and more complex to build. In their report 'Building the Homes and Communities Britain Needs', the Future Homes Commission noted that significant changes need to be made in the way that we provide homes for a growing and changing population. By providing housing that is designed with the needs of older people in mind, we should not only improve their quality of life, with consequent savings to the public purse through the healthcare system, but also free up valuable family homes that could be put to more beneficial use.

In the UK we are not particularly adept at designing homes with older people in mind, and historically other European countries have done it much better. However, this gives us a great deal of scope to improve by learning from these not-too-distant examples. A number of key topics pertinent to the design of housing for older people are touched on in the following section.

Universal Design is a strategic approach to the planning and design of products and environments to promote an inclusive society, equality and participation. Each of us has different abilities, influenced by a wide variety of factors. However, the built environment often fails to take this into account, and all too often design is more influenced by superficial, cosmetic values. For people with disabilities, this can lead to exclusion and unnecessary challenges in the completion of day to day activities.

Put simply, universal design should be usable by all people, to the greatest extent possible, without the need for adaptation or specialised design. This approach is applicable to many aspects of life, but is particularly relevant within the built environment. Older people do not want to be regarded as 'special cases' requiring assistive products and services, but would rather be integrated into everyday life through a more inclusive approach to the design of buildings. The concept of Universal Design is based on seven key principles:

- *Equitable use – The design is useful and marketable to people with diverse abilities*
- *Flexibility in use – The design accommodates a wide range of individual preferences and abilities*
- *Simple use – Use of the design is easy to understand, regardless of the user's experience, knowledge, language skills or current concentration level*

- *Perceptible information – The design communicates necessary information effectively to the user, regardless of ambient conditions or the user's sensory abilities*

- *Tolerance for error – The design minimises hazards and the adverse consequences of accidental or unintended actions*

- *Low physical effort – The design can be used efficiently and comfortably, with a minimum of fatigue*

- *Size for approach and use – Appropriate size and space is provided for approach, reach, manipulation, and use regardless of user's body size, posture or mobility.*

It is estimated that between 10% and 15% of the European population live with some form of disability. Given demographic changes and the likelihood of ongoing investment in more age-appropriate accommodation, it has been predicted that Universal Design will be one of the strongest design trends of the 21st Century[1].

Home zones are a relatively new concept in the UK, extending the principles of universal design to the public domain. They aim to "improve the quality of life in residential roads by making them places for people, instead of just being thoroughfares for vehicles."[2] The principal tool is a shared domain for people and cars, enforcing lower travel speeds and greater care in drivers who are encouraged to feel like they are interloping in the public realm. Now well established, this approach was first introduced to the Dutch city of Delft in 1969 and quickly spread across central Europe.

This approach could yield particular benefit for older residents. In addition to a reduced focus on car ownership, the intention is that the street returns as a place where the community can meet and interact, reducing the degree to which residents become isolated in their homes. Defensible space and privacy are still to be valued and, indeed, prioritised – as is legibility of the public realm. The longer term impact of home zones should be a stronger community identity, one which is more accessible, more integrated, more people-centric and more characterful.

Dementia is an umbrella term for a range of disorders affecting the brain, the most common of which are Alzheimer's disease and vascular dementia. It is more common in older people, and is predicted to rise steadily over the coming years. In 2015, it was estimated that 622,000 people over 65 years of age suffer with dementia.[3] The Alzheimer's Society estimate that by 2021 there will be one million people with dementia in the UK, rising to more than 1.7 million people by 2051.[4]

---

1   Tom Vavik, *Inclusive Buildings, Products & Services*
2   Home Zones – challenging the future of our streets
3   NHS England, Letter from Dr Dan Harwood – London Dementia SCN Clinical Director 2015
4   Dementia 2013: the hidden voice of loneliness, the Alzheimer's Society, 2013

Designing for dementia is a regular subject of discussion at Stirling University's Centre for Dementia Studies. With a similar ethos to that which underpins Universal Design, the Centre advocates that design attuned to the needs of users with dementia *is* good design for all, by virtue of its legibility and its inherent user-friendliness. (The City of London's Dementia Strategy commits to developing a dementia friendly city through better design of the public realm.) Dementia-friendly design principles consistently include:

- *A legible layout – the home should be easy to understand and navigate – even for a first-time visitor. Reference points, such as memorable features and framed views, can be used to improve legibility, prompt memory and reduce confusion*

- *Considered circulation – informal seating places should be combined with points of interest and as few internal dead ends as possible. Similar consideration should be given to the garden, pathways and patios/terraces. External doors should be highly visible and memorable*

- *Good lighting – lighting levels should be high, with limited glare or contrast, and an even spread of light. Natural light should be maximised, to increase light levels and create a stronger relationship between indoors and outdoors. Simple details can assist, such as ensuring that curtain battens are long enough to allow the curtains to gather on the wall without obscuring the window or door*

- *Minimal barriers – floorscapes are an important part of designing for dementia. Changes in material, texture or colour that can be read: as edges should be avoided, due to the risk that they can be perceived as barriers. Conversely, the junction between walls and floors should be well defined*

- *Focus the mind – key features should be highlighted and less important ones played down or hidden. Light switches and other controls should be clearly visible and easy to operate, for example with arthritic hands. Taps, showers and other fixtures and fittings should be legible and easy to operate.*

In conclusion, older people represent an increasingly significant proportion of the UK population. Older people have a broad range of differing needs and aspirations that will influence the location and the dwelling they choose to inhabit. The UK housing stock struggles to accommodate these needs and aspirations successfully, although there are clear improvements that can be made to many existing homes, and recent technological innovations have the potential to offer further solutions. In some cases, specialist or acute needs force older people to make decisions around housing that would otherwise be undesirable. Most significantly, as people continue to demand more from the places where they will spend their later years, there is a clear deficit of accommodation that is appropriate, adaptable and aspirational.

"In 2011, there were 11,700 centenarians and around a third of households in England are 'older person only' households... Because of this longevity, older people need their money to last longer.

They also need to make choices that they wouldn't have had to when life spans were shorter, including the part likely to be spent in ill health. There is an assumption among many that older people will move into retirement housing. Much specialist housing on offer, however, doesn't reflect what most older people want…

In the changing world of housing and welfare policy, gaps in the evidence on older people's housing options ought to be of concern to policymakers and commissioners of housing, care and support because of the effects on existing and prospective residents. The specialist housing currently on offer doesn't reflect the choices that most older people make, so we need new models of specialist housing: flexible tenures in retirement housing and new public and private sector services. We're all aware of the scary numbers – now it's time to do something different."[1]

Further reading

A Better Life – what older people with high support needs value, Joseph Rowntree Foundation http://www.jrf.org.uk/publications/older-people-high-support-needs-value?gclid=CKOr3qew_roCFRIPtAodtA4ACw

Accommodating the Third Age, RIBA Journal July/August Issue (ed. Hugh Pearman), 2011

Building the Homes and Communities Britain Needs. The Future Homes Commission, 2012 http://www.ribablogs.com/files/FHCHiRes.pdf

Design for Dementia: Six Conference Papers. Dementia Services Development Centre, University of Stirling, 1997 http://www.siis.net/documentos/Digitalizados/65095_Design%20for%20dementia.pdf

Designing for Downsizers, Adam Park, Friederike Ziegler and Sarah Wigglesworth, 2017 http://dwell.group.shef.ac.uk

Design Principles for Extra Care, Housing LIN / Department of Health, Care Services Improvement Partnership (CSIP) Factsheet 6, 13.02.2008 https://www.housinglin.org.uk/_assets/Resources/Housing/Housing_advice/Design_Principles_for_Extra_Care_July_2004.pdf

HAPPI reports 1 and 2 (Housing our Ageing Population: Panel for Innovation, All Party Parliamentary group on Housing and Care for Older People), 2009 and 2012 www.housinglin.org.uk/APPGInquiry_HAPPI

Home zones – challenging the future of our streets. Department of Transport 2005 https://www.thenbs.com/PublicationIndex/documents/details?Pub=DFT&DocId=277098

---

1   Aleks Collingwood, It's time for a new model of specialist housing for older people. Guardian Professional, Wednesday 22 May 2013

Housing for People of all Ages, Birkhauser ed. Christian Schittich 2007

Inclusive Buildings, Products & Services: Challenges in Universal Design, ed. Tom Vavik, Tapir Academic Press 2009 http://researchonline.rca.ac.uk/817/

Information for older people, Housingcare.org (Elderly Accommodation Counsel) http://www.housingcare.org/guides-to-elderly-care.aspx

More / better: an evaluation of the potential of alternative approaches to inform housing delivery in Wales, ed. Ed Green and Wayne Forster 2017 http://orca.cf.ac.uk/98055/

Silver linings – the active third age and the city, RIBA 2013 http://www.architecture.com/Files/RIBAHoldings/PolicyAndInternationalRelations/BuildingFutures/Projects/SilverLinings.pdf

The Way We Live Now: what people need and expect from their homes, RIBA / Ipsos Mori, 2012 http://www.housingenabling.org.uk/library-item/way-we-live-now-what-people-need-and-expect-their-homes-riba-research-report

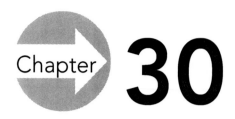

Chapter 30

Financial Advice for Elders

Tony Graham

This chapter should not be considered as investment advice but rather as general guidelines. It is strongly recommended that before embarking on any particular route, professional advice should be sought.

A recent study found that one in eight retired people spent less than an hour calculating how to finance their lives beyond work. The researchers found that more time was spent on researching travel plans and thinking about home improvements. The findings suggest that people are not taking seriously the financial challenge of a long retirement of 25 years or more. The researchers also point to the complexity and paperwork involved. Hopefully these guidelines may help assist with planning for and in retirement.

Principles/Rules of Thumb guidance

- Plan your life and get your finances right to support you. Try to avoid finances running your life

- Plan well in advance as you approach retirement and older age

- Obtain independent financial advice that is personal to you and meets your requirements

- Be economical and shop around, but try to avoid frugality

- If you have saved for retirement, enjoy the proceeds and do not hoard unnecessarily

- prepare and update your will to ensure any assets and possessions are distributed in accordance with your wishes.

Approaching retirement

- Plan at least 10 years in advance

- You may need more money than just the State Pension when you retire. You may be
  able to get money from pension schemes you or your employer pay into. You can get tax
  relief on pension contributions. If you are employed and in their pension scheme your
  employer may also have to help to top up your contributions. The gains from pension
  investments are largely tax free. The longer you save the more benefit is accrued so it is
  usually worth arranging as soon as you can

- Take into account there may be uncertainties such as redundancy, enforced early
  retirement, ill health, unplanned family/friends events

- Prepare a budget of future income and expenditure

- Try to ensure you retire without debt, or have the means to cover debt

- Spend to save in retirement such as making your home and garden easier and less
  expensive to maintain; settlements that you may wish to make on family and dependents;
  life-long subscriptions

- Many best deals are only available online and you can use price comparison sites. If you
  are not computer literate you could consider becoming so. Be aware of the need to keep
  your personal financial information secure and also of fraud and scams.

Tax on your private pension contributions

You can pay into as many pension schemes as you wish. It depends on how much money you
can set aside

- When you pay into a pension scheme the government will automatically add tax relief –
  as long as your pension provider:

  - Is registered for tax relief with HM Revenue and Customs (HMRC)

  - Invests your pension pot according to HMRC's rules

  - You do not pay more than:

    - 100% of your earnings in a year

    - £40,000 a year

    - £1 million in your lifetime

> – If you pay more than that, you usually have to pay tax on the additional amount

- You pay tax when you take money out of a pension.

Income

a) Pensions

This guidance is essentially taken from the government's website **Plan your retirement income** that can be found at the website:

- *https://www.gov.uk/plan-retirement-income/overview*

Information is shown for the 2016/17 tax year. A tax year is from 6 April to 5 April.

Get financial advice

When planning your pension and retirement income you might need help with:

- choosing a personal or stakeholder pension
- planning your savings
- choosing how you want to get your retirement income
- delaying your State Pension payments (deferring).

You can get free guidance on your retirement savings options from:

- Money Advice Service
  - Website: https://www.moneyadviceservice.org.uk/en
  - Telephone: 0800 138 777.
- Pension Advisory Service
  - Website: http://www.pensionsadvisoryservice.org.uk https
  - Telephone: 0300 123 1047.

You can find an independent financial adviser for which you may usually have to pay:

- on the Unbiased website
  - Website: https://www.unbiased.co.uk
- from the Personal Finance Society
  - Website: http://www.thepfs.org

Working past State Pension age

- You do not have to stop working when you reach State Pension age but you will no longer have to pay National Insurance. You can also request flexible working arrangements

- You can claim your State Pension even if you carry on working. However, you have the option to defer which can increase the amount you get

- The law protects you against discrimination if you are over State Pension age and wish to stay in your job or get a new one.

A) State Pension From The Government

You can access the State Pension calculator to find out how much State Pension you could get now – see the Government's website: *https://www.gov.uk/check-state-pension*

A new State Pension system came into effect from 6 April 2016. The way the new State Pension works depends on when you reach State pension age

The State pension age is the earliest age you can claim your State Pension and depends on when you were born. The State Pension ages have been undergoing radical changes since April 2010. the changes will see the State pension age rise to 65 for women between 2010 and 2018, and then to 66,67 and 68 for both men and women. There are plans to change State pension ages further. You can find your State Pension age, your Pension Credit qualifying age and when you will be eligible for free bus travel via this website:

https://www.gov.uk/state-pension-age

If You Reached State Pension Age Before 6 April 2016:

Basic State Pension

The basic State Pension is a regular payment from the government that you can get if you reached State Pension age before 6 April 2016. This applies to:

- a man born before 6 April 1951
- a woman born before 6 April 1953

To get it you must have paid or been credited with National Insurance contributions.

The most you can currently get is £119.30 per week.

The basic State Pension increases every year by whichever is the highest of the following:

- earnings – the average percentage growth in wages (in Great Britain)
- prices – the percentage growth in prices in the UK as measured by the Consumer Prices Index
- 2.5%

This is known as the 'triple-lock'

Eligibility

The earliest you can get the basic State Pension is when you reach State Pension age.

To get the full basic State Pension you need a total of 30 qualifying years of National Insurance contributions or credits. This means you were either:

- working and paying National Insurance
- getting National Insurance Credits, for example for unemployment, sickness or as a parent or carer
- paying voluntary national insurance contributions.

If you have fewer than 30 qualifying years, your basic State Pension will be less than £119.30 per week but you might be able to top up by paying voluntary National Insurance contributions.

Married or in a civil partnership

If you're not eligible for a basic State Pension or you're not getting the full amount, you might qualify for a 'top up' to £71.50 per week through your spouse's or civil partner's National Insurance contributions.

If you qualify for the 'top up' you should get it automatically.

Additional State Pension

The Additional State Pension is an extra amount of money you could get on top of your basic State Pension. You will not qualify for this pension if you are eligible for the new State Pension rather than the basic State Pension. You may still be able to inherit Additional State Pension from your partner.

You get the Additional State Pension automatically if you're eligible for it, unless you have contracted out. You could only contract out of the Additional State Pension if your employer ran a contracted-out pension scheme. Check with them.

There is no fixed amount for the Additional State Pension. If you are eligible for an Additional State Pension, you will automatically get it when you claim your State Pension.

Eligibility

How much you get depends on:

- how many years you paid National Insurance for
- your earnings
- whether you have contracted out of the scheme.

The Additional State Pension is made up of 2 schemes. You might have contributed to both, depending on how long you have been working. The main difference between the 2 schemes is that since 2002 you also contributed to the Additional State Pension if you were claiming certain benefits or had lower earnings.

- State Earnings-Related Pension Scheme (SERPS) applies for the period 1978 to 2002 if you were employed
- State Second Pension (S2P) applies from 2002 t0 2016 if you were employed or claiming certain benefits.

Pension Credit

Pension credit is for older people on a low income to make sure they get a minimum weekly amount. You will have to apply and all your sources of income (e.g. savings) will be checked to make sure you qualify. Getting Pension Credit may mean you're eligible for other benefits too.

Pension Credit is an income-related benefit made up of 2 parts – Guarantee Credit and Savings Credit.

- Guarantee Credit tops up your weekly income in 2016/17 if it is below £155.60 (for single people) or £237.55 (for couples)
- Savings Credit is an extra payment for people who saved some money towards their retirement, e.g. a pension.

You may not be eligible for Savings Credit if you reach State Pension age on or after 6 April 2016.

You do not pay tax on Pension Credit.

You might get more if you're a carer, severely disabled or have certain housing costs.

The quickest way to apply for Pension credit is by phone:

- Telephone: 0800 99 1234

If You Reached State Pension Age On Or After 6 April 2016

New State Pension

You will be able to claim the new State Pension if you are:

- a man born on or after 6 April 1951
- a woman born on or after 6 April 1953.

The earliest you can get the new State Pension is when you reach State pension age.

The full new State Pension in 2016/17 is £155.65 per week.

Your National Insurance record

You will usually need at least 10 qualifying years on your National insurance record to get any State Pension. They don't have to be 10 qualifying years in a row.

This means for 10 years at least one or more of the following applied to you:

- you were working and paid National Insurance contributions
- you were getting National Insurance credits for example if you were unemployed, ill or a parent or carer
- you were paying voluntary National Insurance contributions.

If you have lived or worked abroad you might still be able to get some new State Pension.

You might also qualify if you've paid married women's or widow's reduced rate contribution.

Protected payment

Any amount over the full new State Pension that you get from your National Insurance contributions or credits from before 6 April 2016 is protected. It will be paid on top of the full new State Pension.

Pension Credit

This is similar to the Basic State Pension Scheme – see above

For Either Basic State Pension Or New State Pension

How to claim

You will not get your State Pension automatically – you have to claim it. You should have received a letter 4 months before you reached State Pension age, telling you what to do.

If you haven't received a letter you can phone the claim line. They will discuss with you what you need to do.

There are 4 ways to claim:

- online State pension claims at website:

    - https://www.gov.uk/claim-state-pension-online

- over the phone

    - Telephone: 0800 731 7898
      download the State pension claim form and send it to your local pension centre

- claim from abroad including the Channel Islands by contacting the International Pension Centre

    - Telephone: +44 (0) 191 218 7777.

You do not have to claim it straightaway and you can increase the amount you get if you put off claiming.

There are ways you can **increase your State Pension** if you:

- aren't eligible for the full amount

- want to receive more than the full amount.

- **Voluntary National Insurance contributions**

    - You need 30 years of National Insurance contributions to be eligible for the full basic State Pension.

- If you have gaps in your insurance record, you may be able to make voluntary contributions to increase your pension.

- **Delay (defer) your State Pension**

    - This could increase your payments when you decide to claim. The basic State Pension increases by 1% for every 5 weeks you defer. The extra amount is paid with your regular State Pension and can be claimed on top of the full basic State Pension amount.

- **State Pension top up**

    - Until 5 April 2017 you can apply for the State Pension top up. This lets you add up to £25 per week to your pension in exchange for a lump sum payment. You can get the top up in addition to the full basic State Pension amount.

- If you have gaps in your National Insurance record, it may be cost effective to make voluntary National Insurance contributions before topping up.

- **Other ways you could increase your pension**

  - If you're married or in a civil partnership you may be eligible to increase your basic State Pension to £71.50 per week.

You might also qualify for the Additional State Pension or, if you are on a low income, Pension Credit.

Over 80 Pension

To be eligible you must get either a basic State Pension of less than £71.50 a week, or no basic State Pension at all.

It can give you £71.50 a week

You can get a claim from:

- Your pension centre

- Your local Jobcentre Plus.

War Widow(er) Pension

You may be entitled to War Widow's or Widower's Pension if your wife, husband or civil partner died before 6 April 2005 as a result of their service in Her Majesty's Armed Forces or during a time of war.

If your partner was injured, developed an illness or died as a result of service on or after 6 April 2005, you can claim through the Armed Forces Compensation Scheme.

To claim War Widow's or Widower's Pension you can:

- download a claim form

  - https://www.gov.uk/government/publications/afcs-and-war-pensions-scheme-claim-form

- telephone the Veterans UK helpline.

b) Private Pension Schemes

Workplace pensions and personal, or stakeholder pensions are a way of making sure you have money on top of your State Pension.

For most workplace and stakeholder pensions, how much you get depends on:

- the amount you have paid in
- how well the pension fund's investments have done
- your age – and sometimes your health – when you start taking your pension.

Workplace Pensions

- A workplace pension is a way of saving for your retirement that's arranged by your employer
- A percentage of your pay is put into the pension scheme automatically every payday
- In most cases, your employer also adds money into the pension scheme for you. You may also get tax relief from the government
- You may also be able to make extra payments to boost the pension
- Workplace pensions are protected against risks.

Joining a workplace pension

By 2018 all employers must provide a workplace pension scheme. This is called 'automatic enrolment'.

Your employer must automatically enrol you into a pension scheme and make contributions to your pension if all of the following apply:

- you are classed as a 'worker'
- you are aged between 22 and State Pension age
- you earn at least £10,000 per year
- you usually work in the UK.

Types and Protection for your pension

There are 2 main types:

- defined contribution – a pension pot based on how much is paid in
- defined benefit – a pension pot based on your salary and how long you've worked for your employer.

How your pension is protected depends on the type of scheme.

Defined contribution pension schemes

- Defined contribution pensions are usually run by pension providers, not employers. You won't lose your pension pot if your employer goes bust

- If your pension provider goes bust and was authorised by the Financial Conduct Authority and cannot pay you, you can get compensation from the Financial Services Compensation Scheme

- 'Trust-based schemes' are run by a trust appointed by the employer. You will still get your pension if your employer goes out of business. But you might not get as much because the scheme's running costs will be paid by members' pension pots instead of the employer.

Defined benefit pension schemes

- Your employer is responsible for making sure there is enough money in a scheme to pay each member the promised amount

- Your employer cannot touch the money in your pension if they're in financial trouble

- You are usually protected by the Pension Protection Fund. If your employer goes bust and cannot pay your pension

  - 100% compensation if you've reached the scheme's pension age
  - 90% compensation if you're below the scheme's pension age.

If you change jobs

Your workplace pension still belongs to you. If you do not carry on paying into the scheme, the money will remain invested and you will get a pension when you reach the scheme's pension age.

You can join another workplace scheme if you get a new job.

If you do, you may be able to:

- carry on making contributions to your old pension
- combine the old and new pension schemes

Ask your pension providers about your options.

If you move jobs but pay into an old pension, you may not get some of that pension's benefits – check if they're only available to current workers.

If you worked at your job for less than 2 years before leaving, you may be able to get a refund on what you've contributed. Check with your employer or the pension scheme provider.

Taking your pension

Most pension schemes set an age when you can take your pension, usually between 60 and 65. In some circumstances you can take your pension early. The earliest is usually 55.

Some companies offer to help you get money out of your pension before you are 55. Taking your pension early in this way could mean you pay tax of 55%.

If the amount of money in your pension pot is quite small, you may be able to take it all as a lump sum. You can take 25% of it tax free, but you will pay Income Tax on the rest.

How you get money from your pension depends on the type of scheme you are in.

Personal and Stakeholders Pensions

Personal pensions are pensions that you arrange yourself. You will usually get a pension that is based on how much was paid in.

The money you pay into a personal pension is put into investments (such as shares) by the pension provider. The money you'll get from a personal pension usually depends on:

- how much has been paid in
- how the fund's investments have performed – they can go up or down
- how you decide to take your money.

Types of personal pension

There are different types of personal pension. They include:

- stakeholders pensions – these must meet specific government requirements, for example limits on charges
- self invested personal pensions – these allow you to control the specific investments that make up your pension fund.

You should check that your provider is registered with the Financial Conduct Authority, or the Pension Regulator if it is a stakeholder pension.

Paying into a personal pension

You can either make regular or individual lump sum payments to a pension provider. They will send you annual statements, telling you how much your fund is worth.

You usually get tax relief on money you pay into a pension. Check with your provider that your pension scheme is registered with HM Revenue and Customs – if it's not registered, you will not get tax relief.

How you can take your pension

Most personal pensions set an age when you can start taking money from them. It is not normally before 55. Contact your pension provider if you're not sure when you can take your pension.

You can take up to 25% of the money built up in your pension as a tax-free lump sum. You will then have 6 months to start taking the remaining 75%, which you will usually pay tax on.

The options you have for taking the rest of your pension pot include:

- taking all or some of it as cash

- buying a product that gives give you a guaranteed income (sometimes known as an 'annuity') for life

- investing it to get a regular, adjustable income (sometimes known as 'flexi-access drawdown'.

Ask your pension provider which options they offer (they may not offer all of them). If you don't want to take any of their options, you can transfer your pension pot to a different provider.

Taxes and charges

Your pension provider will take off any tax you owe before you get money from your pension pot.

You might have to pay a higher rate of tax if you take large amounts from your pension pot. You could also owe extra tax at the end of the tax year.

Your pension provider might charge you for withdrawing cash from your pension pot – check with them about this.

Get regular payments from an annuity

You might be able to buy an annuity from an insurance company that gives you regular payments for life. You can ask your pension provider to pay for it out of your pension pot.

The amount you get can vary. It depends on how long the insurance company expects you to live and how many years they will have to pay you.

There are different kinds of annuities. Some are for a fixed time (for example, payments for 10 years instead of your lifetime) and some continue paying your spouse or partner after you die.

You don't have to buy your annuity from your pension provider.

Invest the money in a drawdown fund

You may be able to ask your pension provider to invest your pension pot in a flexi-access drawdown fund.

From a flexi-access drawdown fund you can:

- make withdrawals
- buy a short-term annuity – this will give you regular payments for up to 5 years
- pay in – but you will pay tax on contributions over £10,000 a year.

Capped drawdown is a type of income drawdown product that was available before 6 April 2015. If you already use capped drawdown it will continue under its existing rules, but if you exceed the drawdown 'cap' the tax relief you can get on future pension savings is reduced.

If you have a ' a capped drawdown' fund' and want to keep it, your money will stay invested.

You can keep withdrawing and paying in. Your pension provider sets a maximum amount you can take out every year. This limit will be reviewed every 3 years until you turn 75, then every year after that.

Withdraw cash from your pension pot

You may be able to take cash directly from your pension pot. You could:

- withdraw your whole pension pot
- withdraw smaller cash sums
- pay in, but you will pay tax on contributions over £10,000 a year.

Find a lost pension

The Pension Tracing Service might be able to trace lost pensions that you have paid into.

- Website: https://www.gov.uk/find-pension-contact-details

- Address: The Pension Service 9, Mail Handling Site A
  Wolverhampton, WV98 1LU

- Telephone: 0345 6002 537.

Nominate someone to get your pension when you die

Ask your pension provider if you can nominate someone to get money from your pension pot after you die.

Check your scheme's rules about:

- who you can nominate – some payments can only go to a dependant, e.g. your husband, wife, civil partner or child under 23

- what the person can get, e.g. regular payments or lump sums

- whether anything can change what the person gets, e.g. when and how you start taking your pension pot, or the age you die

- Sometimes the pension provider can pay the money to someone else, e.g. if the person you nominated can't be found or has died

- The person you nominate may have to pay tax if they get money from your pension pot after you die.

Where to get advice

- For questions about the specific terms of your workplace pension scheme, talk to your pension provider or your employer

- You can get free, impartial information – not financial advice – advice about your workplace pension options from:
  - The Pensions Advisory Service
    Website – *www.pensionsadvisoryservice.org.uk*
    Telephone – 0300 123 10477

- You can get impartial advice about workplace pensions from an independent financial adviser. You will usually have to pay for the advice. To find an independent financial adviser, the government's website refers to Unbiased.co.uk
  - Website – http://www.unbiased.co.uk

- If you are over 50 Pension Wise has information about your pension options. You can book a free appointment to talk about your options. Pension Wise does not cover the State Pension, 'final salary' or 'career average' pensions.
  - Website – https://www.pensionwise.gov.uk/

c) Benefits

Up to 1.6 million pensioners are living in poverty, according to Age UK. But many are failing to claim the benefits they're entitled to. Each year up to £3.5 billion of Pension Credit and Housing Benefit goes unclaimed by older people. **Here is a list of benefits you could potentially claim and how to find out if you're eligible.**

Where to get advice

There are many charitable organisations that provide advice including Age UK and Citizens Advice. Contact your local branch.

For UK Government Benefits obtain details of entitlement from the government's website *www. gov.uk/browse/benefits.* or contact your local Jobcentre Plus

Your Local Authority may also be able to help you.

UK Government Benefits

Attendance allowance is for help with personal care because you are physically or mentally disabled and are aged over 65. There are 2 weekly rates, and the rate you get depends on the help you need. You will get:

- £55.10 if you need help in the day **or** at night

- £82.30 if you need help both in the day **and** at night.

Attendance Allowance will not reduce other income and is tax free. If you are awarded it, you may become entitled to other benefits, such as Pension Credit, Housing Benefit or Council Tax Reduction, or an increase in these benefits.

Constant Attendance Allowance (CAA) You can claim CAA if you get Industrial Injuries Disablement Benefit or a War Disablement Pension and you need daily care and attention because of a disability. There are 4 different weekly rates of CAA. How much you get depends on the extent of your disability and the amount of care you need.

Carer's Allowance You could get £62.10 a week if you care for someone at least 35 hours a week and they get certain benefits such as:

- Personal Independence Payment – daily living component

- Disability Living Allowance – the middle or highest care rate

- Attendance Allowance

- Constant Attendance Allowance.

You do not have to be related to, or live with, the person you care for.

You will not be paid extra if you care for more than one person.

Health benefits Everyone aged over 60 gets free prescriptions and eye tests. You may also be eligible for help towards dental treatment, glasses or contact lenses and travel costs to hospital. In Northern Ireland, everyone is entitled to free prescriptions. Ask your dentist, optician or hospital staff for advice

Disability Living Allowance (DLA) and Personal Independence Payment (PIP) DLA is a tax-free benefit for disabled people who need help with mobility or care costs. This is gradually being replaced by PIP. You could get between £21.80 and £139.75 per week. The rate depends on how your condition affects you, not the condition itself. You will need an assessment to work out the level of help you get. Your rate will be regularly reassessed to make sure you're getting the right support. Apply for PIP if you are **under 65. If** you are over 65 and have care needs, you may be able to claim Attendance Allowance.

Blind Person's Allowance is an extra amount of tax free allowance of £2,290.

Housing Benefit (HB) You could get HB to help you pay your rent if you are on a low income. HB can pay for part or all of your rent. How much you get depends on your income and circumstances. You can apply for HB whether you are unemployed or working. You may also be able to get help with your rent if your benefits stop. Benefit cannot be paid for heating, hot water, energy or food.

Bereavement Benefits

- **Bereavement Payment** You may be able to get a £2,000 Bereavement Payment if your husband, wife or civil partner has died. This is a one-off, tax-free, lump-sum payment. The benefits can help ease some of the financial worries you may face following the death of your partner. They are not means-tested and can be paid whether or not you are working

- **Widowed Parent's Allowance.** You may be able to claim if you are widowed under State pension age and have at least one dependent child

- **Bereavement Allowance** (previously known as Widow's Pension). You might be able to claim if you're widowed between 45 and State pension age. You can get it for up to 52 weeks from the date your husband, wife or civil partner died.

Incapacity Benefit and Employment and Support Allowance (ESA) . Incapacity Benefit is gradually being replaced by ESA. ESA offers you:

- financial support if you are unable to work

- personalised help so that you can work if you are able to.

You can apply if you are employed, self employed or unemployed.

You might be transferred to ESA if you have been claiming other benefits like Income Support or Incapacity Benefit.

Income support is a benefit for people under Pension Credit qualifying age and living on a low income. If you cannot work for whatever reason or do not work many hours, you may get some support to top up your income. You must be below the Pension Credit age to claim.

Jobseeker's Allowance is a taxable benefit to support people who are actively looking for work. To claim you must be either unemployed or working fewer than 16 hours a week.

Working Tax Credit is designed **to top up your earnings if you work and you're on a low income.** You could claim if you are 25 or over, with or without children. You must

- work a certain number of hours a week
- get paid for the work you do (or expect to)
- have an income below a certain level.

The basic amount of Working Tax Credit is up to £1,960 a year – you could get more (or less) depending on your circumstances and income.

Child Tax Credit You could get Child Tax Credit for each child you are responsible for if they are:

- under 16
- under 20 and in eligible education or training.

You do not need to be working to claim Child Tax Credit.

Universal Credit is a new benefit gradually being introduced nationally. It will eventually replace the existing benefits:

- Income-based Jobseeker's Allowance
- Income-related Employment and Support Allowance
- Income Support
- Working Tax Credit
- Child Tax Credit
- Housing Benefit.

Other Government and nonGovernment benefits

Heating costs

- Winter fuel payment – Website – https://www.gov.uk/winter-fuel-payment

- Cold weather payment – https://www.gov.uk/cold-weather-payment

- Warm home discount scheme – ask your electricity provider for details

- Insulation and heating schemes:

    – The Energy Saving Advice Service – Telephone
      England, Wales and Northern Ireland 0300 123 1234
      Scotland 0808 808 2282

    – Wales Warm Homes – Website – https://www.nestwales.org.uk/ ; Telephone – 0808 80802244

- Scotland Energy Assistance Package – Telephone 0800 512 012.

Travel and television benefits

- **Free older person's bus pass** If you live in Scotland, Wales or Northern Ireland you qualify for a free bus pass when you're 60 or over. In England, if you are a woman you can get one when you reach State Pension age. If you're a man, you qualify when you reach the pensionable age of a woman born on the same day. Contact your local authority for more information on how to apply

- London Freedom Pass allows free or discounted travel for London residents across London transport networks, including trams, national rail, the underground, river services and buses. Eligibility for this pass is in line with the women's State Pension age. People born on or after 6 October 1954 will have to wait until they are 66 years old to be eligible for a Freedom Pass

    If you are over 60 but not yet eligible for a Freedom pass, you can get a special Oyster card that allows you free travel in London

    You can get more information and check if you are eligible by contacting your Local Authority or on the Freedom Pass website

    http://www.londoncouncils.gov.uk/services/freedom-pass

- **Senior Railcard** is an annual savings card that is available to anyone aged 60 or over. You buy it for a one-off cost and it will allow you to make big savings on most rail fares in the UK. You can order online from the Senior Railcard website using a valid passport or UK driving licence as ID http://www.senior-railcard.co.uk/

You can also apply for a Senior Railcard at most staffed railway stations, where you can also use your birth certificate as proof of age

- **Coach concessions** There is no national concessionary scheme at present, but ask your coach operator if they offer any discounts. For example, National Express offers a Senior Coachcard for people who are 60 or over. It costs £10 and offers a third off your travel throughout the year

- **Regional concessions** Different regions and local authorities may offer additional concessions that apply to local transport, such as trams and ferries, if they operate in those areas. Contact your local council for more information about what they offer

- **Transport concessions for disabled people** If you are disabled you could be entitled to free travel on local buses or discounts on your rail journeys. This includes the disabled person's bus pass, railcard and community transport if you cannot use ordinary public transport and do not have access to a car. Check with your Local Authority

- **Free passport** If you were born on or before 2 September 1929 and are a British national, you could be eligible for a free passport. You will need a full ten-year passport if you want to travel abroad, even if it is for just a day

- **Free television licence** You could be entitled to a concession if you are:

  - aged 75 or over (or your household includes someone who is over 75)

  - registered as blind or severely sight impaired

  - retired or disabled and live in certain accommodation.

Contact TV Licensing Website – https://www.tvlicensing.co.uk/cs/contact-us/index.app Telephone – 0300 555 0286

d) Investments and Other Income

Speak to an independent, or your investment adviser about the investment plan that is best for you in retirement. This can be dependent upon your changing needs for capital and income.

Expenditure

Carefully calculate the cost of:

1 maintaining your home, including any rent or mortgage, council or other local taxes, adequate heating, lighting and water, telecommunications, etc.

2   properly feeding yourself and dependents in order to best maintain your health and energy

3   any essential medication or treatment that you have to pay for yourself

4   maintaining a social life and social networks to maximise the enjoyment of friends and activities, and reduce isolation

5   other essentials for you and your dependents.

Income and expenditure budget

An example is shown in *Table 30.1*. This assumes a couple living together age 70, receiving the joint average retirement income (in 2016), and owning their own home without a mortgage.

However tens of thousands of people approaching retirement will not be in receipt of the average income. Age UK research shows that vast numbers of older people will have debts when they retire and struggle to pay their debts.

The difference between your income and expenditure budget

Expenditure greater than income

It is essential to have a plan to close the gap. In the first instance it is necessary for you to do anything you reasonably can to manage within your means. Options may include:

- Reducing the size and/or location of your home

- Consider an equity release scheme on your property. This is a way of releasing wealth from your home without having to move. You can either borrow against the value of your property, or sell all or part of it for a regular monthly income, a lump sum, or the facility to get equity as and when you like or a combination of these options. If you have a mortgage, it would have to be paid off in full either using some of the equity or using other funds. The income provider will have to be repaid, usually when you die. There are two main types of equity release – Lifetime Mortgages and Home Reversion Plans. Both are regulated by the Financial Conduct Authority and many lenders are signed up to the Equity Release Council code of conduct.

Advantages could include

- Providing a tax-free cash lump sum, or a steady income that can be index linked for life

- Reduce the amount of inheritance tax on your estate

- A no negative equity guarantee that protects you from a downturn in the housing market

Table 30.1 Budgeting for retirement

	January	February	March	April	May	June	July	August	September	October	November	December	Total
Income													
State Pension	1250	1250	1250	1250	1250	1250	1250	1250	1250	1250	1250	1250	15000
Fuel Allowance												200	200
Workplace pension and savings after tax	1200	1200	1200	1200	1200	1200	1200	1200	1200	1200	1200	1200	14400
Total	2450	2450	2450	2450	2450	2450	2450	2450	2450	2450	2450	2650	29600
Expenditure													
Council tax	160			160	160	160	160	160	160	160	160	160	1600
Food and household	420	420	420	420	420	420	420	420	420	420	420	420	5040
Utilities	125	125	125	125	125	125	125	125	125	125	125	125	1500
Communication	80	80	80	80	80	80	80	80	80	80	80	80	960
Insurance – house building and contents	25	25	25	25	25	25	25	25	25	25	25	25	300
Health and personal care	40	40	40	40	40	40	40	40	40	40	40	40	480
Home maintenance													2000
Transport	250	250	250	250	250	250	250	250	250	250	250	250	3000
	1100	940	940	1100	1100	1100	1100	1100	1100	1100	1100	1100	12880
Emergencies 10%	110	94	94	110	110	110	110	110	110	110	110	110	1288
"Cold weather, replacement items, etc"													
Sub total	1210	1034	1034	1210	1210	1210	1210	1210	1210	1210	1210	1210	14168
Further income available	1240	1416	1416	1240	1240	1240	1240	1240	1240	1240	1240	1440	15432

Available for: Recreation and culture; Restaurants and hotels; Alcohol and tobacco; Saving for replacement car, etc; Family commitments and events

Assumptions

General 2 people living together age 70; "Owner occupation, no mortgage, no dependents."

State Pension 2017/18 – 2 people – average of basic Old and full New rate. Will be less if treated as a married couple.

Fuel Allowance – per household if at least one person has reached state pension age. If over 80 increases to £300.

Workplace pension and savings – 1 person – average UK pension and savings after tax

Council tax – 2017/18 paid on an average Band D home – paid in first ten months of financial year from April

Food and household – includes clothing, excludes alcohol

Utilities – gas, electricity, water and sewage

Communication – telephone, broadband, TV licence, stamps, 1 mobile

Insurance – house and contents

Health and personal care – nonprescription items

Home maintenance – replacement of furniture and appliances

Transport – 1 medium size car, 8,000 miles per annum. Excludes depreciation. Rail and other fares

- If interest rates fall, you are free to refinance the arrangement at a lower cost with other providers.

Disadvantages include:

- It may affect the amount of money your family will inherit on your death, and the amount you may wish to give to charities
- It is more expensive than selling the property
- It may impact on means-tested benefits
- Renting out a room/s
- Shopping around for better tariffs for utilities
- Economising in other ways that is not going to have a detrimental effect on your general health and well being.

If there continues to be a gap you need to get help from organisations such as the government's Pension Service, Local Authority, Citizens Advice Bureau, Age Concern, and the Human Resources Department if you are employed.

Income greater than expenditure

You have the luxury of options not available to many others.

Options include:

- planning to spend more on holidays, travel, attending events
- continue to invest in items that are going to make life comfortable and easier for you as you get older, less mobile, and able to look after yourself
- private health care
- residential care
- providing for others including family and friends and charities that give less fortunate people more opportunity to support and develop themselves. Charitable donations are often subject to gift aid and provides tax relief.
- Giving funds or assets away may reduce any capital transfer tax liability
- preparing a will that ensures your assets and possessions are distributed in accordance with your wishes.

It is recommended you use the ongoing services of an independent, or your financial adviser.

Ongoing financial planning and advice

Continue to update your forward financial plans for at least the next five years that addresses your changing needs and requirements. You should consider those changes that best allow you to retain your health, mobility, social contacts, and independence, and are not unduly detrimental to your general physical and mental well being. Some changes may of necessity be drastic and traumatic, so planning in advance can be useful.

Changes may include:

- moving into more suitable accommodation. It is recommended that this is done incrementally if possible to avoid struggling in your home and having no alternative other than going into care

- arranging carers for yourself and other dependents

- planning alternative social activities and support networks as circumstances change

- updating your will.

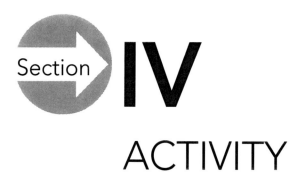

Section **IV**

ACTIVITY

Chapter 31

Remaining Active

A common theme throughout this text is the need for you to occupy yourself, and retain an active mind and body to the end of your days: this is more difficult if you are mentally or physically disabled, but the principles are the same, even if the goals are modified.

Your choice of activity must be something you **enjoy** and are intending to continue. A positive approach of this nature provides you with quality of life, **pleasure** and **satisfaction**, and also contributes to your longevity. If you want to remain physically super-fit, go on the Internet and type in Challenge (take a -; take the-): the choices may change your mind rapidly, but it may be the level at which you want to train. Most of you, however, are more likely to follow some of the lesser activities considered below.

Take some time to explore your options: it is best to have at least **two outlets**, perhaps one incorporating physically activity. Also consider the likely **company**, and whether you know someone who is already involved in the discipline. Joining a new class or group is a step into the unknown and can be rather daunting, but always remember that you are no different from any one else. You have been through similar situations in the past and survived, remind yourself that you are there to learn and for the companionship. Others are there for similar reasons and have empathy with your concerns. Compare the situation with the loneliness and hopelessness of the alternative, and realise that this small step is an entry into a new area of interest, activity, reenergising and enjoyment: it must be fun.

The following lists provide some ideas of what you might already be considering:

Active **exercise**: sport, jogging, walking, gym and exercise programmes (page 245; and don't forget your diet page 70).

Education: is there a subject you have always hankered after, possibly in a previously unexplored field; is there a course to match these aspirations, in a local College or the Open University? You may be someone who is driven by such a challenge, where the journey is as important as the achievement.

Lectures/activities: if you have not previously come across the University of the Third Age (**U3A**) look up their national and local websites to see the enormous range of activities they run, and the gap they fill. Their strap line of 'life is learning' is supported by communal activity and shared skills, all leading to the joys of discovery. Lectures may also be through other universities and societies, and may include history, the arts or sciences, and other areas of interest including debates. Consider classes on public speaking; and clubs such as bridge; board games, scrabble, bingo; and music, art and literary appreciation.

Practical Classes include: gardening; wood/metal work; jewellery; beading; knitting; weaving; tapestry; lace making; art (drawing, life-drawing, painting, botanical); sculpture; pottery; stained glass, photography, bird watching, singing, dance and computing – some of these require dedicated class rooms and equipment. Wine tasting and cooking classes are great fun, but not if you are trying to loose weight (page 78). Search around; you will be amazed what is available in your locality. Local Authorities commonly run classes on falls prevention (page 97) for people with mobility problems.

Visits/outings: libraries; museums; historic sites; theatre (music, drama); cinema; coffee mornings; shopping sprees; pub crawls; sporting fixtures; travel and holidays (the brochures are fun too).

Consider whether you would want to work for a **Charity**, and whether you would do this is as an expert in your field, as a committee member or just as a pair of hands – all are needed. The decision must not be half-hearted – you must take any such appointment seriously, and ask for a written job description. Such positions are likely to be with adults, but do not neglect the contribution you could make to a younger group, as with teaching and training (but remember you need a DBS Certificate to do so).

Many local authorities run **befriending schemes**, they can be telephone calls; visits; walks; wheelchair outings; and car drives. Household tasks include housework; washing; ironing; cooking; archiving; accounting; advocacy; walking the dog; or helping older people communicate with their relatives on Face Time or Skype. All these activities prolong an individual's independence in their own home. Consider if you would be interested in these projects. Take the opportunity of adding **health watch** to the **crime watch** so essential to this section: monitor both your own health and the wellbeing of those around you, whose world of isolation could be opened with a **smile**.

Computing should be a part of everyone's life, regardless of your age. Chapter 34 provides an informative start to your training, but you will probably require some help, if not a grandchild, find a volunteer helper through the local Council, the library or other sources.

Scams (page 263) are all around you, they are considered in this section as the amount of computer fraud is increasing, and becoming more sophisticated and convincing: it is difficult to ignore a message that tells you that your computer account is just about to be withdrawn, or a friend is stranded without any money, credit cards or other means of support in a foreign land. Yet that is what you must do if you do not want to be relieved of a part of your savings. We live our lives with little thought of the dangers that surround us: whereas the previous loss of wallet, handbag, laptop or briefcase was short-lived devastation, you now have to consider the consequences of a security breach and ID fraud.

Music is not just the food of love, it is an integral part of life, supplementing, complementing and changing your state of mind. The ability and need to respond to music appears to be innate, and not dependent on musical training. As Chair of the Music Therapy Charity, your editor has been in a position to appreciate the value of music for the troubled mind, and its importance as a means of communication when other measures have failed. The memories from when you are told, 'today my daughter smiled' or when an unconscious patient stirred, are lifelong. The two articles on music are not prescriptive, but describe the community activities of two experienced musicians. After reading and appreciating the enormous potential for enjoyment in these areas, search for equivalent activities in your own region. Find out whether local musicians run outreach programmes, and whether there are choirs or music appreciation groups you can join – if there are none, consider how you can get them going.

You cannot fail to be drawn by the enthusiasm of the authors of the chapter on **dance** (page 298): their arguments on the need to get your feet involved are very convincing. Similarly, **art** (page 286) can provide you with some of the most intense moments of concentration and absorption of any discipline.

Chapter 38 provides an excellent example of the community activies occurring across the UK. If your local authority does not support such a programme, bring together a group of enthusiasts to initiate one. Ensure that your proposed activities involve all isolated and lonely individuals in your community.

The **library** was probably a great source of fun to you as a child and you may have remained an avid reader and user of the facility. You may not have realised the transformation of modern libraries into remarkable information resources and adaptable public space for multiple activities (page 275). It is a time for inspiration not boredom, but sadly this is easier said than done; change does not happen on its own. Embrace the challenge: vision is about attitude, as this opens your eyes to the many opportunities that are awaiting you – **enjoy**.

Chapter 32

Fitness, Health and Exercise

The term **fit** refers to both your general state of health and your preparedness to undertake specific activities. As 'fit for purpose' can refer to any mental or physical requirement, from the ability to get out of bed to having trained for a marathon, the specific task that you are aiming to achieve must be defined.

This text is not for marathon runners; it is concerned with the mental and physical fitness to meet your needs, expectations and desires in everyday life. These attributes are age related and, sadly, you may also have a physical disability limiting your mobility.

The aim of the text is to help you achieve optimal fitness. This contributes to your independence and helps you enjoy a high quality existence.

Whereas the general concept of fitness is difficult to define, identifying **unfit** individuals is easier. Age has a marked influence on this state. It has been reported that after middle age, your strength, energy, endurance, joint flexibility and bone density decrease by 10% every decade, and muscle power by as much as 30%.

It is also reported that in the over 50s, 20% of women and 14% of men cannot wash their hair without discomfort: while over the age of 65, 12% of the population cannot walk outside on their own and 9% cannot get upstairs unaided.

So, can you do anything to avoid or delay these changes; or are they inevitable and irreversible?

Inactivity

A prime contributory factor to the lack of fitness is a sedentary existence: inertia, immobility and disuse of your muscles lead to wasting, weakness, fatigue and functional incapacity – these in turn reduce your desire and ability to exercise, promoting a vicious circle.

Inactivity leads to joint stiffness and discomfort, with reduced flexibility and range of movement; reduced bone density (osteoporosis) is accompanied by bone fragility and susceptibility to fractures. Inactivity is frequently accompanied by obesity – the body no longer burns off excess calories, and these take the alternative route to become body fat. In retirement, obesity is also promoted by an increased time to eat and enjoy an alcoholic beverage.

Unfortunately, **obesity** not only adds to the load on your deteriorating joints, but is also a cardinal risk factor in the development of cardiovascular disease. Circulating body fat rises, and this is deposited in the walls of arteries (arteriosclerosis/ atheroma) narrowing and eventually blocking them, giving rise to heart attacks, strokes and leg problems. Other obesity related problems are a raised blood pressure, a raised blood sugar and an increased tendency to form clots in your legs.

Lack of exercise is detrimental to the heart and lungs. Both these organs require activity to build up reserve capacity: in the heart, it is a stimulus to produce a more powerful muscle that can rapidly increase its workload to deal more effectively with cardiac problems. Similarly, the challenge of exercise increases the capacity and efficiency of your lungs to take in oxygen.

Inactivity affects the nervous system in many ways. The brain controls movement, where there is already reduced power due to loss of muscle bulk. This is compounded by slower reaction times, reduced reflexes, poor coordination and disturbed **balance**: the latter may also be linked to ear disease, and can lead to **falls** and **injuries**.

All these factors influence your wellbeing: mentally you become less alert, slow and forgetful. They affect your confidence and mood, and in turn, produce tension, anxiety and possibly depression.

Activity

From the above, you can see that **exercise** gives you stronger muscles, more joint flexibility and agility, and smoother controlled movement: these factors guard against heavy foot/ground impact, sudden movements and falls. Improved muscle function reduces the onset and severity of disability.

Heart and lung function are improved with exercise. Mentally, individuals are more relaxed; with reduced tension and stress levels, leading to better sleep patterns, improved morale and reduced anxiety.

Exercise is only one element in the management of obesity. It must be partnered by a well balanced **diet** (page 70), this also supplying appropriate nourishment to tissues, such as bone and cartilage. Other risk factors for cardiovascular disease, such as smoking, must also be controlled, together with a full discussion with your doctor about intended exercise programmes and your medications.

Exercise therefore has important contributions to make to the physical, mental, emotional and social aspects of your health and wellbeing. These factors collectively contribute to the quality of your life style, improved longevity and prolonged independence.

Excuses

Although few people would challenge the importance of exercise to health, many consider it is unrelated to their personal needs – excuses are numerous, diverse, and often creative – I am fit, why do anything; I can do everything I need to do; if something works why fix it; it could do me harm (like in a friend of mine); what is the point; I might fall or faint; I did enough exercise in my youth to last my lifetime; I have no time; I am too old, ill, hot, cold, tired, painful, disabled.

Nonarrival at a session is blamed on the lift, public transport or a chance meeting with a friend. Whatever the excuse, consider turning it into a positive reason for participating: the decision to do some exercise must be your own, or it is certain to fail long term.

Action Plan

To begin with ask and provide answers to the questions: 'Why should I exercise' and ' why bother'? Unless you have the answers to these questions it is not worth starting – exercise is a lifetime undertaking, and not just for (or after) Christmas.

Answers may be 'on doctors orders', as a number of medical conditions benefit from an exercise programme. A **health check** is also advised before starting any exercise regimen, so that measurable baselines are obtained, and unsuspected problems identified and dealt with. Your doctor is aware of any chronic disability and is able to advise on exercise in these situations.

The exercises in this chapter are directed at joint flexibility and muscle power (including heart muscle), and may be postoperative, such as after joint replacement or coronary artery bypass surgery. Arterial disease of the legs can produce pain on walking (intermittent claudication): this can be improved with exercise, as can stroke rehabilitation. In these, and other medical conditions, there are often measurable criteria that can provide tangible goals to work to.

Obesity is another measurable commodity – you (and others) may have noted an unwanted change of your body image. Other motivating factors relate to change in your life style, such as retiring or changing your employment. There may be new challenges; you may have more time on your hands or need for a new social environment.

It is important to identify the stimulus and your **motivation**, so that they are linked to long-term activity – once started the most important factors are commitment and continuity. It is best to establish a routine for the time and place for your exercise. It must become part of your life, given priority, and recognised as valuable use of your time and energy. Unless this is so, you are unlikely to keep it going.

A safe, warm, hospitable **environment** is conducive to regular exercise. This may be at home, in which case ensure there is room, the area is free of obstacles or floor irregularities, and the lighting is good. If joining a Health Centre, take into account the proximity, accessibility and availability. A dedicated centre should provide an appropriate environment with suitable privacy to avoid any embarrassment.

Next consider what advise you need. As with slimming, there is never any shortage of advisors: everyone seems to have an opinion and an intimate knowledge of these areas (as these advisors are often fat and unfit, listen, but do not necessarily follow their suggestions!).

Initially obtain **professional advice**, it is well worth the expense – such individuals are trained, qualified and knowledgeable, they understand fitness and know how it should be achieved by a lifetime commitment. They take into account your current fitness, ability and health, together with any chronic disability, and put in place a tailored programme that meets your requirements, is doable, sustainable, and introduces variety and enjoyment.

Joining a **class** can provide a coach with the above skills at a more affordable rate, since many health centres run special programmes for elderly individuals. Classes enable you to work with like-minded individuals, and build new friendships and mutual camaraderie – the social aspect of exercise can be an important determinant to lasting success.

In this context consider a '**buddy**' system: working with an individual with similar needs, who is aware of the problems you encounter. This can provide valuable support, particularly if you find the going tough at any time. Encouragement from friends and relations is also helpful, although not everyone favors a supporters club.

Starting off

Start off gradually and slowly build up – even short gentle exercises have cumulative beneficial effects. You are not aiming to achieve military or competitive levels of fitness (if you are, hopefully you have been there before and do not need this section!).

If at any time you experience acute pain you must stop, and if it persists seek medical attention. Heart pain is across the front of your chest and may radiate into your arms or neck. Breathlessness and pains from any of your joints or muscles may be related to starting new activities: they are needed, but should be reintroduced at a slower rate.

Stop if you experience dizziness, lightheadedness, are confused or feeling unwell, be sure to hang onto something so you do not fall. All of these symptoms are probably due to trying to do too much too early, but if they persist, check with your doctor before any further activity.

Do not undertake exercise if you are suffering from an acute illness, such as flue, or have a fever, a new cough, vomiting or diarrhoea. With any set back of more than two weeks, start again on your initial schedule, but you will probably be able to advance more quickly to the level you had achieved.

To begin with, undertake a gentle daily exercise for 10 to 15 minutes for the first week: once a **programme** is established you need to introduce five minutes to warm up and five minutes to cool down, both at a slower rate.

Much research has been done on how much exercise is required – but this is mostly concerned with athletic pursuits rather than fitness in the elderly. It is suggested that 200 minutes of hard exercise per week is sufficient to maintain athletic fitness, but that 100 minutes achieves 90% levels, and 60 minutes 70%. This equates to 15 minutes four times a week.

Relating this to your own mild/moderate exercise, three or four, 30 minute sessions/week are sufficient to build your fitness: but do not expect to notice any change for six to eight weeks, and exercise must be at a regular tempo and sessions evenly spaced without any 'catchup' master-classes!

You decide what suites you and works for you: to repeat – this is not a competition, you are aiming to improve your fitness at your **own rate**, modifying activity to your own likes and dislikes, and change or reductions are not failures – so do not give up – it gets easier!

Clothing depends on the activity you are undertaking, but arrange for a change and, if possible, a bath or shower at the end of a session. Outdoor activities may require warmer clothing and a light rain cover if you are walking. If you are jogging, a running vest and shorts or a track suite may be appropriate, and you will probably ignore the rain.

Inside activity is best undertaken with a light shirt and shorts. If you are new to exercise, ladies ask advise on support bras, and gentlemen know if you 'dress' to the right or the left when sitting on cycling or other apparatus.

Footwear needs careful attention in every exercise; there must be room for all your toes to move, but firm fitting over the forefoot and around the heel. Walking requires sound leather soles, but other activities require trainers, and there are more varieties to choose from than there are activities!

The foot impact of running, whether on roads, hard mud or a running machine is transmitted to the ankles, and particularly onto the cartilages of the knees. For these activities trainers should be suitably cushioned to soften the impact. Discuss this with your coach and the sports shop so you buy appropriate and affordable versions.

Trainers for nonimpact exercises should be comfortably fitting, without any toe pressure. Make sure the laces are pulled tightly into bows for all activities, to avoid the risk of catching in equipment or treading on them and tripping over. Socks are advised. If you have difficulty in getting down to do up laces, or your grip is impaired, consider slip on footwear that is done up with Velcro straps.

If laces become undone, stop whatever you are doing and do them up properly – do not try to do this when on the move, as it could produce a fall and an injury. For the inexperienced, the same applies if you wish to adjust clothing, deal with a facial itch, towel your brow, adjust your seating, reset the apparatus you are working on or take a drink. Have a bottle of fluid with you for all exercises, and take a drink every 10–15 minutes.

This text is directed at a wide audience and specific advice is limited. However, if you are frail and unstable, you should only attempt exercise under supervision, or when you know a reliable supporter is close at hand. This is particularly so with apparatus, where getting on and off a machine carries maximum risk of injury.

What exercise

The prime aim of exercise in elders is to increase muscular strength and joint flexibility. This facilitates the optimal range of joint movement and muscle power, and helps maintain mobility and activity. For more active individuals, consideration is given to endurance and cardio-respiratory reserve.

Indoors you may be covering a number of miles a day doing housework, and this may be supplemented by gardening and shopping. If you are manageing these easily, you probably do not need additional exercise, although it can be a social outing and fun.

Stairs add a different kind of challenge to your hips and knees: if this is a chosen exercise, be careful about your balance. You probably already know how well you manage on stairs; take this into account when deciding if additional climbing is appropriate and whether you need supervision. Make sure you have a bannister to hold onto – you only need two or three steps to go up and down (going down backwards is probably safest) to provide one of the most effective (and cost effective) 'exercise machines' available to you.

Walking outside is cheap, easily available, and it is usually possible to identify a safe out-of-doors circuit. It produces less problems of foot impact than jogging or running, and can be undertaken with walking aids, such as walking sticks, frames and walkers. If you do not want to be seen with a walking stick, use one or two ski poles, these can be of adjustable length, and longer poles can help increase your stride – Nordic poles are ideal.

Start walks on flat ground, avoiding rough surfaces, such as gravel, stones, cobbles, pebbles, hard earth or wet sand and mud. Walks can be in a quiet safe urban area, or well-used country trails. If you are used to travelling around by car, try parking some way away from the shops or other destinations, to increase your walking distance.

Increasing activity can be in distance, including hills or by walking faster. When you are ready for the latter examine your length of stride, heel strike and your posture: straighten your back and raise your head, looking forward as you go. A slow steady pace is about 60 – 80 steps/minute, whereas when you start to concentrate, it increases to over a 100. If your legs are short you will be faster than this, but rather than count, decide what are slow, steady and fast for you.

Swimming is another activity that is usually available at low cost, and can be measured. You will know if cold water, water up your nose and chlorine in your eyes are acceptable for a long term fitness programme. These can be modified by choice of venue and walking lengths or widths of the pool.

Water supports your body, eliminating gravity and avoiding ground contact, while allowing resisted limb movement and building muscle strength. Swimming is a good way of building up your endurance. Aim for regular 20–30 minute sessions, varying your strokes: avoid breaststroke if you have neck problems, as this requires exaggerated neck extension. All swimming activity should be carried out in the presence of a lifeguard.

Other milder forms of exercise can be obtained by joining regular **Tai chi, Pilates, yoga** or keep-fit classes. The latter may be undertaken at home using purchased programmes on tape or disc. If you live on your own, consider whether a programme can be undertaken safely, and what means you have of contacting help should you need it.

Jogging is a reliable means of providing you with more vigorous endurance exercise. It is best avoided if you have lower limb joint problems, and note the previous comments on cushioned trainers. You probably wont be able to resist the accessories, such as a head and wristbands, stopwatch, route mapping and measuring apps, and an arm holder for your IPod.

Build up your programme gradually and take time to plan your routes with regard to safety, surface, traffic, obstacles, gradients and distance. Find what pace you can sustain comfortably without a break, and avoid races or running with faster companions.

In early retirement you may well be taking exercise as a continued **sporting activity**. You have probably given up circuit training and contact sports, but racket sports provide good alternatives. When these become unmanageable, think ahead: golf can be bad for your psyche, but provides plenty of walking, or you may prove to be a late prodigy at bowls.

When your sporting days are over explore the great industry that has grown up around health and fitness. This includes the walking, swimming and jogging discussed above, but extends to the Health Centre – the local gym! Many Local Authorities have concessions at a gym for 'Young at Heart' programmes, while others run 'Fall Prevention' classes, to improve your strength, stability and confidence.

Gym

At a Health Centre you will be greeted with a personal trainer and a confusing number of machines, designed to make at least part of you feel good. However, if you intend to follow this (usually expensive) route, protect your muscles with the **stretch techniques,** shown in *Figures 32.1–25*, before and after any vigorous exercise. It is not necessary to do all every time, but discuss and choose an appropriate set, including variations, with your coach.

If you are intent on using your retirement to train for competitive sport, then get down to your pressups, situps, bending to touch those toes, the weights and the roadwork. It is still wise to stretch your muscles before and after such industry as suggested.

Muscle stretching programmes are low intensity maneuvers that tone-up muscles, preventing cramp and muscle injury before and after heavy exercise. They are also valuable as a separate regime addressing flexibility and strengthening muscles for less active individuals.

Stretching is undertaken standing, lying or sitting (including in a wheelchair). It consists of smooth, gentle muscle stretching to the point of tension: this may be on the floor, against a wall or using a stretch band. It must not cause discomfort, and if this occurs, the stretch is reduced, or stopped and restarted – it must be pleasurable rather than painful. Breath deeply throughout.

Once tension is reached, it is retained for 10–15 seconds. The same muscle group is stretched on alternating sides, for up to five times each. The muscle groups targeted are those involved in the heavy exercise. In dedicated stretch programmes, vary the order of stretching, and include all muscle groups in a three-day cycle.

If your mobility is limited, or you are recovering from illness or a stroke, you need an alternative approach. This may include assisted stretching of muscle groups, or retraining, such as fist forming, hand stretching, walking your thumb along your fingertips and doing up a button. Standing balance should be carried out alongside a table or other support, similarly stand on your toes, and try toe and heel walking forwards and backwards alongside a support.

You may find using a **stretch band** or dumbbells helpful. Bands are of different strengths, and a typical size is 5 inches wide and 6 foot long (12.5 x 180 cm); use *Figures 32.26–29* to lead you into their use.

Apparatus

If you have not visited a health centre before, or even observed one through the usually clear glass windows, you will be surprised by the plethora of machinery. You will be shown them all – listen carefully to the advice from the guide and relate this to your own needs: you need to try them all at some point.

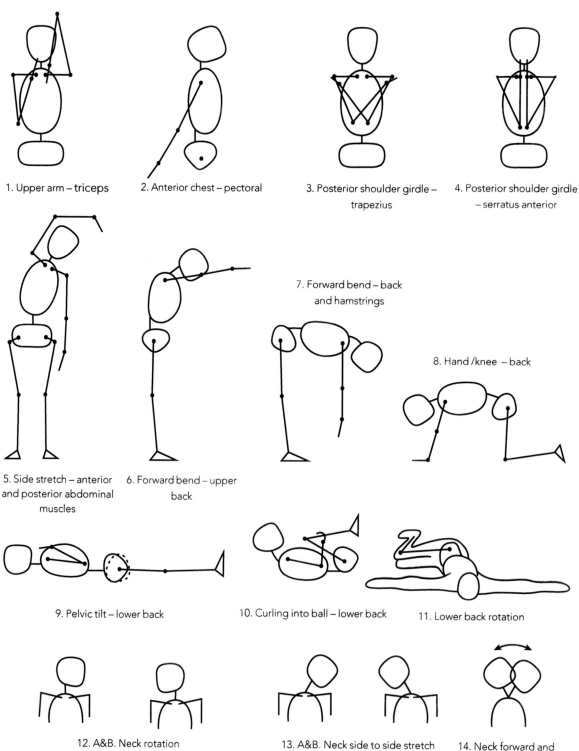

1. Upper arm – triceps

2. Anterior chest – pectoral

3. Posterior shoulder girdle – trapezius

4. Posterior shoulder girdle – serratus anterior

5. Side stretch – anterior and posterior abdominal muscles

6. Forward bend – upper back

7. Forward bend – back and hamstrings

8. Hand /knee – back

9. Pelvic tilt – lower back

10. Curling into ball – lower back

11. Lower back rotation

12. A&B. Neck rotation

13. A&B. Neck side to side stretch

14. Neck forward and back

Figures 32.1-25 Muscle stretching techniques – slowly stretch to the maximum range; hold for 10 seconds; and slowly release; repeat on second side. Neck movements are facilitated by locking the fingers of your two hands behind your neck.

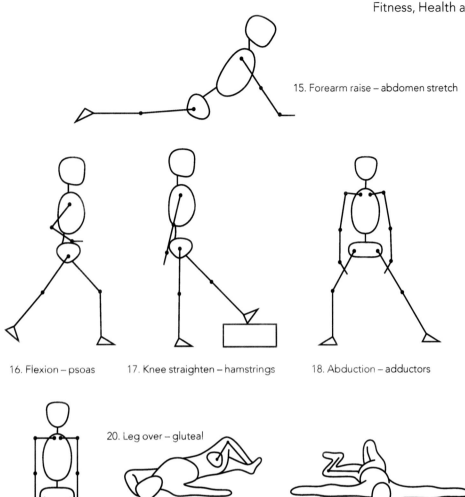

15. Forearm raise – abdomen stretch

16. Flexion – psoas

17. Knee straighten – hamstrings

18. Abduction – adductors

19. Cross-legged – gluteal

20. Leg over – gluteal

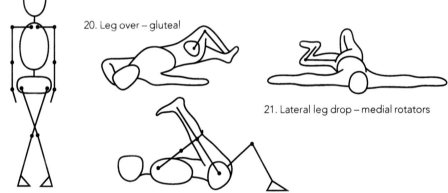

21. Lateral leg drop – medial rotators

22. Hamstring stretch

23. Quadriceps stretch

24. Calf/Achilles stretch

25. Dorsal and plantar foot flexion/extension

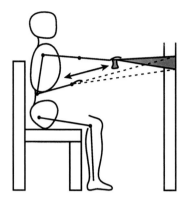

26. The band is passed around an upright, the ends are held in each hand and pulled towards you: strengthening the muscles of the upper limbs.

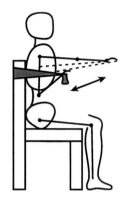

27. The band is passed around the back of the chair, the ends are held in each hand, which are pushed forward: strengthening the muscles of the upper limbs.

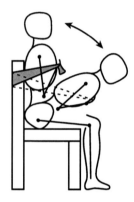

28. The band is passed around the back of the chair, the ends are held in each hand, which are folded across your chest. Forward movement of your upper body strengthening your anterior abdominal muscles.

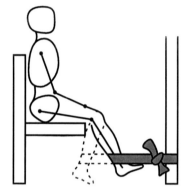

29. The band is tied in a loop around a table leg and each lower leg in turn, and the foot is drawn backwards: strengthening the muscles of the lower leg.

Further improvisation can be introduced by passing the band under your feet or across your back.

Figures 32.26-29 Use of an elastic band for muscle exercises against resistance: the recoil enables the exercise to be repetitive, holding for 10 seconds in each stretched position.

Clothing is a light shirt, shorts and trainers, remember the water bottle and possibly an IPod. Special sportswear may look appealing, but is an expensive and not an essential commodity. A towel is needed and probably provided, together with the desirable postexercise shower.

Be sure you know the details of every apparatus you are going to use, as you can sustain an injury from any of them. They have to be adjusted to suite you. A **treadmill** is a rolling carpet that you can walk or run on and you have to know how to control the rate before you start – otherwise it can eject you off the back.

Modern equipment frequently has a screen that not only tells you the details of your exercise, but also incorporates a television set, easing the boredom that can creep in when you are undertaking repetitive tasks.

You have to strap your trainers securely into the pedals of an exercise **bike,** and adjust the seat, so that your legs can give a full-length push, and your knees do not hit the handlebars. Some modern versions have a comfortable seat, rather than a saddle, and the handles to hold onto are placed low on the sides, rather than in front. This design also provides support to your back.

The bike provides information on the distance travelled and the work done: it is possible to increase the workload by adjusting the resistance to pedaling. Similar consideration should be given to the **cross-trainer**. This exercises both your arms and legs, but also uses rotational forces; it should be avoided if it produces persistent joint discomfort.

A number of other pieces of apparatus are directed at weight training and muscle development, try them all, but take **professional advice** on which ones are appropriate for your current and desired fitness. On all apparatus, you must start slowly, gradually increasing time and resistance, once you have established a rhythmic pattern that suits you.

When you have built up your activity to 30 minutes, you should allow five minutes of lighter activity at the start and finish of an exercise sessions This can be by slowing down, and reducing the rate and the workload setting on the apparatus you are using, by changing to a different apparatus for this purpose or going through a muscle stretching régime.

Home equipment

Exercise bikes have probably been the most frequently sold apparatus for home use; sadly it is not unusual to find them left outside to rust, emphasising the difficulty of sustaining a long-term unsupervised exercise programme.

Before making such a purchase, try a bike in a gym to make sure it is an apparatus that suites your need – it can be hard on your knees, and if it causes persistent pain, it is best avoided. A bike must be heavy and stable enough to take your weight, and not tilt or topple over when you mount and dismount. You must be able to stand on one pedal when this is taking place: turn the pedal so it is at its lowest when you do so and place your foot firmly into the adjustable toe clip (be sure your laces are tied and not at risk of being caught around a pedal).

Adjust the saddle so your heels just reach the lowest position of the pedals; in this way your legs are nearly straight when in motion, with no side-to-side movement of your pelvis. This keeps your body aligned to the bike. Cycle with your head up and a straight back: keep thinking of the pressure you are applying to each foot. It is very easy to pedal gracefully watching TV with minimal active exercise taking place – adjust the tension of the apparatus and your speed so that you know you have had a proper workout over about 10 minutes.

A **rowing machine** is another favorite – try one in a health centre before any purchase. They can be quite slim and have a folding limb to elevate when not in use. Be sure the limb is secure when elevated, let it down carefully and don't trip over it: it is heavy and can easily injure you or anyone nearby.

Sitting down on a rower can be difficult as there is not much to hang onto – stand well forward of the seat, otherwise you may miss it! Once seated, position your feet fully on the foot holders and strap them in firmly: unstrap them fully to release the foot and lift it clear at the end.

In the stroke, push first with your legs – they should be straight but not locked back – and then pull with your arms and shoulders. The rowbar should end up somewhere between your belly button and your nipples. To begin with do not use too much back movement, but this can be increased once you know it does not produce any persistent discomfort.

Pay particular attention to getting up at the end of a rowing session. If your legs are too weak to stand easily, work out how to lean forward, placing the weight of your shoulders over your feet, and pushing downwards on one or both knees. Alternatively, consider rolling off sideways, onto your hands and knees and reaching adjacent furniture to help.

To increase flexibility and muscle strength, it is more important to undertake regular **rhythmic** activity, than to reach exhaustion. If you are aiming for more endurance, aerobic style, exercise, it is possible to increase the workload adjustments on the bike and rower, but be sure there is adjacent furniture to steady yourself afterwards, and take account of the finishing and **stretch** exercises considered above.

Heavier apparatus, such as treadmills and cross-trainers, require much more room and an important consideration with apparatus at home is the potential lack of the supervision that is always present in a health centre. Know whether help is available or whether you are fit enough to be on you own.

The risks from an apparatus are concentrated at times of mounting and dismounting, particularly the latter, when your legs are tired and weak. Keep this in mind, as the apparatus may have to be placed up stairs: you have to be particularly careful going down after a full session, as you may be unsteady on you feet.

Once exercise becomes routine, fun and part of your life, you can experiment with apparatus **settings**. Read (you may need your glasses) the measurements on the machine and set yourself targets – there is still no need for more than 30 minutes a day. You can dream of Olympic medals, adjusting you wrist positions during strokes on the rower and adding pressure and rate to your pedaling, but do not stand on the bike to receive applause, and avoid bruises across your belly from the rower!

Boredom and rewards

Thirty minutes of exercise, 3–5/week may not seem a lot, but when it requires longer than that time to reach a gym, and then a similar period of time to cool down, shower and reach your next destination, you either have to get up very early, or it can take a large part of a morning or evening. Thus unless the time is looked on as productive, the project is doomed to failure.

It is essential to cut down the time before and after exercise, and this must be addressed by using a conveniently placed gym or by undertaking exercise at or from home. An additional approach is to constructively make use of the exercise time, which can be boring and depressing, particularly when progress is slow.

The introduction of **TV screens** onto some gym apparatus makes an enormous difference, as you can use the time to keep up to date or access a channel of your choice. Gyms usually have piped **music** as a background, but this is not necessarily to your taste. Taking your own headphones with radio or personal music is an important step to address boredom.

Your choice of music may be powerful and rhythmical, but it is unlikely that its metre matches the rhythm of your activity: you may be speeded up by rapid passages and loud passages may stimulate an increased workload. The supervision, camaraderie and mutual support in a gym, and the variety of apparatus available, are all determinant factors in maintaining a programme.

At home you may have to buy an extra TV. There is currently no way to read a book, as this requires breaking your rhythm to advance the pages, even in electronic format, and pages may go in and out of focus with a rower. You can use the time to ponder, meditate, plan your day/life, or calculate progress from the continually changes figures presented on the screen in front of you. If you are listening to music, it helps to know how the time of a musical collection relates to that of the exercise.

Rewards must be primarily a positive outcome of wellbeing. This develops with increased muscle power and improved joint mobility, overcoming joint stiffness and leading to greater mobility. Strength and stability improve balance and can have a remarkable effect on confidence, and fulfillment in your quest for fitness – the feel-good-factor is important in determining the long term success of an exercise programme.

Records

Maintaining interest and long term momentum in an exercise programme can be difficult – you therefore need to add extra items. One of these is to record your activity. Use a large diary to document events, note: the frequency (perhaps 3-5/week); the type of activity or apparatus used; the duration; the distance travelled (and route if out-of-doors); the rate and the load – the latter should be in your comfort zone, and a record kept of any pain or difficulty.

Include all clinical **measurements** you have access to. Learn to take your own pulse (heart) rate (if it is irregular, discuss this with your doctor), and note any shortness of breath. Documentation of your progress enables you to see trends and set realistic targets for weight and activity. If appropriate, add comments on your diet.

Feel your pulse on the front, outside of your forearm, just above the wrist (*Figure 32.30*). The recommended range for your **heart rate** in exercise is from 0.6 to 0.8 X (220 – age). If you do not like arithmetic, count your pulse rate for a minute at rest (i.e. before starting any exercise)

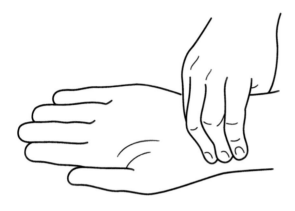

Figure 32.30 Feeling and counting the pulsations of your radial artery: on the front of the forearm, just above the wrist

– moderate exercise should increase the rate by 60% and rigorous exercise by 80% – you should ease up before the heart rate reaches double its resting value.

Shortness of breath on exercise is common, but it should match the amount of activity. It may be accentuated by chest disease, such as spasm of the airway passages in asthma. The **talk test** is that you should be able to talk in moderate exercise; when this is increased, you should still able to talk, but wont want to; in severe exercise (which must be avoided), talking is with single words.

The above measurements are useful to assess fitness at the level we are aiming for in this text. To assess athletic potential, more sophisticated tests of the heart output and oxygen consumption are used, such as the maximum volume of oxygen (VO$_2$max): your basal metabolic rate (BMR) estimates the amount of energy you use up in a day, at rest.

Fitness is not about exercising to exhaustion; even competitive athletes have to build up their muscles gradually to prevent injury. If we consider exercise on a scale of 1-10: one, is breathing comfortably at rest, while ten, is the most extreme you can imagine. For our target audience – all exercise should fall between 6 and 8 on this scale.

Aim to get slightly out of breath; have at least a 50% rise in pulse rate; and to raise a sweat. Do not expect an obvious change in fitness for at least 6-8 weeks from the start of a programme.

Exercise can therefore be divided into low-cost, walking, running and climbing stairs or the more expensive gym option: however, in the latter you do get a personal and professional advisor. By exploring the various pathways you will find out what is best for you; but never forget your underlying search for fitness is to achieve a better quality of life and remain independent for as long as possible.

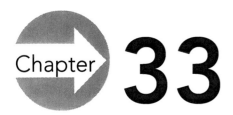

Chapter 33

Health Related Activity

A gym may bring back bad memories, be against your strongest held principles or just not locally available. There are, however, a number of other ways of addressing your **physical and mental wellbeing**: the former to retain a healthy heart and lungs, optimal mobility and to control your weight, and the latter to combat the tensions and stresses of everyday life.

Communal classes such as Pilates, T'ai chi and Alexander technique combine activity with social involvement – an important factor in encourageing social engagement and overcoming loneliness.

Pilates is an exercise programme: it aims to strengthen muscles, particularly those of the trunk, including breathing. **T'ai chi** is a Chinese martial art, related to both defense and health benefit: the latter (t'ai chi chuan) involves low stress, slow sequence movements, through normal ranges, emphasising a straight spine and abdominal breathing.

The **Alexander technique** (like Pilates) is named after its originator: it was initiated to combat bad postural and breathing habits, and, by addressing mental and muscular tension, remove habitual discomfort. All these techniques concentrate on activity, address cardiovascular fitness, flexibility and improve balance, and by so doing guard against falls. Regular activity also burns up calories, helping in the control of obesity. **Yoga** adds meditation and a spiritual element to these forces.

Other techniques involving physical contact, such as reflexology, auricular therapy, acupuncture, acupressure and massage, aim to relax you mentally and physically, and focus on specific areas of discomfort or disability. Tactile contact introduces communication between the therapist and subject in these various activities: an important personal addition in manageing your wellbeing, while verbal communication through **hypnosis** can markedly help some individuals.

Reflexology involves firm pressure over areas of the hands and feet, linked to related zones of the body. Manipulation in theses areas can improve problems in the related area. **Auriculotherpy** is also based on the body being represented as a microsystem within the ear, and that manipulation or acupuncture in these areas can improve problems in associated areas, such as the mind or discomfort in parts of the body.

Acupuncture and **acupressure** are traditional Chinese medical techniques for treating disease. The procedures are based on the principle that disease is due to an imbalance of energy flowing though channels (meridians) in the body. Needling or pressure applied to points on the body linked to meridians aims to correct this imbalance, and associated problems.

The various techniques described above, together with homeopathy (treatment with vary small doses of usually naturally occurring ingredients), Chinese medicines and osteopathy are widely available in the UK, they provide different approaches, originating from many different cultures, but are usually referred to collectively as **complementary medicine**. They provide invaluable relief for many ailments. Your choice may be limited by availability and relative cost.

Be sure to go to qualified and experienced therapists, as they will not only provide optimal management, but will also recognise conditions that need referral to a physician for specific medicines and, occasionally, surgical management.

Massage

We all tend to rub and massage a local are of tenderness or an aching muscle. However, massage applied by a professional masseur, has a much wider application, and can be markedly beneficial to your general wellbeing as well as local physical ailments.

Massage has its origins in a number of ancient civilizations, including Chinese, Egyptian and Greco-Roman; each had specific traditions. Japanese traditional massage was applied by blind ladies, and focused on the head and neck, while Chinese techniques were linked to acupressure and acupuncture, controlling the meridian pathways through the body.

Modern massage techniques are primarily based on the Swedish School and involve whole body massage. The physical elements are directed at the muscles, joints, the skin, and any excess fluid beneath it.

Massage can markedly improve muscle tone, and passive movement reduces wasting and contractures following injury, inactivity and strokes. It reduces tension, fatigue, cramps and spasm after hard muscle activity, and speeds up recovery after sprains and tears. It reduces muscle mediated headache, and shoulder and back pain.

In joint disease, such as arthritis, massage and passive joint movement prevent joint adhesions and maintain an optimal range of joint movement in these conditions. Fluid accumulates under the skin in inactive and dependent parts, and this swelling can be reduced by massage, as can unwanted skin folds, such as on the face and belly.

Body massage also relieves mental stress, having a soothing effect, relaxing and releasing both mental and physical tension. The whole body gains a feel-good effect, with reduced fatigue and it initiates reinvigoration. **Aromatherapy** uses fragrant oils for massage, adding further relaxing sensory stimulation, to this situation.

With care and practice, the relaxation achieved by the professional masseurs can be created between carers and loved ones: the effects being enhanced by verbal communication. If you wish to develop such a relationship, also consider the optimal environment. This should be warm, draft free, dimly lit, secluded, and peaceful, possibly with quiet appropriate background music.

Your hands should be smooth, clean and warm. Movements should be regular and rhythmical – initial gentle pressure is increased when requested by the subject. Massage may be delivered onto bare skin or over light clothing. Massage techniques can be greatly appreciated, but require practice and patients – they are otherwise tiring to apply, and it is self defeating if the subject becomes too demanding. All these factors must be taken into account when considering such an approach.

Chapter **34**

Computers

David Wilcox

The Internet is the world's library, conversation and learning space, created through a vast network of linked computers. It is also the place to shop, play games, find friends, watch TV and movies and discover lots of free programmes to help with health and fitness. You can shoot and edit movies and photos and share them with others, and hold video conversations across the world for free.

However, the Internet can also seem like a foreign country with its own language, customs, institutions and risks.

Where to start, if you are new to the online world, or helping someone begin to use digital technologies like computers, tablets, smartphones or smart TVs?

The Internet is evolving very fast, so any specific advice is likely to date quite quickly. This chapter explains Internet and computer language, and suggests where to explore further.

Computers used to be big machines with separate keyboards and screens, and then they became laptops, opening like a clamshell with the screen hinged to the keyboard. These days' computers may be tablets, smartphones, smart TVs, games consoles and many other devices. They all enable access to the Internet, with different pros and cons, and run software **programmes**. These are sets of instructions, written in programming code, that make a computer carry out certain functions and behave in a particular way.

Computers have always run programmes – like those for word processing that allow us to type up letters and reports. They can't operate without them. Connecting to the Internet means you aren't limited by what your computer can do on its own.

Online means using the Internet. To **stream** content, like TV, videos or audio, is to view it without transferring it to your device. To **download** is to make the transfer to your device.

The fastest growth in use is in tablets and smartphones. Tablets are like electronic slates with touch sensitive screens, where a finger tap will open an application or "app" as it is popularly known. Apps are software programmes that run on mobile devices. The iPad is perhaps the best known, although others using the Android operating system are cheaper, and retailers have launched their own versions to help promote online shopping. Some of the larger smartphone are like small tablets.

The **apps** are usually specific to a particular task: finding weather reports, bus times, ordering shopping, choosing recipes, taking notes, reminding you which pill to take, or what exercise might be beneficial. Many of them are free, or cost just a pound or two. Some come preloaded on the tablet or smartphone (phone with Internet access), while others are available to purchase from an online **app store like iTunes or Google Play**.

A **browser** is the programme or app you are likely to be using when looking at a page of content online – known as a **web page.** The **World Wide Web** is the term used to describe these trillions of pages offering an enormous range of content on the Internet connected by **hyperlinks.** These links are the bit of magic by which a touch or click on a page hotspot allows you to jump from one piece of content to another, usually somewhere else on the Internet.

Tablets and smartphones these days can do most of the work of personal computers because they also have the more familiar email and word processing programmes, and browsers to view and engage with web pages.

Email is a message that can be sent to one or more people over the Internet. You can also attach documents, photos or video to an email.

The advantage of tablets is that they are light and portable, and in many ways more intuitive than a personal computer or laptop. You can type into an on-screen keyboard, or attach a more traditional one.

Smartphones like the iPhone were developed before the tablets, but these days there is some convergence, as phone screens get larger, and tablets get smaller. You can do many of the things on a smartphone that you can do on a tablet, again using apps. The main challenge is typing onto a screen rather than a keyboard, although you can connect one to a tablet. Programmes are also available that increase the size of keys and buttons on a phone or tablet.

What makes all of these devices useful is the **Internet**, with its vast access to people, communities, information and services all connected through a global network of networked computers. You connect your own computer, tablet or smartphone to the Internet in a number of ways.

If you have a fixed phone line or cable connection, you may choose a broadband package from BT, Sky or another provider, and then connect a computer directly by wire to a **router**. That's the box that connects to the phone line or cable to deliver broadband.

These days most people choose a router that also enables wireless connection via **wifi**. That means your computer, laptop, tablet, phone or other device can access the Internet without a direct wired connection in your home. You can also use wifi hotspots that are increasingly available in cafés, trains or hotels. Some of these are available for you to use freely (with a sign in a window to promote that), whilst others may require payment.

If you want to ensure an always-on connection wherever you are, you can get a **SIM card** to provide 3G or (faster) 4G mobile wifi to your smartphone, tablet or laptop. The cards, that slip into the phone or tablet can be bought for a few pounds. The catch is that this isn't a one-off cost – you are charged by the amount of content that you stream or download. There are also mobile data plans that give you a set amount of data per month at a fixed cost.

At the time of writing – spring 2017 – you can buy tablets for under £100, and get home wifi including line rental for a first year cost of about £200. You should be able to get 4G for under £10 a month, but there will be a limit on data use, so beware watching movies online.

The options can be bewildering, but fortunately BBC WebWise (link below) has a good range of guides and videos, together with links to other sites. They have a guide to Internet safety, to protect your personal information and avoid harmful viruses coming from email or other content.

Like everything else in this field, much of the best information is online … which is a bit of catch if you aren't connected. However, local libraries can usually provide access and initial guidance that's enough to get started. There are also a lot of books that provide more detailed guidance than I can give here.

Although I've focussed on the technical issues first – to explain the language – that isn't the place to start in practice. What's important is why you may want to get online and use the Internet.

You can carry out the basics of sending and receiving email, and viewing web pages, from any device – although typing is more difficult on a phone as the screen is small. Tablets are ideal for viewing TV, live or through the catch-up sites, and movies – with headphones if you wish to improve the listening experience.

You can download and read books, some of them free, using any of the devices, although again tablets are best unless you want to sit at a desk.

One of the major benefits of the Internet is connection with other people, and communities online, not just accessing information. Skype and other similar apps – like Face Time for Apple devices – allow you to make free video calls.

Social networks like Facebook provide a shared space (which can be made private to friends and family) for sharing links and messages, photos and videos, and comments. It can also be used more publicly with a larger audience if, for example, you wanted to share more public information or support causes.

Although Twitter may be derided by those who don't use it – "who wants to know what someone is tweeting about their breakfast" it is like a global meeting room, and you can choose to follow conversations with interesting people in that room, even if they are not your 'friend'. This link to a stream of messages from people you are interested to follow can (often with links to other content) be personally and professionally invaluable.

At this point it should become clear that you can do pretty much anything you want to with a tablet and the Internet … although it remains the case that a computer with a standard keyboard might be better for writing a book. Incidentally, if you want do that with others there are lots of programmes that enable collaborative online writing and editing of documents.

The best approach to finding out what might work for you is ideally to try a computer, tablet or smartphone with someone who can be your guide. The BBC WebWise site not only has its own guides, but also lots of links to other sites. Some of the main ones are listed below, and include databases to search for volunteer digital champions or local centres.

Which computer, tablet or phone to buy? I wouldn't presume to offer detailed advice, because it all depends on your specific needs, and budget. My suggestion is to find someone who will act as guide and adviser, and perhaps help you explore some of the links below. Even if you do get started on a computer or tablet, keep in touch with your adviser, and make sure you review issues of privacy and safety. There are online scams that will try and solicit payments from you, and there is a risk that your computer may become infected by a destructive programme – a virus.

Is it worth the effort of getting online? I believe so. How else can you visit the rest of the world without leaving your home?

Further reading

Myageingparent http://www.myageingparent.com/ is a site dedicated to helping people with older relatives, and it has a technology section including guidance on the pros and cons of computers or tablets, the top apps for older people, and gadgets to assist the elderly with dementia.

BBC WebWise http://www.bbc.co.uk/webwise - guides, videos and link
Safety and privacy http://www.bbc.co.uk/webwise/topics/safety-and-privacy/

Digital Unite http://digitalunite.com/ has a range of guides to devices and online activities, with a focus on older people

UK Online Centres http://www.ukonlinecentres.com/ help people develop online skills.

Community How To http://www.communityhowto.com/ - suggests digital tools for community use

AbilityNet http://www.abilitynet.org.uk/ - provides free help for disabled people using computer and the Internet

Helpful Books https://www.helpfulbooks.co.uk have developed a range of publications backed up by lots of hints and tips online and through newsletters

Webopedia http://www.webopedia.com/ provides concise definitions of Internet terms

Chapter 35

Scams

Steve Playle

Every year, consumers lose staggering amounts of money to fraudsters who bombard us with online, mail, door-to-door and telephone scams. The true scale of the problem is unknown but it is estimated that mass marketing mail scams alone, which often target vulnerable and disadvantaged consumers, cause £3.5 billion worth of detriment. Doorstep crime which involves cold calling doorstep traders offering home repairs and maintenance are estimated to cost consumers something like £440 million. The detriment caused by investment scams where fraudsters persuade consumers to purchase items such as diamonds, wine and land as a surefire way of generating 'fantastic returns' is unknown but runs into billions of pounds with some individual losses often exceeding £100,000.

No one likes to feel that they've wasted or, even worse, been conned out of their money. Unfortunately, there are plenty of situations in which you can act in good faith and suddenly find you've come off worse from a transaction.

The word 'scam' is a little unfortunate because it fails to recognise the fact that it is caused by highly organised criminals. However, the word 'scam' can be used to describe anything from criminal fraud to sharp, but legal, selling practices designed to cheat someone. Fortunately, a lot of scams and bad purchases can be avoided if you know what to look for.

Scams do not discriminate

Scams target people of all backgrounds, ages and income levels. However, some of the worst cases that I have encountered are deliberately targeted at vulnerable consumers and, in particular, those of more senior years. One of the reasons for this is that the elderly generation are perhaps more trusting and less likely to believe that there is hard core of criminals who want to financially abuse them. In addition, the elderly tend to be a little more socially isolated and therefore far more likely to respond to phone calls or knocks on the door from friendly sounding fraudsters. Very few scams are ever reported to the law enforcement community with best estimates putting the reporting levels at something between 5 and 10%. A consumer who has been scammed is often embarrassed about what has happened and, sadly, elderly victims may think that admitting to being defrauded may be their ticket to a care home because family members may think they are no longer able to look after themselves.

The impact of scams on the elderly can be absolutely devastating with studies showing that the quality of life for victims can deteriorate rapidly and lead to premature death. Fraudsters also know that elderly and vulnerable consumers do not always make the best witnesses if they are asked to assist law enforcement agencies such as the Police and it must also be remembered that bringing a case to trial at Crown Court can often take three years or more

New varieties of these scams appear all the time

Trading Standards and The Police have seen the devastating effects scams can have on people and their families. One of the best ways to fight scammers is to help you take steps to prevent yourself from being caught out in the first place. Some adults may be especially vulnerable to financial abuse. **Consider liaising with your local Social Services safeguarding adults department if you are concerned about someone** you know who may be vulnerable (when contacting your local Social Services, ask for adult social care).

Remember these 10 golden rules to help you beat the scammers:

1 There are no guaranteed get-rich-quick schemes: an early scheme promised enormous rewards for helping to move money (originally from Nigeria, now many copy-cat schemes from elsewhere)

2 Do not agree to offers or deals straight away. If you think you have spotted a great opportunity, insist on time to obtain independent/legal advice before making a decision

3 Do not hand over money or sign anything until you have fully checked the credentials of the company that you are dealing with

4 Never send money or give bank or personal details to anyone you do not know or trust. This includes sending money abroad and using methods of payment that you are not comfortable with

5 Log directly on to a website that you are interested in **and not clicking on links provided** in an email

6   Do not rely on glowing testimonials, from lawyers and Government departments; find solid independent evidence of a company's success

7   Always get independent/legal advice if an offer involves money, time or commitment

8   If you spot a scam or have been scammed, report it and get help. **Contact Citizens Advice consumer helpline on 03454 04 05 06 or Action Fraud on 0300 123 2040 or you can call Crimestoppers anonymously on 0800 555 111**

9   Always remember: scammers are cunning, highly organised and clever. They know how to manipulate you to produce the response they want

10 Be suspicious. If you are unsure about anything, seek independent/legal advice.

Perhaps the simplest advice is to NEVER deal with cold callers on the telephone or who knock at your door. The sad news is that you need to treat anyone who cold calls you unexpectedly as a fraudster. It isn't rude to put the phone down and it isn't rude to ask someone on your doorstep to leave – it is your right.

Protect yourself

Protecting your Address:

- If you start to receive post for someone you don't know, find out why

- Register to vote at your current address. Lenders use the electoral roll to check who is registered as living at a particular address. When registering to vote, tick the box to opt out of the 'Edited' register to prevent unsolicited marketing mail. (This does not affect credit checks)

- Sign up with the Mail Preference Service to help prevent you receiving marketing letters. Go onto this website http://www.mpsonline.org.uk to find out how to register or get a trusted family member to do it for you. It won't stop all unsolicited mail but it will help

- Protect mail left in communal areas of residential properties

- Redirect your mail when moving home by filling out a form at your Post Office.

Protecting your Bank Accounts:

- Regularly check statements and chase up any statements that are not delivered when expected

- Securely shred, using a cross cut (confetti) shredder or tear up into small pieces anything containing personal information

- Consider signing up to American Express SafeKey, MasterCard SecureCode or Verified by Visa when you receive your cards, even if you do not intend to use your cards online – this protects you if your card or details are lost or stolen

- Beware unsolicited phone calls, letters and emails pretending to be your bank, or other financial institution and asking you to confirm your personal details, passwords and security numbers. Banks will **never** ask you to do this

- If you think someone is misusing your bank account details then report it to your bank.

Protecting your Phones:

- Go onto the Telephone Preference Service web site http://www.tpsonline.org.uk to find out how to reduce the number of unwanted calls or get a trusted family member to do it for you. This won't stop all calls but it will help

- There are clever call blocking devices that can now be purchased that will screen out all unwanted calls. One particular device is called 'truecall' http://www.truecall.co.uk but there are now some telephones available from BT with the 'truecall' protection already built in

- Never reply to unsolicited texts, e.g. texts referring to accident claims, even to get them stopped. Simply delete them

- Banks rarely telephone you: one scam asks you to ring back, but stays on the line, when you think they have hung up. Subsequent discussions may result in you keying in the pin number of a credit card and even someone coming to collect it because of alleged fraud.

Protecting your Computer:

- Keep your computer security programs (antivirus, antispam) up to date

- Restrict the amount of personal information that you disclose when online

- Don't fall for online scams, scam letters via email, advance fee or other internet-related frauds

- Know how to verify secure web sites if making financial transactions. You can do this by looking at the address line. Normally it will start with http but when you log into a secure site this will change to https for example; http://www.mybank.com is the address of mybank, but if you want to go to the transactions page you log in and the address bar will change to something like https://mybank/login. com. The address bar may also change colour. A padlock also appears in either the bottom left or bottom right corner of the browser, not in the website

- If you have received an email claiming to be your bank, requesting that you contact them, consider the legitimacy of such an email. If you are unsure, do not use the link in the email you have received

- Open another window in your browser and visit your bank's website using your normal method

- One of the most difficult scams to reject is when the mail comes from a trusted email account that has been hacked (phishing). The mail may have come from a bank, web-provider or a friend. It usually has a scaremongering message (credit card used illegally; mail account hacked or due to be closed; friend been robbed and stranded in a foreign land), all messages require the release of information and cash. Check through another source before clicking on a given website or any other requested response.

Mass Marketing Fraud – Scam Mail Big Scams

Many people in the UK and overseas are drawn by the thrill of a surprise win and find themselves parting with large amounts of money in order to claim fake prizes. Large numbers of victims, often the elderly and vulnerable, fall for Mass Marketing scam mail.

What you should know

You cannot win money or a prize in a lottery if you have not entered it. You cannot be chosen at random if you do not have an entry. Many Mass Marketing scams will trick you into parting with money or providing your banking or personal details in the belief that you will win a cash prize. You do not have to pay a fee to claim a legitimate prize. It only takes one time to respond and you will be inundated with scam mail. Your name and address will be included on what's known as a 'Sucker's List' and you will receive large amounts of mail on a daily basis. A fake prize scam will tell you that you have won a prize or competition. You may receive 'confirmation' of this by post, email or text message. There will often be costs involved in claiming the prize. Even if you receive a prize it may not be what was promised to you. You may be offered a dream job but prior to starting, you may be asked to pay for taxes, visas, 'antiterrorism certificates' or any other advanced fee.

An alternative to the lottery scam is where you have been told that you have won a guaranteed prize and all you have to do to claim it is to purchase of goods. These are normally things like vitamin pills, cosmetics or tacky housewares but if you are tempted to make a purchase, you won't win anything and you will quickly be consumed by lots more unsolicited letters.

Investment Fraud

The average victim of an investment fraud loses £32,000 and recent research shows that a third of people aged over 75 years have been targeted. Also known as boiler room frauds – the 'boiler room' refers to a rented space from which salespeople call hundreds of potential victims each day, using high pressure sales techniques. Investments where fraud is commonplace involve the sale of land (including car parking spaces and burial plots), wine, carbon credits and diamonds. Fraudsters cold-call you normally by telephone and try to sell you investments that supposedly lead to huge financial gains. In reality they either do not exist or are worthless. In one recent case, the City of London Trading Standards has come across consumers who have purchased diamonds costing £35,000 which, although they exist, are virtually worthless. Often the scammers give you details that you might think only a genuine investment company will have. They may have details of previous investments you have made, shares you hold and know your personal circumstances. Be aware the scammers do their homework and make it their business to know as much about you as possible. The scammers often call you a number of times slowly developing a friendly relationship, effectively grooming you to give them a large sum of money. Having obtained some money from you, they will probably call again and try to persuade you to 'invest' further money, perhaps in a different commodity. Scammers may say they are from a well known and reputable investment company and will often have persuasive looking glossy brochures and impressive web sites, often using a 'head office' address in the City of London.

Never deal with cold callers offering to sell you investments like this. Simply say that you aren't interested and always put the phone down. Remember – it isn't rude, it is your right. The promised returns never materialise and it may be several years before you realise that you have been defrauded out of your life savings. These investments aren't regulated by the Financial Conduct Authority and you will get nothing back. Even after you may have lost significant sums of money to an investment fraud, you will probably find you are then subjected to what is termed a 'recovery room' fraud where more criminals will contact you, claiming that they can recoup your previous losses but only after payment of a fee or after investing in yet more products.

Frequent Scamming Tools

Scammers often use one or more of the following to help them commit fraud and hide their true identity.

Money Transfer Agents

Using a money transfer agent is a way to send money to people that you know and trust. Money transfer agents offer fast, convenient and reliable options for customers to send and receive money worldwide. However, they are often used by scammers in order to commit many types of fraud such as advance fee, identity theft, investments and mass marketing fraud to name a few.

WHILST THE SENDER OF THE MONEY HAS TO PRODUCE IDENTITY DOCUMENTS, THOSE THAT COLLECT THE MONEY DO NOT.

This is why scammers often try to get you to send them money using a money transfer agent. This method enables them to hide their identity.

You should:

- Never let a scammer educate you on how a money transfer service works – only take advice from the money transfer agent

- Read the warnings on money transfer documents. The information is there to protect you

- Do not pay for items bought online, including auction sites using a money transfer agent. Money transfer agents are not responsible for the satisfactory receipt of goods or services paid for by means of a money transfer

- Never share details of a money transfer with anyone else to prove the availability of funds. Doing so may enable the money transfer to be paid to that third party. This is known as a 'Proof of Funds' fraud.

Bank transfers

A lot of people now have bank accounts that allow you to ring up to make money transfers or to go online and do them yourself. It is very quick and easy but if you are subjected to a fraud which results in you making a bank transfer to a fraudster, you will not get any money back. The bank will say that you authorised the payment and that they have no responsibility over how you spend your money. In contrast, if a fraudster hacks into your account or clones your credit card and steals money, you are protected provided that you haven't been negligent.

One major flaw with the current banking system is that when you make a transfer, your bank is only interested in the account number and sort code of the payee and NOT their name. This means that you can think that you are sending money to a particular person or business but the reality is that their bank account hasn't actually been set up in their name. This is something that is due to be corrected by 2020 but, in the meantime, if sending money to a new payee, just send them a pound first and ring the person you think you are dealing with to check it has been received.

Banks have a duty of care to their customers but they can't check every transaction. Great steps have been made by the banks to question large 'over the counter' cash withdrawals but more work is needed with telephone and internet transfers. One idea currently being pursued by

Trading Standards is to allow customers to opt for a slower payment service of three days to all new payees. At the start of the three day period, a trusted representative of the customer would receive a text or email alert that a transaction is being attempted which gives the opportunity for an intervention to be made to stop the money being lost.

Virtual Offices

A virtual office is an address where any person or business wishing to use an alternative address to their own can use office facilities, telephone answering services or a postal address. You might think you are dealing with a well established, professional individual or business with a prestigious address in the City of London. However, the reality can be very different. Many businesses using 'virtual offices' are honest and legitimate. However, fraudsters may often use a virtual office address instead of their own in order to receive mail and conduct business using a false ID to obtain the virtual office facilities. In reality, the fraudsters may be working from overseas and beyond UK law enforcement or in other locations that are very difficult to find. Lots of work has been carried out under the 'Operation Broadway' banner by Trading Standards and the Police to clamp down hard on virtual office providers and it is now getting increasingly difficult, but not impossible just yet, for fraudsters to operate from a virtual address.

If you see a website or an advert for a website that has a telephone number and address on it, be aware that the address could well be a virtual office address. Victims of many scams have been known to visit the address shown on a fraudulent website or on a letter in order to remonstrate and try to get back the money they have lost. They are often surprised and dismayed to find that the office was a virtual office, used by a fraudster who has provided the virtual office owner with false ID and that now there is no trace of them. Additionally, it is also worth remembering that a fraudster may just use a virtual office address without the virtual office owner's knowledge or permission. This is known as 'squatting' and is becoming more common.

General

Be suspicious of EVERYTHING and remember: If it sounds too good to be true it probably is.

Lots of people who end up getting defrauded are normal, intelligent individuals. When they look back at what they have done, they always say "I can't believe I was so stupid". If I had a fiver for every time I have heard that expression, I would have retired many years ago. Fraudsters are clever and manipulative but you must simply learn to say "no" every time you get an unsolicited phone call or knock on the door. In the case of unsolicited emails, delete them – and in the case of unsolicited mail, destroy it.

Always think very carefully before parting with any money and perhaps consult with a trusted family member or friend who may quickly be able to spot that you are about to be another victim of a scam.

It is natural to be embarrassed and reluctant to admit that you have been scammed, particularly over sensitive financial or personal issues, such as online dating. Nevertheless, you are not alone in these matters, and reporting real or suspected scams can really help to protect others and to help law enforcement agencies target their resources against the worst criminals.

Chapter → 36

Connecting with the Arts in Later Life

The Arts Council of Great Britain was founded after the Second World War with the aim to provide great art for everyone: it is currently celebrating its 70th anniversary. Whereas the mission has not changed, the institution has gone through many reincarnations. The initial emphasis on London-based events was expanded by devolution into national and regional bodies. In 2002, 10 regional arts boards merged with the Arts Council of England to become the Arts Council England (ACE). In 2011 this body assumed new responsibilities for the support and development of museums and libraries. The expanded remit included supporting the Cultural Olympic Programme, and led to the current strategic framework of **Great Art and Culture for Everyone**.

Funding for the organisation has been primarily from national and local government, but since 1993, this has been substantially boosted by national lottery funding, and it also encompasses many partnerships across the public and private sectors. Both Government and Lottery policies have defined the distribution of ACE funding. Forty percent provides core National Culture Infrastructure funding for over 700 institutions across England, such as the British Museum and the London South Bank Complex. The remaining funds are divided equally between Sport, Heritage and the Arts.

ACE has prescribed five goals for the funding of art and cultural activities: holistic, education and health, society, and economy. Funding for children and youth activity is a dominant feature, encourageing exposure and experience to all art forms, promoting understanding and appreciating of cultural heritage, including cross-cultural awareness and integration. The programmes stimulate imagination, creativity and self expression. The results are improved academic performance, better university degrees, successful job hunting, and active inspired community involvement, in volunteering and pioneering change. The overall aim is to produce well-rounded adults with sound social skills and confident social mobility.

Public engagement in artistic and cultural experience is directed at enriching peoples' lives, while recognising and releasing the talent within our diverse society. The performing arts feature high on the ACE agenda. Support ranges from theatre – digital art; reading – dance; music – literature; and crafts – collections. The broad canvas has no cultural or geographic barriers across the country, and every effort is made to balance this wide spectrum with the mission of art and culture for everyone; maintaining the highest of standards in all the ventures that the ACE supports. The aim is to make England a better and happier place to work and live in.

ACE, like all funding bodies, recognises and understands the changing demographics of the English population: people are living longer. Whereas, when the pension system was introduced at the turn of the twentieth century, the life expectancy was only a few years over the retirement age, it is now over twenty, and rising. Thus people currently in their middle age, will have to adapt their life and work-style to match these changes, in particular they will have less disposable income for art and cultural activities. Nevertheless the population will continue to expect and demand a full cultural life; ACE and other funding bodies has to adapt to meet these expectations.

Change is a driver of invention, and ACE is expanding its policies to celebrate age, introducing a more open, wider and flexible approach to funding, and incorporate health and wellbeing. It is seeking initiatives and opportunities that can be explored, rewarding creativity, and breaking through previous boundaries, such as those between education, performance, sport and health.

ACE is looking for cross-fertilisation and merging of disciplines, and transferrable skills. It is funding research initiatives that assess outcomes, identify learning requirements, and public involvement, engagement and participation in activities that search for excellence and promote best practice.

Ageing brings on its own problems, with increase of disease and disability. It also creates an increasing population of vulnerable, lonely and socially isolated individuals that are subject to marginalisation, discrimination and exclusion. The trauma of these changes, and the potential loss of partners and friends, increase depression and anxiety, and highlight any preexisting psychoses.

Whereas ACE funding is mainly to established bodies that have already demonstrated achievable goals, usually across different geographic areas, ageing problems are local in nature and require a community response. These often result from the entrepreneurial activities of an enthusiast who has taken on a specific mission. Such small beginnings, however, can lead to valuable skills that are transferrable to a wider population, be these education, art or health initiatives.

ACE can provide a great deal of nonfunding help to such ventures. It may be able to recommend alternative funding streams, and links to skill sources, experts, potential partners and networks in the same field. ACE can add support and advocacy to a project, providing insight into its strengths and weaknesses, and help with business planning and commissioning. Such help adds to the credibility of a project, and also facilitates publicising successful outcomes.

ACE is charged with the responsibility of obtaining the maximum value for a large public investment. This has included research and development in delivery of a wide range of diverse projects across the arts and culture, ensuring operability, resilience and sustainability. It has played an important role in shaping the future of the arts nationally and internationally, laying down its own history, and ensuring a long term legacy of excellence.

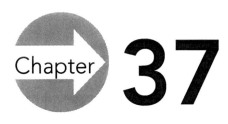

Chapter **37**

Love Your Library

Carol Boswarthack

If you are no longer a regular user of your local library, do look again because our public library service is an amazing resource for people of all ages.

Libraries are safe, neutral community spaces, open to all. Step inside and you will be able to find out about social groups and other local events or maybe attend a talk or join a reading group. Library membership is free and there are currently 3850 libraries in the UK[1]. The free lending of books is still very much the core service offered but many libraries also have CDs, DVDs and talking books for customers to borrow. And that's not all…

The Society of Chief Librarians (SCL) has defined the modern public library offering via 5 Universal Offers: Digital, Information, Reading, Health and Learning. A brand new Culture Offer is coming soon.

The Digital Offer

The Internet is now key to modern life and people of all ages use it for all kinds of reasons: to keep in contact with friends and families; to share photographs; to pay bills; to shop for goods including weekly groceries; to fill out official forms and much more. Despite this, it is estimated that approximately 10% of adults in the UK (5.3 million people) have never used the Internet, 20% of adults have not used the Internet in the past 3 months and only 38.7% of adults aged 75 years and over are regular Internet users[2].

If you fall into any of these categories and you want to know more, your local library could be the solution. Most public libraries have computers that you can use for no or very low cost and if you need some help in getting started, library staff will be able to help you get online. Most libraries provide one to one help and all can point you to classes where you can develop your skills.

Once you are comfortable with using the technology, you can begin to enjoy a range of online library services such as eBooks and eAudiobooks, which you can download whenever and wherever you wish. They even return themselves at the end of the loan period so there are no fines! You can also start to explore what else is on offer such as learning a language online, reading eMagazines, streaming music and video and consulting online reference services including dictionaries and encyclopaedias.

The Information Offer

Libraries support people to access information and services in vital areas. You can either use the library catalogue or browse the books on the shelves to search for the information you need yourself or you can ask the staff to help you. Library staff are trained in answering enquiries whether they be simple, complex or confidential and they are used to being asked questions on anything and everything! They will try to find the answers you need using library stock, the Internet and other online services or maybe by referring you to a more specialist agency.

The Reading Offer

Books and reading are at the heart of the public library service. People read for a number of reasons including reading for pleasure, to improve skills, for relaxation and to improve one's knowledge. All public libraries offer customers a huge choice of fiction and nonfiction books which, by law, can be borrowed free of charge. If the book you need isn't in stock or is on loan to another customer, libraries also offer a reservation service (there is usually a small cost involved). The UK public library service is an effective network and this may involve borrowing the book from a completely different local authority or from the British Library.

We are creatures of habit and readers tend to stick to what they know they like but there can be so much pleasure to be gained from breaking out and trying something completely different. Reading groups encourage you to do just this and are a fantastic way to challenge yourself and try new reading experiences. The basic premise is that a group of people read the same book and come together, usually once a month, to talk about it. Sometimes the groups meet in libraries and some meet in members' homes. If you would like to join a group or set one up, do talk to the staff at your local library.

Another way of introducing people to new reading experiences is by checking out the displays and promotions in your library or asking staff for suggestions. They will be delighted to help you.

The Health Offer

It may surprise you to know that there is strong evidence that proves that Public Libraries make a real contribution to the health and wellbeing of communities. A report commissioned by Arts Council England on The health and wellbeing benefits of public libraries, estimated that *it is possible to aggregate NHS cost savings across the library-using English population to estimate an average cost saving of £27.5 million per year.*[3]

That's an impressive figure so how do libraries make such a difference? The answer is "in many ways". Here are some of those ways.

Book stock

If you want to learn more about how to control a diagnosed condition, if you are looking for some new recipes to improve your eating habits or maybe you want to learn how to support a family member or friend with their ill heath, somewhere there will be a book that will answer your questions. Ask at your local library.

Books on Prescription

The Reading Well, Books on Prescription scheme, endorsed by health professionals and delivered by The Reading Agency in partnership with the Society of Chief Librarians, helps you to understand and manage your own health and wellbeing. There are currently three book lists available: Reading Well Books on Prescription for common mental health conditions, Reading Well Books on Prescription for dementia and Reading Well for young people. A fourth book list, Reading Well Books on Prescription for long term conditions is due at the time of writing. Most Library authorities stock the books on all of the lists – ask at your local library for more information.

Talks and more

Find out if your local library offers a programme of clubs, talks and events. Most public library services will programme regular activities in at least one library venue. Some events may specifically focus on Health and Wellbeing topics such as talks about living well with dementia or arthritis. Other activities, especially those focussing on culture, learning skills or sharing hobbies will help to contribute to your general wellbeing.

And this leads us neatly on to

The Learning Offer

Learning doesn't stop when formal education ends. The phrase *you learn something new every day* is so very true and for hundreds of thousands of people, libraries play a huge role in lifelong learning. Whether you want to learn new skills or brush up on old ones, take a look at your local library and see what is on offer. Some libraries host formal classes but, as discussed already, with books and more about all manner of subjects that you can borrow, language courses, music, talks, events, one-to-one computer assistance… all libraries offer multiple opportunities for you to expand your horizons. The sky really is the limit!

Volunteering opportunities

Do you have a skill or some expertise on a subject that you could share with others? Do you have some time to spare and want to commit to something that will benefit your community? If you do, maybe you could help to improve somebody else's life as well as your own. Why not consider discussing your ideas with library staff and find out what volunteering opportunities are available? Hundreds of adults up and down the country are helping to improve their local library services by listening to children read, assisting staff with events, helping with surveys and much more. Volunteering is incredibly rewarding and there are so many things with which you could get involved. Ask your local library staff for more details.

In conclusion, libraries are gems that can improve lives. They can improve **your** life. Be sure to take another look!

Further reading

[1]CIPFA figures for 2015/16

[2] Internet users in the UK: 2016, Office for National Statistics, May 2016

[3] The health and wellbeing benefits of public libraries, Daniel Fujiwara, Ricky Lawton, Susana Mourato, March 2015

[4] https://reading-well.org.uk/

38

A Village Community Life

Graham Peiser

By way of background, my village is in a parish of 1,849 adult residents, but this includes not only the village itself but also the surrounding hamlets. It is within spitting distance of the M25 and only five miles from stations with rapid access to central London, and is central to a dozen well documented country walks. In view of the location in particular, over the last half century there has been a marked shift from a predominantly farming community to more of a commuting community.

Three things are primarily pertinent to our village community life: firstly our Community Centre, secondly the host of volunteers in the village, both 'leaders' and unsung heroes, and thirdly our village shop.

The location of both the Community Centre and the shop is crucial – being in the centre of the village, close to two of the four village pubs, and adjacent to a large Village Green, the village Church of England primary school, and the doctor's surgery. These facilities, and their location, provide a powerful community hub.

The Community Centre is very versatile with five different rooms of varying size. The main hall is 17.5m x 10.2m (58ft x 33ft) and is licensed for 200 people, 170 when seated. Both round and rectangular tables are available, plus upholstered chairs, all to match these requirements. The main hall has a hardwood floor and includes an amazingly versatile stage, which can be adjusted for both height and dimensions. The hall can be blacked out for film and other entertainment, and appropriate lighting, projection, PA and sound equipment, including an induction hearing 'loop' system, is also in place. The area of the hall can be increased by opening a 'musicians gallery' from one of the two upstairs rooms, and there is an adjoining well appointed kitchen plus a separate bar area.

Three other rooms can provide separate meeting areas for 20 – 50 people. There is an additional kitchenette for the rear and upper rooms, plus of course storage space and toilets, including two with disabled access.

The whole building is licensed for music, dance and performance, and similarly holds a license for the playing of prerecorded music and for the showing of films. Alcohol consumption is permitted on the premises, however no alcohol is housed on site.

Two rooms are permanently let for the offices of the Parish Council and the parish church administration.

Whilst the facility started life as a Village Hall between the wars, it was completely rebuilt in the year 2000, plus an extension added in 2005, both funded from multiple sources, including local council contributions, various grants and from hard earned and gratefully received charitable donations.

Strict fund management is in place to run the centre. Part-time employment is provided for hiring administration, cleaning and furniture moving, but an extensive network of volunteers runs the building and most of the activities therein. This ensures that local events are available at acceptable, and where necessary supported, rates.

As well as the events organised by the local CARE organisation, umpteen other events regularly take place at the centre. Dinner dances for both St George's Day and the local branch of the British Legion; an annual Music Festival; an annual local am-dram pantomime; regular film club nights; regular Zumba and Pilates classes, a local quilting group; biannual local horticultural flower and vegetable shows; plus regular fundraisers for the centre itself.

Two countrywide community organisations that also use the centre are the local branches of both U3A (the University of the Third Age) and NADFAS (the National Association of Decorative and Fine Arts Societies). But more of both CARE and U3A below. A Sunday morning market once a month with an extensive bring-and-buy section and book exchange raises funds for the centre.

The Parish Council uses the centre for its meetings and parish activities, and similarly, the parish church uses the centre for many of its events, as it lacks a Church Hall. The centre also serves as the local Polling Station.

So, as can be seen, the centre is very well used, to the extent that local societies have to ensure they book well in advance.

One of the prime contributors to the care of the village community that needs special mention is the village CARE organisation. This amazing team of people was started some 25 years ago and, from small beginnings, has grown into a volunteer group providing a helping hand to the people of the village.

It currently delivers meals-on-wheels to those in need at lunchtime on Mondays to Fridays; a three course lunch is provided in the Community Centre on the third Monday of every month; and a 'Coffee Corner' meeting point in the Community Centre on alternate Wednesdays including subsidised chiropody, hairdressing and head-and-neck massage, plus a bring-and-buy sales table and a book exchange, and is timed to coincide with the Mobile Library visit to the village.

CARE also arranges varied activities at regular intervals of a Friendship Club mostly, again, at the Community Centre, and a team of volunteers undertakes regular transport of individuals to hospital and out-of-village doctor's appointments, and other similar events. Day-to-day help is provided for anyone of any age who has a problem they cannot overcome unaided – no problem is too trivial to deal with.

The local U3A (the University of the Third Age), which regularly meets in the Community Centre as referred to above, provides a remarkable array of activities. As well as a series of lecture, the U3A runs groups on art, painting, crafts, knitting, bridge, music, literature, languages, history, heritage, stamps, singing and dancing. Outdoor activities cover gardening, bird watching, walking, rambling, cycling, racket ball, golf and sailing.

An important recent development in village life has been the community taking over the ownership and running of the only residual shop left in the village (there were six shops in the village some only thirty years ago, the remainder sadly having closed over the years). The shop sells a wide range of products, ranging from fruit, vegetables and groceries to cigarettes, own-baked bread to stationary, and medications to daily papers, which are also delivered within the village. It also sells lottery tickets, takes in cleaning, hands out prescriptions delivered by the local doctors' surgery (also located within the village) and you can even top up your prepaid mobile phone.

The shop also most importantly incorporates the local Post Office – which not only deals with postal matters and local banking but also, significantly, the facility of handling state pensions.

Whilst there are paid managers of both the shop and the Post Office, the staffing of the whole venture is predominantly by volunteers.

So far I have focused on the caring-for-the-elderly aspects of the village, however the other community aspects mustn't be forgotten as many of these also cater for the elderly and their families.

We have a 'traditional' type local family-run garage and filling station close to the centre of the village; the doctor's dispensing surgery referred to above; a very successful Church of England primary school right in the centre; a pre and post school activity organisation; a mothers and toddlers group; cubs, scouts, guides; the parish church; and a local WI group catering for other residents. The large Village Green referred to above is host to various activities including a Boxing Day classic vehicle meeting.

We also have a recreation ground with football and cricket pitches, two floodlit hard tennis courts and a children's play area plus a large pavilion used, amongst other things, for short-mat bowling.

Crime is fortunately low in the village, but a Neighborhood Watch is well established to keep us all informed and to combat problems in this area.

A unique village feature is the running of two vintage buses for community purposes. One of the buses was purchased by one of the then residents approximately twenty-five years ago for this express purpose. When he left the village some ten years ago he 'gave' the bus to the village for this purpose to be continued. Following that a group of thirty or so local residents now manage and fund this continuance, doing all the maintenance and driving from within themselves. The value of the bus for outings and transport for groups within the community can be judged by the purchase of the second bus five years later.

Apart perhaps from the buses, this community life is probably replicated in towns and villages across the country, but documenting here the importance of a Community Centre, the various organisations run predominantly by volunteers, and latterly the emergence of a community managed shop, may stimulate others to explore all potentials for voluntary care of the elderly, much of it on a self help basis.

In this day and age it is particularly relevant to fill this current deficiency in our central governance.

Chapter 39

Music

Connecting to Music

Sean Gregory

Much of my work over the years as a composer has focused on giving people of all ages, backgrounds and experiences the opportunity to **make music** in a creative workshop environment. The **workshops** and projects have involved a range of participatory activities that facilitate the development of new musical ideas within a collaborative context. This encourages a '**team' approach** to all activities, instilling a sense of ownership and responsibility both in the creative process and in the final product. The exchange of ideas and skills amongst the participants is an integral part of the process, collectively giving people the freedom to interact and to respond intuitively to what is going on around them.

The development of my own practice as a musician working in the community has coincided with the evolution over the past three decades of a rich variety of tied to orchestras, opera houses, theatres, galleries and museums across the UK. More often than not the projects are held in local spaces, such as schools, sixth form colleges, arts centres, community halls, hospitals and youth clubs. Some of these projects can also lead to large-scale performances in major venues such as the Barbican and South Bank Centre. Their inclusive approach embraces everything from classical to popular music, western and nonwestern genres, and set repertoires, as well as new works created through **collaborative** workshops, often involving other arts disciplines.

Much of my work – both as a musician and now as Director of Creative Learning at the Barbican Centre and Guildhall School of Music & Drama – is about making **connections**, putting people, organisations and cultures in touch with each other and enabling them to do better together what they would do less well alone. It places an equal emphasis on process and performance for project leaders, professional musicians, students and community participants. As a result of this, boundaries are broken down between musical genres, arts disciplines, 'specialists' and 'nonspecialists', enabling people to 'open up' and feel better about themselves as human beings – individually and collectively.

Collaboration and **creativity** lie at the heart of this work. This is an environment in which the voices of all participants, experienced and less experienced, are heard, listened to and acknowledged. Although the musical contexts are generally nonformal and the approach to learning informal, the way in which the music is created, shaped and performed is both organised and goal-directed. All participants quickly grow in **confidence**, gain **self discipline,** develop their creative and performance skills, acquire an awareness of artistic standards and strengthen their ability to communicate with each other and with audiences.

The opportunity to be able to connect, to make sense of another person's world, is fundamental to making music in a creative, collaborative environment. This can be particularly powerful for older people who may be dealing with a growing sense of isolation from family, friends and the wider community. Music is a freer **language** than words, and being able to express yourself through your voice, percussion or an instrument you already play, can be quite liberating and empowering. It is the participation in such activity that is so empowering that brings out both the integrity of artistic engagement and the spirit of human engagement, which in turn leads to making a difference in people's lives.

Music in Public Libraries

Chris Huckle

The word 'library' is nearly always synonymous with books and reading. Libraries, however, are about much more than this, they are often a hub for the local community; a place of quietness, private study and lifelong learning.

Libraries provide a wealth of **information** in the form of: newspapers, journals, reference material and community literature. Information **technology** is a feature with PCs providing: Internet access, office software and e-government services. Digital material including: film, music and spoken word is also a significant part of the stock available to customers.

When people say that libraries are simply about books and reading they are perhaps forgetting music, which has been a part of libraries for decades from when vinyl collections first appeared in the 1960s. Music is important, not only because of its popularity with children and young people but because it speaks to all age groups and cultures.

In recent years, I have been focused on maintaining and **promoting music** in the public library service. The classical music stock in terms of books, CDs, printed music and scores had to be revitalised. Purchasing new stock and improving the presentation and accessibility of this stock has helped to turn things around. The music CD collection has also been expanded to include the audiovisual element of DVDs. The music section has been developed to include music displays for both popular and classical music, making things more interesting and promoting stock. A **music notice board** has been introduced to advertise: local musicians, concerts and events.

In contrast to books and reading groups, I took the step of starting a **Classical Music Appreciation Group**, possibly the first of its kind in the service. The group meets once a month and spends some of its time listening to and discussing the works of anniversary composers. The use of questionnaires has enabled me to gauge interests in the group and to introduce variety by inviting guest musicians to come and talk or play to the Group. The attendance figures are encourageing and now average about ten per session.

With the promotion of music in libraries I have found it important to constantly develop the music section and its stock. The Classical Music Appreciation Group has proved to be successful, paving the way for groups in other musical genres. The printed music section can be enhanced by the introduction of an electric piano with headphones. Further developments involve working more closely with local schools and colleges to provide new music stock to support the musical activities of children and students.

In the last few years, my local library statistics indicate that issues for music CDs have remained constant. An interesting fact to consider when there is competition from the Internet and the downloading of music. We appear to have a stable user base to build on, where the CD remains a popular music stock item.

In future, it is important to remember that the word 'library' encompasses a sense of reading and listening for both words and music.

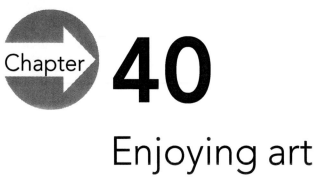

Chapter **40**

Enjoying art

Will Cooper

There are two main ways to enjoy art: by appreciating art made by others or by creating your own. These two activities are completely distinct and you might choose to pursue one or the other. However they can be mutually beneficial if enjoyed together. An interest in art appreciation might lead you to try your hand at making your own work. And if you are thinking of taking up art, you will learn a great deal from studying the work of others. Both activities can often seem intimidating to a beginner, but neither making nor appreciating art requires any previous experience, training or knowledge. Art is a world of pleasure that literally anybody can enter, and I hope in this article to show how you can take your first steps.

Appreciating art

Here in the City of London we are extremely lucky to be within easy reach of several world-class art galleries, as well as the crucible of new and cutting edge art that is the contemporary East End. There are few better places in the world from which to begin a journey into discovering art. If you're new to art you might want to start by going to see some well known paintings in the flesh. The permanent collection at the National Gallery in Trafalgar Square contains some of the world's most well known paintings dating from the thirteenth century up to 1900. The story of art continues across the Thames at Tate Modern, which houses famous works of art from the twentieth century onwards. Explore the rich heritage that exists in you own locality, throughout the UK.

If you are new to art you may find "modern art" more off putting or confusing than the traditional, representational work of earlier artists. My advice would be to dive in and try a bit of everything. See what you like. Art can be appreciated on many different levels, and obviously the more you learn about it the more enjoyment you will get. However, I will let you into a secret: *you don't have to know what any of it means.*

We may never know who the woman in the Mona Lisa was; why Leonardo chose to portray her, or the secret of her enigmatic smile. But this has not stopped millions of people enjoying this painting for hundreds of years. Many historical paintings from as recently as the nineteenth century are full of symbols, codes and references whose meaning are now lost to all but the keenest scholars. This does not stop the rest of us from enjoying their beauty. Modern art is no different. For example it is not necessary to know the theoretical reasons why Picasso chose to paint in the various styles that he did, or why Dan Flavin chose to make his art out of nothing but coloured neon strip lights. This needn't stop anybody enjoying the beauty of their work. Art is created in order to provoke a response in the viewer, and all responses are valid. You might like a work of art or you might not, however little you might know about the artist's intentions in making it.

If you do choose to look deeper into the meaning of works of art you will experience greater and deeper levels of enjoyment. You may even find yourself liking something that you previously disliked. Most of the major art galleries offer personal electronic audio guides that provide explanation and commentary about some of the pieces in their exhibitions. These can be a great way of enhancing a visit to a gallery. You may also choose to join a live, guided talk from one of the gallery's staff, giving you the chance to ask questions.

Further reading

These books provide an excellent introduction to art history

- The Story of Art, Ernst H Gombrich, 1950
- The Art Book, Phaidon, 1997

Making art

When it comes to making your own works of art, the same rules apply: there are many levels at which you can practice art and none of them are wrong. Lack of experience should be no barrier to enjoyment, but the more you learn about art and the techniques involved in making it the greater your enjoyment will be.

You may already have an idea of the sort of art you want to make, but again I would recommend trying out lots of different techniques and approaches. I happen to believe that drawing is at the heart of all art practice. Whatever medium or style you choose to work in, the regular practice of drawing will underpin everything you do.

Some people are naturally good at drawing but most say that they "can't draw". In fact nearly everybody can be trained to be competent in drawing at a basic level and I would recommend taking classes with a qualified instructor if you are keen to develop your draughtsmanship.

Learning how to draw does not only improve the quality of your artwork it can also benefit your physical and mental health in all sorts of ways. The act of drawing is extremely good practice for your hand-eye coordination, but the most important skill you develop when drawing from life is *looking*. Our eyes scan the word around us all the time and much of what we see is taken for granted. In order to successfully draw what we see it is necessary to look in a deeper and more intense way than we would ever normally take the time to do. Attempting to draw even the most simple, mundane object such as a teacup engages the eyes, hand and mind to such a degree that you never look at that teacup in the same way again!

This way of looking at the world is infectious, and the more you draw and paint the world around you the more you will find yourself appreciating the shape and colours of things; how they are made and how they interact with the objects and spaces around them.

If you don't feel inclined to take classes in art, there is no reason why you can't still make satisfying pictures and sculptures. There are numerous books and magazines that give you tips on materials and techniques. Sharing your experiences with other artists can also be encourageing and inspiring. Look for local art clubs and societies near where you live so you can share your enjoyment of making art with others and learn from their experiences.

To a beginner, the world of materials and equipment can seem as intimidating as any other aspect of art. My advice is to start with simple materials that you understand. A small range of pencils for drawing; pastels or acrylic paints if you want to use colour. These kinds of materials can be used without any particular training. If you do choose to take classes you will be shown how to use more advanced media by a trained instructor. Picking up a set of oil paints without first being shown how to use them is likely to result in little more than a disappointing mess!

Good quality art materials can be expensive. However I would always recommend using the best quality materials you can afford. You will be rewarded with paintings and sculptures that look better, endure longer and are much more pleasant to work on.

Equipment suppliers

- Cass Art www.cassart.co.uk Branches throughout the UK
- Atlantis Art Supplies www.atlantisart.co.uk Basement, 16-28 Tabernacle Street London EC2A 4DD

Local art classes

The Art Class and Art in the Guildhall Art Gallery

adulteducation@cityoflondon.gov.uk

Drop-in life drawing

www.londondrawing.com

Search for your local classes through your library, Local Authority and the Internet

Chapter **41**

Dance

Stella Howard & Kate Wakeling

From attending a preperformance talk at Sadler's Wells to joining your local salsa class, there is a myriad of ways to develop your interest and pleasure in dance as an audience member and/or participant. Dance is for everyone, regardless of age or physical ability, and its value in promoting health, wellbeing and social inclusion for people of all ages is increasingly recognised by arts venues, community organisations and educational institutions, with rising numbers of outreach programmes seeking to support older people to get involved in dance.

This brief introduction to dance for older people firstly explores the appreciation of dance in performance then considers opportunities to be an active dance participant, be it at a local arts centre, community event or in your own living room.

Appreciating Dance

There is a wide range of categories of dance widely available to experience as an audience member. The term **social dance** covers a large number of dance forms, all designed to be enjoyed as part of broader social interaction. Social dance includes forms like ballroom dancing, salsa, flamenco as well as 'tea' dance styles, and the room set up for social dance is often 'conversational' in style, allowing attendees to enjoy refreshments and interact with other audience members as the dancing takes place. While social dance forms are sometimes presented with a clear distinction between performers and audience members, they are also often interactive, providing open opportunities for anyone to participate in dancing in a relaxed and informal setting.

Perhaps the most well-known form of dance experienced by spectators is **ballet**, but there are also large numbers of theatre spaces and dance venues which present other **theatre dance** forms, including **contemporary dance** and **physical theatre** which provide a vibrant contrast to the rigours of classical ballet. Venues across the country are also increasingly committed to what might be termed '**cultural dance**': dance forms based on cultural traditions from Ireland to

India, Mali to Bali. The extraordinary diversity of dance (and music) found across the globe can make for a particularly inspiring audience experience, offering a rich means of gaining insight into another culture.

Dance venues always offer concessionary rates and frequently discount ticket prices further still for group bookings of, e.g. ten people, so gathering together a party to attend can be a good way to save on costs, as well as creating an immediate discussion forum for reflecting on the performance together afterwards. Venues are also increasingly keen to engage their audiences, gather feedback and support attendees to get the most out of performances, so look out for free pre- and postshow conversations. These events often provide audience members with a chance to discuss the show with a panel of the work's performers and creative team and can be an excellent way of finding a 'way-in' to new works, particularly for more challenging contemporary or abstract works. Certain dance forms can also be even better appreciated with a little preparation before arriving at the venue: if attending classical Indian dance consider looking online or in your local library for the meaning behind the form's intricate hand movements (mudras); brush up on the plot to *Giselle*; or explore other works by a particular choreographer on YouTube. Crucially though, appreciation of dance is entirely subjective. While there are many ways to enhance your understanding and appreciation, do not be put off by the idea that one must be an aficionado to enjoy certain kinds of dance performance. Remember too that the cross-arts element to dance performance (the use of music, costume, set and lighting) means that there are many elements to enjoy, consider and absorb, so it is always worth taking the odd risk with what you might decide to view.

Participatory Dance

Dance is for absolutely everyone. While certain outmoded views of dance may hold it as an art form primarily executed by the young, dance is a profoundly inclusive activity and the opportunities for older people to participate in dance in community programmes are growing exponentially. This growth is supported by a expanding body of scientific, sociological and psychological research pointing to the intense benefits of participating in dance, including marked improvements in lung capacity, memory, balance, fall-prevention, sense of social inclusion and many more. Furthermore, and perhaps most crucially, taking part in dance can build or reinstate confidence in one's own body. There is no need to feel you must be at a certain level of fitness or mobility to dance. As with many other art forms, much of dance is fundamentally about personal expression. While an older body may have new physiological limits, it also contains a wealth of knowledge, experience and movement skills that younger bodies cannot have developed, and which growing numbers of dance venues and companies are now keen to celebrate.

There are numerous kinds of participatory dance opportunities available specifically for older people, from creative dance (involving improvised and newly devised movement) to flamenco.

As well as regular dance exercise classes offered round the country for older people, there is a growing number of performing dance companies comprised entirely of older people, often performing at anywhere from international arts venues to local community events. Sessions run for older people tend to be highly sensitive to different levels of ability and will likely incorporate a range of activities that encompass this diversity, often, for instance, providing options for seated movement or modifications in case of additional pain in a particular body part. If you are in any doubt about a movement, mention your concerns to the class' facilitator who will be able to suggest modifications to suit your physicality.

Alongside group dancing, there is also wide scope to explore dance and movement within your own home. While watching television or listening to music, gently rotate your feet at the ankles and try small stretches and extensions from the knees. Rotations are excellent at helping to keep the body mobile, so when sitting in a chair find ways to rotate the spine to give your lower back (often an inactive and hence painful part of our bodies) a gentle twist. Rotating your hands at the wrist and lightly stretching and wiggling the fingers is also a great way to restore and maintain manual dexterity. Find a piece of music you enjoy and listen carefully for a short period, concentrating on the feelings or sensations it awakes. Explore using your body as a mirror for these dynamics in the music then try to capture the energy of the music in the movement of the hands and arms or in the whole body.

Above all, dancing in any shape or form can offer a fun and inspiring means to engage with others, rediscover one's body, and invigorate one's health and wellbeing.

Where to dance: The Foundation for Community Dance website (**www.communitydance. org.uk**) provides good listings of classes and companies working with older people across the country.

The age of creativity website (**www.ageofcreativity.co.uk**) is another great platform listing numerous opportunities for older people to engage creatively with the arts, including dance.

Your local Age UK branch (**www.ageuk.org.uk/about-us/local-partners/**) can also offer listings of regular classes in your area.

Equipment: It's worth remembering that dance rarely requires any specific clothing or equipment of any kind. So long as you have clothes you are comfortable and can move freely in, there is seldom any need for special clothing or footwear, and participatory dance groups rarely have any specific form of 'dress code'.

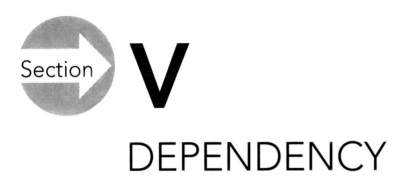

Section V

DEPENDENCY

Chapter **42**

Needing Help

The vast majority of us want to stay in our **own home** to the end of our days. Two-thirds of us think we are as happy in later life as we ever were, and a third think that these years are the happiest they have encountered. Factors promoting this contented state are being active, disease free, a satisfactory home environment and being surrounded by good social support: selfsufficiency and independence rule!

Regrettably, however, as your disability increases, the need for some **help** becomes unavoidable. There are a number of medical reasons for this change of status and, as medical students (perhaps like everyone else) love lists, the great and the good of Elderly Care have obliged us with all the 'Is' – they are worth a visit (even if only a brief one).

Immobility: difficulties of mobility are present in 18% of individuals over 65, while in those over 70, 20% cannot leave the house unaccompanied. Immobility heralds **Isolation**, and leads to muscle wasting, joint stiffness and the risk of venous thrombosis. Possible causes include all forms of arthritis, neurological problems (such as stroke and dementia), visual loss, breathlessness from cardiac and respiratory disease, debilitating conditions, such as cancer and malnutrition, and certain medications.

Instability: all of the conditions giving rise to immobility can make you unsteady on your feet, and to these can be added specific neurological problems affecting balance. Instability puts you at risk of **falling**; it prevents you going out alone, and may lead to **Inactivity** at home, with **Inability** in such tasks as getting safely to the toilet, particularly in the middle of the night, when it is dark and you are half asleep.

Incontinence: this may be of urine or faeces. This is linked with the immobility and instability of the last two paragraphs, but also problems of urgency and poor control of your urine. The bowel problem may follow tablets for various ailments, and constipation itself produces another 'I' for **Impaction**, where altered diet and reduced gut motility, interfere with normal evacuation. Sadly you may have to throw in **Impotence**.

Impaired cognition: the decline off your higher cortical function is considered with the nervous system, and although you are probably worried about dementia, the changes are usually subtle and unrelated. They may also be linked to the change in your circumstances – an awareness of the imminent loss of your **Independence** is a powerful factor in the onset of depression: other links to these changes are **Insomnia** and **Isolation**. If you can no longer spell exhaustion, you may have to throw in **Inanition**.

Insufficiency: expresses a gradual decline of all systems, albeit at different rates. These include cardiac, respiratory, renal and endocrine systems, as well as the neurological, reduced vision and hearing, and the musculoskeletal changes considered above.

Irreparable: your body is continually repairing tissues by replicating cells and repairing your DNA, these actions decline with age – one theory concerning ageing is that replication may be limited to about 50 such cycles.

Infection: your resistance to infection declines with age, as does your **Immunological** response to foreign proteins and organisms – both supporting various theories of ageing.

Iatrogenic: this is a term that may be new to you – it implies medically induced disease. In this case due to the large number of drugs that tend to be prescribed for the elderly, and the supplements you might have added on your own volition. This **polypharmacy** leads to confusion and the constipation already alluded to. Dossett pill delivery boxes help to keep a check on your medication, but you should go through this list regularly with your doctor, as some tablets do not work together.

While reading a list of this type may be of interest and provide some background information, what is probably more relevant is the following list of risk factors that can influence your independence, when you are fragile and elderly:

a. Over 80

b. Living alone

c. Lost spouse within the last 12 months

d. Changed residence within the last 12 months

e. Terminal illness

f. In hospital within the last 12 months

g. Needed medical care at home within one month

h. Cognitive difficulties

i. Depression

j. Insecure finances

Even with a sound temperament and a supportive family, sudden changes of this kind can have a profound impact on your resilience. These effects also depend on your existing agility and abilities. Assessment of these abilities can be judged by examining a typical day's activity:

Can you get out of bed in the morning unaided; has there been any incontinence of urine or faeces; do you need help undressing; are you safe going to the toilet on your own; do you wash, groom and dress unaided; are you safe going downstairs; do you need a walking aid or a wheelchair; do you cook for yourself; do you need help feeding and drinking; do you go out on your own to shop, and undertake activities and hobbies?

Your dependency can be graded:

Grades of dependency

1 Entirely self sufficient

2 BDAs OK, but complex travel difficulties

3 BDAs some difficulty, mobility impaired: walking aids or wheelchair

4 Permanent walking help needed

5 Two carers

6 Bedridden – continuous care, incontinent

[BDA – basic daily activity]

Help comes in many different packages, ranging from someone telephoning you to have a chat, to full-time nursing care. It may be from professional care workers, or more commonly (85%) from family, friends and volunteers. Subsequent chapters consider these options, while *Table 42.1* outlines the types of help that may be appropriate.

The arrangements for your care must try to avoid conflict and tensions between family members, or potential emotional disruption. If these relationships were previously good, problems are less likely, but understanding is needed if you develop illness and/or personality changes.

Safety and mobility

As your instability increases, you must be sure to **avoid falls**. Wear firm safe **footwear**, even around the house: remove loose rugs, loose leads, unsecured objects and projecting furniture, and avoid wet floors. Your living area must be free of obstacles and the approach to the bathroom and toilet must be **unhindered**, with all necessary mobility **aids** and structural supports in place. **Lighting** must be optimum in all areas.

Table 42.1 Systems of Support: they must be desirable, doable, reproducible, robust and sustainable

Personal Support	Communal Support
Getting up	Mutuality/company
Mobilising	Buddying/befriending
Dressing	Good neighbor
Bathing	Networking
Personal hygiene	Information sharing
Skin, hair, nails, feet	Newsletters
	Radio/Computer links
Warmth	Pendants/24hr Emergency number
Meals/nutrition	Advice on scams
Mental/physical health problems	Builders
Managing medicines	Banks
Fitness/exercise	Computing
Sitters and Companions	Advice reliable providers
Shopping	Computer help
Errands	Electrician/TV
Transport	Plumber
Cleaning	Builder
Sewing	Medical
Repairs, heavy tasks	Social
Electrical/electronic	Pendant schemes
Home improvement/adaptation	Physiotherapy
Shared accommodation	Chiropody
Respite Care	Complementary medicine
Computer/email/scams	Social Clubs/daytime/evening
Skype/Face Time/Facebook/Twitter	Tea/coffee
Newspapers, books, magazines	Lecture programs/courses
Sort diary	Gym
	Art/Photography
Vulnerability – safety/security Travel/holidays/	Music
insurance	Bridge/ Bingo
Advocacy – legal and moral rights	Visits
Bills/accounts/tariffs	Library
Pensions/benefits/tax/insurance	Theatre
Wealth management, investments	Museums/Historic sites
	Shopping sprees
End of life issues	Sporting events
Archiving	Pub crawls
Bereavement	Walks
Power of Attorney	Pets
Wills/living wills	Travel/holidays
Funerals	Volunteering

Mobility Aids

A **walking stick** is the first aid: this must be adjusted to your height, and it must be used inside as well as out of doors. A second stick can be of great help, but the next stage is a **three** or **four-**

legged support, adjusted to your height: both provide excellent stability. Some have wheels (and brakes!) that help mobility. Crutches are designed for fit young people with fractures and are not for supporting an older generation.

A walking frame (the **Zimmer**) is a light four-footed structure that has proven stable features, although replanting with each step means slow progress. With all these aids, a lot of effort is required to **stand up** to use them. Place them against your chair, and push up from the arms of the chair until you are upright. This is helped with a high, and sloping seat, and may require an addition push from a helper.

When using a **wheel chair**, make sure the breaks are on, the footrests up and you are standing with the backs of your legs against the seat: put your hands back and take a firm hold on each side before sitting. Slide back until your back is resting against the backrest, and lock any safety belt. If you are too weak to sit down on your own, it is wise to have two assistants control your descent.

Once you are sitting firmly and comfortably in the chair, your assistant should put down the **footrests** and place your feet firmly, pointing forward on them, strapped if these are present. Any blanket must be tucked in away from the wheels and not floating free: your elbows must never project outside the armrests.

You should be pushed **facing forward**, to see where you are going, if you encounter anything more than a gently hump, the assistant should turn round and pull the larger back wheels over it, before turning and proceeding. Do not let the assistant leave you looking at a blank wall, but turn you round so can see what is going on, ensuring the **brakes** are on.

When **getting out** of a wheel chair, ensure the brakes are on and your feet are clear of footrests and firmly on the ground, before gripping the arm rests and pushing yourself up. Again two assistants may be necessary to lift you up by each shoulder. A single assistant can pull you up or provide some forward pressure against your lower back, or with one arm under your shoulder to lift, while steadying the chair with the other hand: the carer must make sure their own back is straight when pushing at this awkward angle.

Bathrooms

A bathroom is a place where you value your privacy, but as your mobility decreases, your safety becomes equally important. A tiled wet floor becomes a skating rink; use **nonslip** mats or a carpet is preferred for safety, even if the latter is not so hygienic. **Toilets** can be difficult to get on and off, consider rails to help and a raised clip-on seat: if properly fitted these are very effective, and can be cleaned efficiently.

Getting in and out of a bath if you have impaired mobility can be hazardous. Bath seats within the bath are an initial aid, and later those placed across a bath, enable you to soak yourself all over. The latter, however, require some assistance, and a **shower** is an essential solution for most homes, possibly with a plastic chair within it and plenty of handrails. Walk-in showers at floor level are desirable, but all adaptation is costly.

The shower controls must be easily adjusted, if you have limited hand movements, extra attachments may be needed. **Handrails** are an essential safety feature, both in the shower and around the bathroom. Dry yourself near one of these, or sit on a stool or the toilet seat to steady yourself. If you are bedbound a **hoist** is an important addition to enable you to have the joy of a bath, also to get you in and out of chairs and wheelchairs. They must be well maintained and cleaned, and you must be safely strapped in during use.

Immobility

Professional skilled help is needed in the later stages of immobility, particularly if you are bedridden, whether at home or in care. At home, however, professional help may not be available 24/7, and home-helpers have to decide whether some of these skills can be learned. To take on such a responsibility requires dedication and determination, together with love, care and attention, if you are to maintain your dignity.

Difficulties are related to moving you safely, without risk of a fall, and maintaining adequate **skin care**, particularly if you are incontinent. Such a carer must be observed by a professional to ensure they are not putting themselves at risk: if there is doubt, alternative measures, including a change of accommodation, must be considered.

Carers

The decision to be a carer may not have been your choice, but possibly a family responsibility that has come your way. It requires a great deal of **time** and **commitment**: it can destroy your leisure time and your private life, as well as being physically demanding.

Effects on your health relate to physical and metal **fatigue** and presentation can be with minor symptoms from many systems, such as headaches, breathlessness and constipation. Mental **exhaustion** can lead to mood swings from anger to depression, and markedly influence your quality of care.

It is essential you report problems, and that the professionals monitoring your situation recognise these problems, and discuss them with all concerned. If there is consensus that the cared for individual should continue home care, and this is also your personal wish, arrangement must be made for additional help, and for you to have regular **rest periods**, either from help at home or a temporary **respite** admission to hospital for the cared one.

Some hints for carers:

- Respect privacy and dignity

- Be cheerful, positive and show affection

- Encourage communication and friendship

- Be careful with use of names and respectful language

- Listen carefully

- Speak loud enough to be heard, while retaining respect

- Determine what a subject likes and deliver it

- Encourage activity (reading, writing, TV, radio = information)

- Encourage helping and being useful

- Encourage independence

- Encourage getting out and exercising

Physical Care

If you are undertaking any **lifting**, take particular care of your back. Keep it straight and lift by bending and then straightening your knees, rather than leaning forwards. If you do a lot of lifting, it is wise to use a supportive body **belt**, and well fitting **shoes** with nonslip soles. In any lift, make sure your feet are apart and firmly on the ground.

When moving a subject from a **bed to a chair**, sit the subject on the side of the bed, lock any bed wheels, and bring the target chair, or wheel chair alongside the bed, locking all wheels. Stand in front of the subject, with your feet in front of theirs to prevent slipping. Place your arms under their armpits and place your hands over the back of their shoulders to apply a lift to the upright position. Once this has been achieved, rotate yourself and the subject in line with the chair, and let them down slowly.

Use the same lift to get a subject out of the chair and back to bed. When making a bed, again take care to keep your **back** as **straight** as possible, and carry heavy objects close to your body, neither leaning back or far forward.

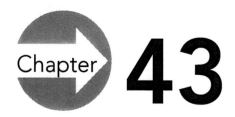

Chapter 43

The Importance of Frailty, Living Well and Population Ageing

Martin Vernon

What is frailty?

Frailty is a particularly problematic expression of human ageing. It is relatively easy to identify when advanced but more difficult to spot in the early stages. It is characterised by an accumulation of health issues over time, which gradually increase the risk of needing health and social care support.

Frailty is more common as you get older but **not all older people are frail, and not all frail people are old**. For people over 65, half of them will be classified as fit (i.e. not frail) while 3% will be severely frail. In England there are just under 2 million people aged over 60 living with frailty, and just under a million people aged over 80 living with frailty. Over 90% of these people will have problems with their mobility, over 60% need a walking aid and over 70% receive help from other people to live their lives.

Typically someone who is frail will notice that they are slowing up, less able to do what they could before and need more help to accomplish day to day tasks including looking after themself. Someone who is frail may be losing weight and his or her muscles may be wasting away. This can lead to slowed walking or loss of grip-strength. While this can be associated with individual serious illnesses such as cancer or diseases of the nervous system, it is commonly associated with having several long term conditions at the same time, such as diabetes, heart, lung or kidney disease.

Importantly, frailty is also a condition which makes it much more likely that when you suffer from a relatively minor stressor event such as an infection, you may deteriorate physically much more quickly than you might expect. In these circumstances your recovery might be more prolonged than expected or even incomplete. This means that you can be left needing more care and support than you planned for had you not been living with frailty.

Most importantly, living with frailty becomes part of many people's life stories. Because it progresses over time, for someone who has even mild frailty, compared to someone of the same age who is fit, it is twice as likely each year that they might require admission to hospital, admission to a care home, develop a disability or that this will contribute to their end of life. For people with severe frailty these risks are over four times those for people who are fit at the same age.

What causes frailty?

Frailty has been described in human beings across the world. A key feature of the condition is loss of skeletal muscle function (known as **sarcopoenia**). The strongest risk factor for that is rising age. It is also associated with poor social and economic circumstances, being female and having depression. Poor diet and shortage of vitamin D have been associated with frailty and it may also be linked to obesity, particularly when other features of an unhealthy lifestyle such as inactivity and smoking accompany this. The prescription of multiple medications may also be contributory to the development of the condition in some people.

Frailty is also associated with the presence of other long term health conditions including diseases of the heart and circulatory system, diabetes, chronic lung disease, stroke, dementia, disability and arthritis or other diseases causing inflammation. For these reasons there is a close association between frailty and the presence of multiple long term health conditions.

Multiple long term health conditions

A **long term health condition** can be diagnosed and treated, but cannot usually be cured and so will persist and tend to get worse in the long term. **Multimorbidity** refers to the simultaneous presence of 2 or more long term health conditions. These include physical and mental health conditions, ongoing conditions such as learning disability, symptom complexes such as chronic pain, sensory impairments such as sight or hearing loss, or alcohol and drug misuse. On this definition **frailty is itself also a long term condition**, which contributes to multimorbidity and vice versa. Multimorbidity is associated with advancing age, poverty, being female and having a mental health disorder. The most frequent patterns of multimorbidity include arthritis together with heart and circulatory disease and/or diabetes.

In 2016 the National Institute for Clinical Excellence (NICE) set out guidance for optimising care for adults with multimorbidity by reducing treatment burden associated with multiple medications and multiple health care appointments. Its aim is to improve quality of life by promoting shared decisions based on what is important to each person in terms of treatments, health priorities, lifestyle and goals. Beginning a conversation with a person to tailor the approach to their care can be triggered by:

- Request from the person themself

- Difficulty manageing treatment or day to day care

- Receiving care and support from multiple services and needing additional services

- Having both long term mental health and physical conditions

- Having frailty or falls

- Frequently seeking unplanned or emergency care

- Being prescribed multiple (10 to 14) regular medications.

Identifying people with multimorbidity can occur opportunistically during routine care or proactively using electronic health records. Best practice guidance supports the use of validated tools to identify adults with multimorbidity who are at risk of adverse events such as unplanned hospital admission or admission to care homes. This can help ensure they continue to receive optimal treatment while also providing an opportunity to plan for and make decisions about their future care and treatment.

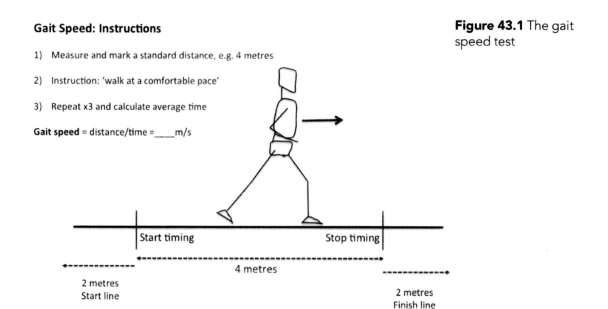

Gait Speed: Instructions

1) Measure and mark a standard distance, e.g. 4 metres

2) Instruction: 'walk at a comfortable pace'

3) Repeat x3 and calculate average time

Gait speed = distance/time = _____m/s

Start timing   Stop timing

4 metres

2 metres
Start line

2 metres
Finish line

Figure 43.1 The gait speed test

Greater than 5 seconds to cover 4 metres gait speed <0.8 m/s) suggests frailty

Timed Up and Go Test (TUGT): Instructions

1) Person should sit on a standard chair, back against chair, resting arms , walking aid nearby for use if needed, usual footwear
2) Say 'GO': Stand, walk to line 3 metres away, turn around, walk back to chair and sit down
3) Start timing on 'GO' and stop when sat down again
4) Test ends when firmly sat down

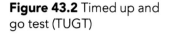

Figure 43.2 Timed up and go test (TUGT)

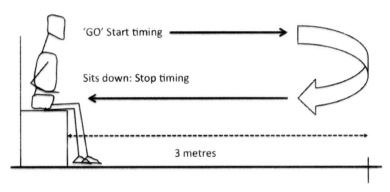

Greater than 10 seconds to complete TUGT suggests frailty

1. Are you more than 85 years?

2. Male?

3. In general do you have any health problems that require you to limit your activities?

4. Do you need someone to help you on a regular basis?

5. In general do you have any health problems that require you to stay at home?

6. In case of need can you count on someone close to you?

7. Do you regularly use a stick, walker or wheelchair to get about?

3 or more YES answers suggests frailty requiring further assessment

Figure 43.3 PRISMA 7 self-completed questionnaire

How can frailty be recognised?

The British Geriatrics Society (BGS) 'Fit for Frailty' guidance recommends that older people should be assessed for frailty at all healthcare encounters using a validated tool such as gait speed, the timed up and go test (TUGT) or the PRISMA 7 questionnaire [see *Figures 43.1, 2, 3*].

These three tests are highly sensitive but only moderately specific for identifying frailty, meaning that they may identify more patients with frailty than actually have it. By combining these tests it may be possible to reduce the number of false positive results. If two or more of these tests suggest frailty is present you should seek the advice of a health professional such as your GP who will be able to organise a more specialised, comprehensive and holistic assessment. This should include:

- Identification and optimisation of any long term health conditions
- Consideration of referral to a specialist which might include a:
    - Geriatrician (medical specialist for older people)
    - Therapist or other member of the community health team
    - Specialist nurse for older people
    - Member of the older people mental health team.
- Setting Individualised goals to stay well
- Medications review
- Assessment of risk of falling
- Care planning to document your preferences for care in anticipation of a health crisis and/or end of life.

Routine frailty identification in the NHS

In 2016 an electronic frailty index (eFI) which uses routinely available electronic health data from GP records was validated as a means of easily identifying populations of people aged 65 or over who have varying degrees of frailty. These groups of people are at varying degrees of risk of adverse health outcomes and knowing about this helps to direct key interventions more effectively to reduce the risks of frailty for individuals. This tool makes it possible to identify mildly frail people, comprising 35% of the population aged 65 or over who, compared to their fit counterparts, are twice as likely over the coming year to require unplanned hospital admission, care home admission or die. For severely frail people comprising 3% of the population aged 65 or over, the risk of these adverse outcomes compared to their fit counterparts is increased by over four times.

From 2017 GPs in England will **routinely** use this (or any other validated frailty identification tool) to diagnose moderate and severe frailty in all people aged 65 and over. For all those with **severe frailty** there will be a routine **review of medications** at least once per year and identification of the **risk of having future falls**. All of this information will be coded onto your electronic health record for future reference. If you give permission, this information can also be shared with other health and social care professionals via your summary record to help them plan and deliver your care.

Can frailty be treated?

Frailty varies in severity from one person to the next and for this reason, people should not be labeled as 'being frail'. Instead someone with frailty should be viewed as **living with the frailty condition**. It is also important to note that frailty is not an inevitable part of getting older and that it is not static condition but can vary in the way it affects an individual.

If we think about the possible causes of frailty there are a number of potentially modifiable factors to either prevent it or reduce the risk of a person's frailty condition progressing. These include, wherever possible:

- Improving levels of daily activity
- Improving nutrition
- Improving lifestyle such as stopping smoking or drug misuse and reducing alcohol intake
- Strength and balance training to reduce risk and fear of falling
- Optimisation of medications to ensure benefits remain in excess of burdensome effects
- Treatment of mental health disorders including depression.

The best way to do this is through proactive routine identification of frailty, followed by comprehensive professional assessment. This importantly enables proactive treatment and provision of support to older people with frailty through the provision of preventative and Individualised care to help avoid or reduce the impact of crisis events.

Why is frailty identification so important?

The key problem with frailty is that it can lead to serious outcomes such as hospital or care home admission or death after a comparatively minor stressor event. By finding the people in the population who are developing or already living with frailty, we can improve the way we organise and deliver their health and social care. And by finding those people who are still fit we can try to prevent frailty.

When thinking about **ageing well** we should set ourselves a triple aim:

1 Keep older people who are fit, healthy and active

2 Delay the onset of poor quality ageing

3 Meet the needs of those who are not ageing well through to the end of their life.

To do this we need to understand a few things about ourselves, and the people who live along side us:

1 Who has managed to remain fit despite their advancing years?

2 Who is at risk of not ageing well?

3 Who already needs greater support and help but is not having their needs recognised?

By understanding the frailty condition you can start to address these questions both for yourself, and for those close to you. This is particularly important now because of population ageing.

Population ageing and the importance of frailty

You may have heard of this, but what does it actually mean? Across the world, declines in fertility and improved life expectancy are thought to be the main reasons driving changes in the population age structure. Fewer children are entering the population and more adults are living longer, meaning older people represent an increasing proportion of the total population.

Between 1960 and 2015 the proportion of older people in the world population rose steadily so that now around 1 in 12 people are aged 65 and over. If we then consider that the world population itself is expanding, we can begin to understand how the number of people in the world aged 65 and over has risen from 249 million to 690 million. A key reason for this is that global disease burden has shifted from communicable (infectious) to noncommunicable diseases and from premature death, to a greater number of years lived, but sometimes with disability.

Of course successful ageing is something to celebrate. However one of the consequences is that greater numbers of people than ever before now survive to later life with multiple long term health conditions and increased levels of social care need. This poses significant challenges for governments, health and social care systems around the world. In consequence the present and future care of older people, especially those nearing the end of natural life in greater numbers, has begun to assume greater prominence in health care policy.

In 2010 the leading causes of **disability adjusted life years** (the number of years lost due to ill health, disability or early death) were heart disease, chest infection and stroke. Rising levels of mental health problems, bone and joint disease and diabetes are now expected to put health systems under even greater pressure. By 2050 the worldwide prevalence of Alzheimer's dementia is expected to quadruple from an estimated 26.6 million in 2006. This means that there will be an estimated 1 in 85 people living with dementia.

Current predictions suggest that across the world we should be preparing in particular to meet the needs of older people whose leading causes of disability will be depression, hearing loss, joint disease, dementia, falls, chronic lung disease and diabetes mellitus. In the coming years prevention and early identification of people living with frailty is going to become increasingly important in helping us to sustain our current health and social care system.

Frailty in an Ageing society

In the UK there are now just under 12 million people aged 65 or over. By 2040 nearly 1 in 7 people will be aged over 75. The proportion of the working age population aged between 50 and state pension age will increase from a quarter in 2012, to a third in 2050. Challenges facing the ageing UK workforce include supporting older people to lead fuller and longer working lives, through maintained fitness and lifelong learning.

Current estimates for female life expectancy at birth are around 83 years and 79 years for men. Healthy life expectancy in the UK is 66 years for women and 64 years for men. At age 65, women in the UK can expect to live on average for another 12 years in good health and men just under another 11 years. Put another way, men and women aged 65 can expect 60% of their remaining life expectancy to be in good health. This means however that for women aged 65, on average just under 10 of their last years of life, and for men 7.5 years will be spent living with a disability.

By 2037 there are projected to be 1.42 million more households headed by someone aged 85 or over. Poor housing has been estimated to cost the National Health Service £2.5 billion per year and so maintaining housing and communities suitable for an ageing population has become an increasing priority. Families play a major role in maintaining support across generations: over 70% of older people living with disability do so with support of a spouse or family member. The shape of families is diversifying with an increase in lone parent households in the last 10 years to 3 million and more generations alive simultaneously in the same family unit than ever before. There are currently 2 million people, the majority women, aged over 75 and living alone. There are estimated to be 14 million grandparents in the UK.

A key consequence of these complex issues and the expected rising numbers of people living with frailty mean that it will increasingly become the business of everyone in our society to recognise and actively address the condition for themselves and those around them.

Healthy ageing

Reassuringly current UK government policy is focused on addressing the needs of a society whose age structure is changing. This includes improving recruitment and retention of an ageing workforce by encourageing a positive attitude to working into later life and removal of the default retirement age, which means that in most cases employers cannot force people to retire just because they reach the arbitrary age of 65.

This will mean that people will be encouraged to stay healthier and fitter as they age to enable them to remain employed and contribute positively to the economy. This is important when considering the expected rising levels of need for care and support for increasing numbers of older people in the last few years of life. While some of this will need to be met by an ageing care workforce in paid employment, family members and those in their social networks will also meet some of it informally.

Talking about frailty

One final issue, which is important to bear in mind when talking about frailty, is the word itself. 'Sounding Board' work undertaken by NHS England and Age UK in 2017 found that older people were able to appreciate the positive benefits of routinely identifying a condition, which then helped everyone to anticipate and plan for the future. However there were concerns that the **'frailty label'** might be misapplied or be used pejoratively.

Many were reassured that routine frailty identification will be undertaken methodically and has the dual benefits of distinguishing those with greater needs who might benefit from proactive care, from those who remain and can be encouraged to stay fit. For many talking about the presence or absence of **'resilience'** landed better while for others being focused on **maintaining wellbeing** was at the root of **ageing well**.

However we also need to bear in mind a potential **'fear of frailty'**. For some there might be concern that diagnosing the condition will become a self fulfilling prophecy or lead to denial and disengagement. When talking about frailty it is important to remain focused on the benefits of understanding the condition. People will be reassured to know that frailty identification in its early stages provides many opportunities for **promotion of good quality ageing**.

Further reading

British Geriatrics Society Fit for Frailty: http://www.bgs.org.uk/campaigns/fff/fff_full.pdf

National Institute for Clinical Excellence (NICE Guideline 16) Dementia, disability and frailty in later life – midlife approaches to delay or prevent onset: https://www.nice.org.uk/guidance/ng16

National Institute for Clinical Excellence (NICE Guideline 56) Multimorbidity clinical assessment and management: https://www.nice.org.uk/guidance/ng56

NHS England Supporting routine frailty identification and frailty through the GP contract 2017/2018: https://www.england.nhs.uk/wp-content/uploads/2017/04/updated-supporting-guidance-frailty-identification-may-17.pdf

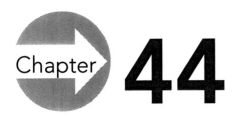

Chapter 44

Care Act 2014; Addressing the Mental and Physical Needs of the Individual

For the first time in nearly 70 years the Care Act 2014 created a single, modern law, providing the principles that should be expected for adult social care in England. It defined duties for local authorities and partners, and new rights for service users and carers. The act provides **clear, fair care** and **support** for those most in need, and defines high-quality **standards**, with tougher penalties for those who do not provide the expected care and support. The act emphasises that local authorities should promote health together with housing, welfare and employment, in a collaborative, cooperative and **integrated** fashion.

The act puts you, the **individual** receiving care, in control, considering that you know what is best for you. Greater emphasis is given to personal budgets, enabling you to spend allocated money on tailored care that suits your individual needs as part of a support plan. Everyone is entitled to a free assessment and, if necessary, you may appoint an independent **advocate** to promote your wishes, feelings and beliefs.

The main concern of the professionals should be for your **wellbeing**, i.e. your physical, mental and emotional needs. Professionals should protect you and other people from abuse and neglect: to facilitate this, each local authority has to establish a **Safeguarding Adults Board**, equivalent to that already in place to protect child welfare.

Another key factor in the act is **prevention** and **delay** of the need for care, encourageing and assisting people to lead healthy lives, which in turn, will reduce the chances of them needing more support in the future.

One of the biggest changes introduced by the act means that **carers** who look after an adult relative or friend with care needs will have the same right to assessment and support as the people they care for. National guidance has been issued in the form of eligibility thresholds for both individuals in need and their carers. Many of these are still evolving and some are not due come into effect until 2020. The subsequent sections provide more detail of some of these areas.

Addressing the Mental and Physical Needs of the Individual

Gwilym Tudor Jones

Assessing the Physical needs of Older People

Community care assessments

The community care assessment, carried out by the social services department of local authorities, assesses the needs of older people in order to establish what, if any, community care services they might need, and whether the local authority can meet this need. Community care services may be necessary to deal with a specific disability or health condition, or because of fragility due to old age.

As the NHS guidance explains, the nature of the assessment can vary according to the particular needs of the person. An assessment is required to provide certain basic information and to be able to draw up a **care plan**. However, if concerns are raised about the process of the assessment or the care plan itself, it can be challenged.[1]

The provision of services by local authorities

Under normal circumstances, the social services department of the local authority do not provide any services until a full assessment has been carried out. Where there is an urgent need, however, the assessment can be bypassed and the service provided immediately.

Once the needs of the older person have been established, the local authority has a duty to provide that service. Local authorities should not then refuse the service on the grounds of cost, but if there are different ways to meet a particular need, they are allowed to choose the most cost effective option.

Depending on the outcome of the community care assessment, a wide range of services is then available, ranging from aids and adaptations in the person's own home to care workers or residential care.[2]

---

1   http://www.nhs.uk/choiceintheNHS/Rightsandpledges/complaints/Pages/AboutNHScomplaints.aspx

2   http://www.nhs.uk/CarersDirect/guide/assessments/Pages/Communitycareassessments.aspx

Carer's assessment

A community care assessment is different from the assessment available to a carer, which is called a carer's assessment. Most carers are legally entitled to an assessment of their own needs, offering the opportunity to discuss the possibility of receiving help that would maintain your own health, and balance caring with other aspects of your life, such as work and family.[1]

Carers are entitled to an assessment if they look after someone on a 'regular' and 'substantial' basis. However, as the NHS guidance states, there is no clear legal definition as to what regular and substantial mean.[2]

The right to an assessment does not depend solely on the number of weekly hours spent looking after the person, but also the overall impact on the life of the carer and the type of care delivered. For example, looking after a person with severe mental health problems may give the carer additional rights to a carer's assessment.

Following the assessment, the needs identified in the assessment are expected to be met. While this may be directly by the local authority that carried out the assessment, legally it is entitled to ask another authority or the NHS to assist in planning services for the carer and person they are caring for. An example of such collaboration could be social services asking the NHS to provide aids and adaptations to assist the carer.[3]

Allowances

Carer's Allowance

At the time of writing, Carer's Allowance is £59.75 a week to help the carer look after someone with substantial caring needs. To be eligible, the carer must work at least 35 hours per week, and the person they are caring for must receive one of a number of benefits, including Attendance Allowance, Disability Living Allowance (DLA), or the Personal Independence Payment (PIP) daily living component. Carer's Allowance is not, however, available for carers in full-time education or earning over £100 a week.[4]

Carer's Credit

Carer's Credit is a National Insurance Credit available for carers, under State Pension age, providing care for at least 20 hours per week. To qualify, the person being cared for must, again,

---

1   http://www.nhs.uk/CarersDirect/guide/assessments/Pages/Carersassessments.aspx
2   http://www.nhs.uk/CarersDirect/guide/assessments/Pages/Carersassessments.aspx
3   http://www.nhs.uk/CarersDirect/guide/assessments/Pages/Carersassessments.aspx
4   https://www.gov.uk/carers-allowance/eligibility

receive one of a number of benefits including DLA, Attendance Allowance and the PIP. Carers who are ineligible for Carer's Allowance may qualify for Carer's Credit. Carers can still be eligible if they take breaks from caring of up to 12 weeks.[1]

Attendance Allowance

Attendance Allowance is intended to help older people to stay independent and continue to live in their own home. People over 65 who, whether through physical or mental illness or disability are unable to look after their own personal care, may be eligible for Attendance Allowance. People receiving DLA or PIP who turn 65 will continue to receive DLA or PIP rather than claim Attendance Allowance.[2]

Attendance Allowance is based on the help the person needs, rather than the help the person actually gets,[3] and it is entirely up to the recipient to decide how to spend the money – there is no obligation to spend it on paying for care.[4] It is paid at 2 different levels – £53.00 per week or £79.15 per week – depending on the level of care needed because of the disability. The lower level is available to those who fulfil either the day or the night conditions – in other words if, because of a disability or health condition, frequent help is required with basic bodily functions either throughout the day or night – while the higher payment is for those who need help both during the day and night. In order to receive Attendance Allowance, the claimant normally needs to have first satisfied the conditions for six months.

Specialist secondary care for older people

With the demographic shift in the UK towards an ageing population – one in which more than 10 million people are now aged over 65[5] – a significant proportion of people in hospital are aged over 65. The current Government has recognised that better community facilities and intermediate care have the potential to speed up hospital discharge and avoid emergency hospital admissions.[6] Nevertheless, multiple specialist services are provided within secondary care, tailored to the complex needs of the elderly population.

In addition to gerantologists and consultants who specialise in care of the elderly, many hospitals have established specialist multidisciplinary teams led by nurses, focusing on specific needs of the elderly whilst in hospital and on discharge.[7] This section looks at the levels of specialist care

---

1   https://www.gov.uk/carers-credit/eligibility
2   http://www.ageuk.org.uk/Documents/EN-GB/Factsheets/FS34_Attendance_Allowance_fcs.pdf?dtrk=true
3   http://www.ageuk.org.uk/Documents/EN-GB/Factsheets/FS34_Attendance_Allowance_fcs.pdf?dtrk=true
4   http://www.ageuk.org.uk/Documents/EN-GB/Factsheets/FS34_Attendance_Allowance_fcs.pdf?dtrk=true
5   http://ageing-population-conference.co.uk/
6   http://www.nhs.uk/nhsengland/NSF/pages/Olderpeople.aspx
7   http://www.patient.co.uk/doctor/Elderly-Patients-in-Hospital.htm

provided for three vital services for older people: stroke treatment, fall and fracture services, and palliative care (pages 44, 97 and 371).

Stroke treatment

Evidence suggests that stroke patients fare best when admitted to specialised stroke units. While the specialist care provided for stroke patients has been described as 'patchy', the National Institute for Health and Clinical Excellence (NICE) guidelines on stroke in 2008 has helped to standardise care across the UK. Figures from 2011 reveal that over half of all patients (55%) with suspected stroke were admitted directly to a specialist acute stroke unit and assessed for thrombolysis. This is in line with the NICE stroke quality standard.

Fall and fracture services

One in three people over the age of 65, and one in two of those over 80, suffer from a fall each year, the physical – as well as psychological – impact of which can be devastating. Falls and fractures among the over-65s take up four million hospital bed days each year in England, costing an estimated £2 billion.[1] Hospitals are therefore increasingly providing specialist treatment for patients who have had a fall, including multifactorial fall risk assessments.

However, while government policies over the last 20 years – and in particular since the 2008 report 'Fair Society Healthy Lives' (The Marmot Review) by Sir Michael Marmot[2] – have increasingly focused on prevention, studies have found significant gaps in a patients' care after falls and fractures, a lack of integration between falls and fractures services, and inadequate levels of secondary prevention for both falls and bone health.[3] A 2011 report by the Royal College of Physicians found that of 385 patients who fell in hospital, 28% were not reviewed by medical staff within 24 hours of their fall, and 22% of the 142 patients who may have experienced a head injury did not have neurological observations taken after their fall.[4]

In cases such as this, where gaps appear in patients' care, the Health and Social Care Act 2012 presents a unique opportunity for commissioners in the NHS, social care, public health and local government to collaborate in order to establish a more comprehensive care pathway. This means ensuring that falls and fracture services are integrated across community, primary care, social care and specialised health services.[5]

1   http://www.nhsconfed.org/Publications/Documents/Falls_prevention_briefing_final_for_website_30_April.pdf
2   http://www.instituteofhealthequity.org/projects/fair-society-healthy-lives-the-marmot-review
3   http://www.nhsconfed.org/Publications/Documents/Falls_prevention_briefing_final_for_website_30_April.pdf
4   http://www.rcplondon.ac.uk/sites/default/files/documents/inpatient-falls-final-report-0.pdf
5   http://www.nhsconfed.org/Publications/Documents/Falls_prevention_briefing_final_for_website_30_April.pdf

Palliative care

When there is no cure for an illness, palliative care attempts to maximise a person's comfort towards the end of their life. This is done by attempting to relieve pain and other distressing symptoms while providing psychological, social and spiritual support. Carers and family are also offered emotional and spiritual support.[1]

Palliative care (page 371) can be received in a hospice, at the home or residential home, as a day patient in a hospice, or in a hospital. Despite the array of services available to patient, carer and family, the Palliative Care Funding Review (commissioned by the Secretary of State for Health Andrew Lansley in 2011) identified gaps in the system. The review revealed that up to 457,000 people need good palliative care services every year but around 92,000 people are not having their palliative needs met. It also concluded that access to services, including round-the-clock nursing care, depends on where people live.[2]

Provisions for the treatment of mental health illnesses

In the UK, mental illness accounts for a third of all illnesses and, at any given time, one person in six experiences anxiety or depression.[3] Mental health services can be provided through GPs, other primary care services, or through more specialist care. There has, in the past, been a clear distinction between frontline, primary care for mental conditions, such as GPs and community mental health nurses (CMHN), and more specialised services, such as psychiatrists.[4] However, following the national services framework (NSF) report,[5] there has been a shift towards providing specialist services within community settings, such as day centres and within the home.

Mental health trusts

Mental health services are organised by specialist mental health trusts in many parts of the country. There are 59 mental health trusts in England, 41 of which have become foundation trusts (not-for-profit, public benefit corporations).[6]

The most common route to accessing mental health services provided by trusts is through a GP.[7] Mental health trusts provide inpatient care, community and rehabilitation services,

---

1   http://www.nhs.uk/CarersDirect/guide/bereavement/Pages/Accessingpalliativecare.aspx

2   https://www.gov.uk/government/uploads/system/uploads/attachment_data/file/215107/dh_133105.pdf

3   http://www.nhs.uk/NHSEngland/AboutNHSservices/mentalhealthservices/Pages/Overview.aspx

4   http://www.nhs.uk/NHSEngland/AboutNHSservices/mentalhealthservices/Pages/Availableservices.aspx

5   http://www.nhs.uk/nhsengland/nsf/pages/mentalhealth.aspx

6   http://www.nhs.uk/NHSEngland/thenhs/about/Pages/authoritiesandtrusts.aspx#mentalhealth

7   http://www.nhs.uk/NHSEngland/thenhs/about/Pages/authoritiesandtrusts.aspx#mentalhealth

psychotherapy (commonly Cognitive Behaviour Therapy), community drug and alcohol clinics, residential care centres, day clinics and drop-in centres.[1]

Community mental health teams

Trusts may operate community mental health teams, which aim to provide the necessary day-to-day support to enable a person to remain living in the community. They particularly focus on helping people with complex mental health conditions such as schizophrenia and bipolar disorder.[2]

Crisis resolution teams

Crisis Resolution Teams (CRTs) provide an alternative to inpatient care by offering intensive community support.[3] Their aim is to treat people with serious mental health conditions in the least restrictive environment possible, ideally near to home. Without the involvement of the CRT, they would require hospitalisation. Due to the nature of their work, CRTs offer a 24-hour service, and cases are often referred to them via A&E departments or the police.[4]

Loneliness and social isolation in the United Kingdom

In the UK, over half (51%) of all people aged 75 and over live alone.[5] According to the Campaign to End Loneliness, there are 800,000 people in England who are chronically lonely.[6] Moreover, 5 million older people say the television is their main form of company.[7]

Moreover, loneliness and social isolation are harmful to physical health. According to the Marmot Review, social networks and friendships not only have an impact on reducing the risk of mortality or developing certain diseases, but they also help individuals to recover when they do fall ill.[8]

Loneliness also adversely affects mental health. Research finds that lonely people have a 64% increased chance of developing clinical dementia.[9] Indeed, about one-third of all people with

1 http://www.nhs.uk/NHSEngland/AboutNHSservices/mentalhealthservices/Pages/Availableservices.aspx
2 http://www.nhs.uk/NHSEngland/AboutNHSservices/mentalhealthservices/Pages/Availableservices.aspx
3 http://www.mhsc.nhs.uk/services/help-in-a-crisis/crisis-resolution-home-treatment.aspx
4 http://www.nhs.uk/NHSEngland/AboutNHSservices/mentalhealthservices/Pages/Availableservices.aspx
5 https://www.gov.uk/government/uploads/system/uploads/attachment_data/file/141895/uk-advisory-forum-230512-tackling-loneliness-isolation.pdf
6 http://www.campaigntoendloneliness.org/wp-content/uploads/downloads/2013/10/FINAL-Jeremy-Hunt-Response-17.10.13.pdf
7 http://www.nhs.uk/Livewell/women60-plus/Pages/loneliness-in-older-people.aspx
8 http://www.instituteofhealthequity.org/projects/fair-society-healthy-lives-the-marmot-review
9 http://jnnp.bmj.com/content/early/2012/11/06/jnnp-2012-302755

dementia in the UK live alone.[1] Furthermore, loneliness puts individuals at greater risk of cognitive decline.[2]

Support for lonely older people

The transfer of responsibility – and funding – for public health to local government, together with the creation of health and wellbeing boards (HWBs), which provide strategic oversight of the entire health and social care system in local areas,[3] has enabled local authorities to take more coordinated action to tackle loneliness. Loneliness is rightly being treated by some councils as a public health concern: it is clearly correlated with socioeconomic deprivation, housing status, and societal factors, all areas which fall within their wider public health remit.[4] Moreover, where local authorities are prioritising the tackling of loneliness, it has been proven to reap benefits: one study showed that a cost saving of £300 per person per year resulted from 'befriending' someone at a cost of £80 per person.[5]

Despite such evidence, a study by 'The Campaign to End Loneliness' in November 2013 showed that only 51% of the strategies published by HWBs (71 of the 147) recognise that loneliness and/or isolation are issues that need addressing. Indeed, only 11 of the 76 published strategies commit to measurable actions/targets to address loneliness in older age.[6] In formulating their strategies, HWBs should therefore take greater account of the impact of loneliness on wider health and wellbeing.

A number of charities do, however, devote themselves to tackling loneliness among older people. Contact the Elderly is the only national charity dedicated solely to tackling loneliness and social isolation among older people. They organise monthly Sunday afternoon tea parties for small groups of older people aged over 75 who live alone. Members of the group are collected from their home by a volunteer driver and taken to a volunteer host's home for the afternoon.[7]

Age UK has developed befriending services, through which each older person is assigned a 'befriender', who provides friendly conversation and companionship on a regular basis over a long period of time. The idea is that the befriender serves as a vital link to the outside world and a gateway for other services and valuable support. The charity also runs a telephone befriending service, 'Call in Time', consisting of a prearranged daily or weekly phone call.[8]

1 http://www.alzheimers.org.uk/site/scripts/documents_info.php?documentID=550

2 http://www.campaigntoendloneliness.org/threat-to-health/

3 http://www.nhsconfed.org/Publications/Documents/guide_to_governance_for_health_and_wellbeing_boards210612.pdf

4 http://www.campaigntoendloneliness.org/wp-content/uploads/downloads/2012/03/A-guide-for-local-authorities-combating-loneliness.pdf

5 http://www.campaigntoendloneliness.org/wp-content/uploads/downloads/2012/03/A-guide-for-local-authorities-combating-loneliness.pdf

6 http://www.campaigntoendloneliness.org/blog/just-over-half-of-englands-health-and-wellbeing-boards-now-acknowledge-loneliness-and-isolation/

7 http://www.contact-the-elderly.org.uk/about-us-3/what-we-do/

8 http://www.ageuk.org.uk/health-wellbeing/relationships-and-family/befriending-services-combating-loneliness/

Poverty in older age

Poverty remains an issue for a significant minority of older people. 1 in 6 pensioners (1.8 million or 16% of pensioners in the UK) live in poverty, defined as 60% of median income after housing costs. While the number of people living on low income fell between 1997/98 and 2004/5, since then there has been little improvement.[1]

Support for older people living in poverty

The Government had pledged to keep the 'triple lock' pension system, which ensures that the state pension goes up by whichever is higher – inflation, wages or 2.5% – until 2020.[2]

Pension Credit is also available for about 4 million older people across the country. Pension Credit is an income related benefit consisting of 2 parts – Guarantee Credit and Savings Credit. Guarantee Credit tops up your weekly income if it is below £145.40 (for single people) or £222.05 (for couples). Savings Credit is extra money for people who have an income higher than the Basic State Pension or who have a small amount of savings.[3]

Safeguarding Adults Boards (SABs)

Adult safeguarding is the process of protecting adults with care and support needs from abuse or neglect.[4] While local authorities have long had responsibility for safeguarding, there have never been clear laws or regulations behind them. The Care Bill, which, at the time of writing, is at report stage in the House of Commons, requires local authorities to set up a **Safeguarding Adults Board** (SAB) in their area, giving them a clear basis in law for the first time.

The Bill requires the SAB to include the local authority, NHS and the police, who should meet regularly to discuss and act upon local safeguarding issues. SABs will work with local people to decide how best to protect adults in vulnerable situations. They will be statutorily required to carry out a formal **case review** if an adult at risk in their area experiences serious abuse or neglect or dies as a result of abuse or neglect.[5]

---

1   http://www.ageuk.org.uk/about-us/international/livelihoods/

2   http://www.bbc.co.uk/news/uk-25609485

3   https://www.gov.uk/pension-credit

4   https://www.gov.uk/government/uploads/system/uploads/attachment_data/file/198104/9520-2900986-TSO-Factsheet07-ACCESSIBLE.pdf

5   https://www.gov.uk/government/uploads/system/uploads/attachment_data/file/198104/9520-2900986-TSO-Factsheet07-ACCESSIBLE.pdf

Financing care

Under the Care Bill, which comes into force in April 2017, the means-test threshold for residential care will be raised to £123,000. This means that people entering a care home with less than £123,000 – including the value of their house – will not have to pay the full cost of their care. This represents a substantial increase from the current threshold of £23,250.

Furthermore, under the Bill the amount an individual has to pay for care over their lifetime will be capped at £75,000. This will mean that all individual care costs will effectively be 'metered', and once £75,000 is reached, the state will pay for all remaining costs. Under the current system, no cap exists, leaving many people facing potentially limitless care bills. The Government expects the cap to benefit women in particular, who are more likely than men to both need care and be a carer.[1]

The reforms follow the publication of the Dilnot report in July 2011, commissioned by the Government in 2010, which proposed capping individual care costs at £35,000.[2]

Funding home adaptations

Under the Regulatory Reform Order 2002, a local authority has general powers to improve living conditions in its area in the ways it consider the most appropriate. This may include assistance for the repair, improvement and adaptation of housing. Examples of adaptations and equipment provided by local authorities include grab rails, ramps, and kettle tippers. Such disability equipment and small adaptations costing less than £1000 are generally provided free of charge if, through assessment, the local authority deems the person eligible.[3]

Larger adaptations may be funded through a Disabled Facilities Grant (DFG), which aims to enable a disabled person to live as independently and comfortably as possible. Under the Housing Grants, Construction and Regeneration Act 1996, a person qualifies as disabled if their sight, hearing or speech is substantially impaired, if they have a mental disorder or impairment, or are physically disabled by injury.[4]

---

1   https://www.gov.uk/government/news/landmark-reform-to-help-elderly-with-care-costs

2   http://webarchive.nationalarchives.gov.uk/20130221130239/http://dilnotcommission.dh.gov.uk/

3   http://www.ageuk.org.uk/home-and-care/adapting-your-home/ways-to-make-tasks-easier-around-the-home/

4   http://www.ageuk.org.uk/Documents/EN-GB/Factsheets/FS13_Funding_repairs_improvements_and_adaptations_fcs.pdf?dtrk=true

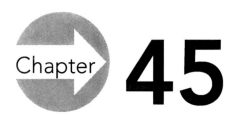

45

Community Care

Peter Tihany

Community Care is usually the provision of activities, or providing companionship or assistance to individual frail older people, enabling them to access services and activities in the local community, which they may not be able to do alone and without help.

The single largest social problem faced by older frail people is loneliness. Although practical daily living problems and attention to health issues are more acute, once some of these have been solved to the person's satisfaction, loneliness becomes a major issue, particularly if the individual is housebound. As a person becomes older and frailer, the friends and contacts they had in earlier healthier life tend to diminish. This is partly because of death among their contemporaries, partly because retirement causes a disruption in many individuals' social as well as working life, and partly because friendships and contacts tend to diminish when a person becomes increasingly frail and is no longer able to go out into the community.

A lot of older people live with others in the home, often one person being the **carer**, or **care workers** come in to assist with daily living tasks. However, the carer is often very busy preparing meals and running the home, and those who are not frail and housebound, possibly having partners, require the opportunity to partake in stimulating activities outside the home, and to have the companionship of their own friends. Where an individual is sharing their home, loneliness is possibly less acute, but it nevertheless can still be a major problem. Care workers coming into someone's home mean that at least a housebound individual sees a friendly face; but care workers (especially in the current economic climate) are allocated the minimum of time to carry out the physical help that the housebound individual requires, and are often on a tight schedule, sometimes as little as 15 minutes per visit. Therefore, even with care workers coming into the home, loneliness remains a significant problem.

Community Care activities can be provided in two ways:

By **organisations** that are often incorporated as charitable companies, sometimes local authorities and sometimes organisations that do not specialise in providing activities for older people, but provide activities to the wider community, such as education, swimming, concerts and theatre visits. A lot of these organisations provide their activities by using volunteers or sessional teachers and activity leaders.

The other way that community care is facilitated is by the use of **volunteers** to visit individuals in their own home, or take them out to participate in activities that occur in the wider community. Some volunteer visiting, transporting and taking individuals out for tea and/or meals, is facilitated by organisations who recruit the volunteers, provide training and do the necessary administration. The latter includes DBS checks (disclosure and barring service; previously criminal record bureau – CRB), which are required by all volunteers visiting vulnerable adults alone or spending significant time with them in their own homes. Individual volunteers not organised by organisations, are often neighbours, or friends with someone who knows the situation of the vulnerable adult, so DBS checks are not undertaken. However, administrative issues, such as insurance, DBS checks and other safeguards, such as health and safety, and other forms of training, are protection both for the vulnerable frail older person and for the volunteer. Therefore, unless there is a personal connection with the older person who is being assisted, it is advisable to do one's volunteering with and through an organisation. If a new volunteer visiting service is being set up, it is a wise precaution to form an organisation (which need not be a registered charity) to provide the necessary protection for both the frail older person and the volunteer.

The most important service provided by volunteers to frail older people is companionship. This can be provided by home visits. A home visit undertaken on a regular basis is a friendship. The volunteer can talk, or undertake other home leisure activities that combat loneliness, such as playing parlour games or cards. A home visit should not be geared to undertaking too many tasks, although making tea and providing treats, in the form of cakes and scones should not be too onerous, and might well be a welcome break for the housebound older person. Visiting a neighbour or a local person who one knows is frail and housebound should not require too much organisation; although if the person is not known before home visiting begins, steps must be taken to check whether the individual wants a visit, and prearrange an introduction by someone known to both parties. Although a housebound older person may be lonely, you as a volunteer are going into their home and you must be an invited and welcome guest.

There are many groups and organisations that organise schemes providing volunteers to visit older people at home. The advantage of doing the voluntary visiting through an organisation is that they not only carry out administration and training (if needed) for you as a volunteer, they have also interviewed the housebound older person. They therefore have the agreement of the older person to have a voluntary visitor, know what they want during a regular (perhaps weekly) visit, and, knowing something about the older person and the volunteer, are able to do a matching of personality and interests.

Many organisations provide other solutions to loneliness and lack of activity, such as nutritious meals, and day care centres. Local authorities and established charities run the most formal.

However, they often recruit volunteers themselves to help run their service. Less formal are friendship clubs that provide an afternoon's entertainment and a good tea, and tea clubs, which do the same. These informal clubs are run entirely with the help of volunteers. If you work with just one individual, they often need to be introduced to a friendship service in community premises by someone they know, and need driving to these facilities and returning home. A volunteer so minded can also stay for the duration of the club session and act as a volunteer both to their individual "friend" and also to others attending.

Accompanying and assisting a frail older person to attend events, and do other activities in which they are interested is very important to enable them to participate in their wider community. This may entail taking and accompanying individuals shopping (not necessarily food shopping, which is often done by carers and care workers). Outings to theatres, concerts, education sessions and sporting events, which they had done in their younger healthier days, are often very welcome. However, make sure the older person wants to do the activity and can pay for it: this is important, as paying for entertainment is usually above and beyond the remit of a volunteer. Also check access for disabled frailer people, special parking if driving, and the suitability of transport if other methods are being used. Often taking an older frail person out requires some physical effort, perhaps pushing a wheelchair or giving assistance up stairs; the volunteer must ensure they know what is required and are physically able to provide such help without endangering or harming their own health.

If there is no family around, the volunteer might also consider assisting with administrative tasks, such as home insurance, providing information on what services may be available to make life easier and more pleasant for the person they volunteer with, and arranging holidays and other breaks.

There are many organisations that provide **holidays/respite** for older disabled or frail people and carers. Helping the older person access holidays and finding sources of funding, if they cannot afford it, is a valuable community service. If someone is very frail and needs special help, a break in a residential holiday home, with the specialist staff and facilities able to cope with their difficulties, may be the best option. These are often run by local authority adult social care services or big national charities, such as the disability charities that cater for the blind, the deaf and people with multiple sclerosis. Smaller local charities also offer facilities for holidays or short breaks for people with special needs. Many local authorities provide funds to enable people who cannot afford to go on holiday, and they may also provide funds for carers to have a holiday. There are many organisations that cater for disabled older people or carers that organise group holidays and short breaks, and helping older lonely people to access these is a very worthwhile activity.

The chapter on caring discusses the provision of necessary daily tasks, cooking or provision of meals – the provision of one home cooked meal a week or other cooked treats is often something a volunteer would like to do. There may be other light tasks within the person's home that a volunteer has the appropriate skills, and is willing to undertake, such as light sewing;

but the tasks that the volunteer can and cannot do, must be made clear at the beginning of the relationship. The volunteer must always be aware of safeguarding him/herself and must resist tasks requested if they feel unsafe, unable or unwilling to undertake.

Volunteers are a very valuable resource in providing community care for older frail disabled people, for finding out and providing information and for helping to access activities, both within the person's own home and out in the wider community. Volunteering for an organisation that provides community care services for individuals, and helping deliver the service, is a valuable resource. However, continuity and commitment are important in volunteering and so great care must be taken to negotiate the voluntary work and to undertake a volunteer role that is within your competence. It is also important to be able to resist pressure to do more than you feel safe and able to do.

Chapter **46**

Caring

Peter Tihanyi

The United Kingdom has a universal system of Health Care, free at the point of delivery, operates a Welfare State and has a universal benefits system.

Benefits System

There is a retirement pension from the Government which is payable to all men over the age of 65 and used to be payable to all women over 60 but this is now being revised and in the near future will be 65 for women as well. There is pension credit (if the older person's income is just the basic pension, either full from paying contributions during a lifetime of work or reduced because there are less than 35 annual contribution payments). There is housing benefit if the older person is on a limited income and rents a property and other universal benefits, such as a winter heating allowance. There are also two benefits which can be applied for if there is disability: the one applicable to people over the age of 65 is called **Attendance Allowance** and there is a daytime rate for those people who need help or supervision in their own home during the day, and an additional night time allowance if someone needs help or supervision during the night (even if this is a partner, who needs to be awake when the disabled older person uses the toilet at night). Currently the benefits system is undergoing change led by the Department of Work and Pensions and there is an attempt to reduce the benefits bill. Unfortunately the benefits system is very complex, but there is comprehensive advice available from national charities, such as The Citizens Advice Bureau, Welfare Rights Centres, sometimes operated by local authorities sometimes by charities, and also on the Internet from the Government. It is quite easy to access the Department for Work and Pensions and make applications by telephone or email, but it may sometimes be prudent to seek an independent source for advice before applying.

Welfare State

Many of the provisions of the Welfare State and the laws, which confer rights on individuals, are operated by Local Authorities, which make provision through Adult Social Care Departments. After an assessment of needs, help can be given in money and the individual must use this to purchase the services they need, although there is some flexibility in the individual determining what their needs are. The downside of direct payments is that the system is complex to operate and needs to conform with employment law if employing an individual to provide care, and needs to be organised by the person receiving the direct payment, although there is some provision for using a relative, a social worker or a charity to help with the organisation of accessing help through direct payments.

There is also help provided in kind. Some local authorities operate domiciliary care services directly or have contracts with specific private caregivers and do the commissioning of services for the needy older person. Some local authorities also provide direct services, such as day care, or pay for the services provided by charities or private companies. There is a means test for the provision of all services provided by local authorities or commissioned by them and, depending on the income and income from savings of the individual, a weekly charge is made. It is worth commissioning services directly if the recipient of services is assessed to pay the full charge, it is cheaper that way.

There are also many charities (voluntary organisations) that exist to help the older person and his/her carer. Some charities are commissioned by local authority to provide a service for an individual and some charities provide services to the individual, always free at the point of delivery. Charities are often supported by local authorities and also raise funds privately from commercial organisations, charitable trusts or private individuals. There are many National Charities that provide some services nationally, but have local branches that provide a range of different services. These need to be checked out in the local area in which the prospective beneficiary lives. Age UK is the largest national charity for services for the elderly. There are specific disability charities such as the Royal National Institute for the Blind and the Royal Society for the Deaf. There are also national and local charities catering for the carers of older individuals: nationally the Carers Trust and Carers UK and locally affiliated to the Carers Trust and Carers Centres.

Local Authorities Social Care Services are financed largely by Central Government, and they finance charities from this income. However, income from Central Government is very seldom ring fenced and, as decisions are made locally: the type and range of social care provided and funded by local authorities varies tremendously. Local Authorities have some statutory obligations to provide services, but the quantity and criteria for access is seldom determined centrally. In addition the current Government is cutting all services, and Local Authority social care services and the funding they provide for charities is being severely reduced: this is threatening the provision of some services altogether. In 2016 there is now great concern that the money from Central Government goes to the Department of Health> The Department of Health finances the NHS and there is currently less and less money for the provision of services to the Elderly in the Community.

Caring Services

Within the United Kingdom there are a wide range of caring services available both at the individual's home and in appropriate premises within the local authority.

Emergency help is available by telephoning 999 and the options available once through are The Police, Ambulance/Paramedic Services and the Fire Service. There are also other telephone numbers, such as 101, which can be used to access the same services when the situation is urgent but not acutely so. The ambulance service also provides services (only in an emergency), which do not necessarily mean admission to hospital. The ambulance responds if an older person has fallen, cannot get up themselves and there is no one in the Home capable of helping the person up. If injury from the fall is suspected, a trip to hospital is recommended, but if there is no injury and the paramedics have checked this, helping the person up is the only service provided. The main role of the Police is to do with crime, but they have access to resources and provide assistance in a range of other ways. Dialling 999 is only for emergencies, but in other situations police can be contacted though a range of other telephone numbers. The Fire Brigade's major role is to fight fires but they also provide preventative services, such as installing smoke alarms for older people, and assisting when someone is trapped and cannot free him/herself and removing dangerous obstacles. Unfortunately, there is no National Police, Ambulance or Fire Authority,it is therefore difficult to be specific about what these services provide in an emergency,as it varies according to local regulatory authorities.

NHS services, other than through a doctor or hospital, are also provided in the Home, and include District Nurses, who provide visits at Home and are accessed through GPs, and Health Visitors: both professions provide preventative advice and nursing services in the Home. Certain voluntary organisation such as Macmillan Care and Admiral Service provide nurse visits in the person's own home if they have cancer/dementia.

Home visits from the NHS can be requested if someone is housebound, for services such as chiropody, aids for hearing, physiotherapy and occupational therapy. Services for the maintenance of good health can also be accessed at Home privately, and paid for if the person requiring the services has more than a basic income. The NHS provides nursing advice at Home for incontinence and provides equipment, such as commodes, incontinence pads, water bottles and other types of protection. Mobility aids, such as frames, wheelchairs (if the person cannot walk) can also be provided. It is the right of each older person when discharged from hospital, after a life changing illness or operation, to have a home assessment carried out by a professional from the hospital, and subsequent provision of the necessary gadgets to help them cope. Additionally they are entitled to six weeks of free domiciliary care with getting in and out of bed, washing, eating and other necessary tasks: this is provided by special teams. The object of this is to assess someone's need for help, and to teach them to start doing again as many of the daily living tasks that they used to do for themselves, thus giving them the maximum possible independence.

The Local Authority, sometimes together with domiciliary health services or voluntary organisations, provides a range of services in the person's own home. In order to access any of these services, one needs to request an assessment of needs. Everyone is entitled to request an assessment of their needs, either as an older or a disabled person, known as a **users' assessment**. Also a carer providing care for an older or disabled person, who cannot manage their daily lives without this help, is entitled to a **carers' assessment**.

The most common service provided to older persons in the home is through visiting **care workers.** This service is provided to enable frail older people or those with severe disability to get in and out of bed, have a wash, bath or shower, access the toilet or commode, get dressed and be prepared for the day. If they live alone they are also provided with breakfast, and settled for the day. If someone is totally alone, care workers visit to provide meals and reverse the procedure, to get into bed and help with undressing, in the evening. These services are sometimes provided by the Local Authority directly, or sometimes by private/voluntary sector companies, funded from payments to older people by local authorities or commissioned directly by adult social care departments. There are voluntary agencies who provide care workers to relieve family carers of some of the practical difficulties of caring, or to provide cover to enable the carer to go out, and attend to their own health and other needs. This type of service enables many older people to continue living in their own homes either within a marriage, with family or alone.

If the older person is very disabled or frail, then, provided they have less than £23,500 worth of assets and wish to do so, Local Authorities can place and pay for residential care. With greater than the above amount in assets, older people can access and pay for private homes.

Local Authorities or private companies can provide **emergency call buttons** accessed by pull cords within specialised flats, or pendants worn around the neck by frail individuals who can then access help if they fall or have other mishaps whilst alone in their own home.

Personnel: The above services are usually provided by the Local Authority or other formal organisations (private or voluntary): they arecarried out by paid care workers because of the skill and effort required for this sort of help. There are however some services that provide light meals, cover for the carer, when they want or need to absent themselves from home, and companionship; they recruit and provide volunteers to carry out these functions. Unfortunately, since 2008 there have been economic problems causing the Government to cut local authority income, and there is now considerably less money to provide the above services to the frail elderly. This has meant a tightening of the criteria of disability or frailty,for frail older people to be eligible for such services, or alternatively that a lower level of service is provided to frailer people in their own home.

Volunteers: With the exceptions already mentioned, paid professionals carry out most of the above services. Nevertheless, there is still a role for volunteers to make referrals, and help implement services for the older frail person living alone. Theoretically, services should be readily available and easily accessible, but although this varies between local authorities, it is a complex system and to get the right sort and the right amount of help can sometimes be very difficult.

Carers: Many frail older people do not live alone but live with spouses, partners or relatives. Not automatically, but in most cases of increasing frailty, one of the coresidents becomes a carer. A carer is defined as a person who assists an older frail disabled person with the tasks of daily living, when the person cannot cope without that assistance. It is reckoned that the majority of caring, in a situation where there is a carer, is carried out by that person. Sometimes skilled or heavy tasks can be carried out by paid care workers, but the majority of caring is done by the carer, and they are often on duty 24/7. In 1995 the first act was passed, giving carers the right to an assessment, and this has been amended by later acts to give carers **rights to an assessment**. This gives them the choice to care, and within the assessment their wish/need for employment, education, and recreation are taken into account. The various **Carers Acts** have also enabled local authorities to provide services to carers, and given them a duty to consider carers, in a situation where a community care assessment is required for an older, frail, disabled person.

Benefits can be claimed in the form of Carers Allowance for a carer under retirement age, where they are providing care for more than 35 hours a week and where the person they are caring for receives a qualifying disability benefit if under 65, and an Attendance Allowance if over 65. This is known as the **Carers Allowance**.

Although **discretionary**, local authorities can provide other services for carers after an assessment has been made, either in the form of necessary equipment to assist in the caring process (e.g. a washing machine) a holiday, training courses for a return to employment or direct payments to purchase items to assist the carer either in their caring responsibilities or to give them an opportunity to have some education and recreation. Many local authorities run **a carers' register** and provide services such as a **carers' card**, which provide carers with a range of goods and services at discounted prices. Although assessments are a right for carers to receive, the services provided are discretionary, and vary between local authorities. A point to note is that respite care services provided by a local authority are considered a service to the frail older person rather than a service to the carer.

There are also voluntary organisations (charities) that provide a range of services to the carer. These organisations are usually local, within a local authority area, although some organisations provide a national lobbying service and advice on telephone helplines for the carer.

Volunteers involved within a family where there is an older frail person and a carer, need to know and advise where they can access services to assist them with their caring role, and give them a greater measure of freedom and independence. It is often useful to offer to stay with a frail person when the carer goes out to shop or look after his or her own health, or even to have some recreation or education. Further help can be given in the provision of light meals and teas/coffees to the frail older person, always being careful not to offer help with tasks that are beyond the physical strength or skill of the volunteer.

Conclusion: As can be seen from the chapters on community care and caring, there is a range of provisions available from local authorities, voluntary organisations and private companies, with money given to pay for them. It would be nice to believe that this social care system makes the family carer and the volunteer redundant, but this is still a dream. There is not enough provision to meet all the needs for frail disabled people, nor the money to pay for all the services required. A 2014 report from Age UK estimated that there were 800,000 frail disabled people, living in their own homes who could not get in and out of bed, use the toilet, wash themselves or provide food for themselves, who were not receiving any help from the social care services, as there was insufficient money to provide these essential services. The carer and the volunteer are still very much in business.

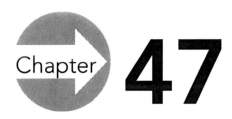

Chapter 47

Safeguarding Adults

John Binding & Ilona Sarulakis

The Care Act 2014 has replaced the previous government "guidance" in respect of adult safeguarding and has placed it on a statutory footing. The Act has introduced a new definition of an "adult at risk", increased the safeguarding domains and introduced the concept of Making Safeguarding Personal which promotes person led approaches and outcomes to safeguarding concerns.

Who Is An Adult At Risk

The Care Act 2014 (14.2) states that the safeguarding duties apply to an adult (18yrs or over) who:

- Has needs for care and support (whether or not the local authority is meeting any of those needs) and

- Is experiencing, or at risk of, abuse or neglect; and

- As a result of those care and support needs is unable to protect themselves from either the risk of, or the experience of abuse or neglect.

The Pan-London Safeguarding Adults Policy and Procedures, was revised in Dec' 2015 in order to comply with the Care Act 2014. It enables different agencies and individuals to promote the following principles:

Empowerment:
Adults are encouraged to make their own decisions and are provided with support and information.

Prevention:
Strategies are developed to prevent abuse and neglect that promotes resilience and self determination.

Proportionate:
A proportionate and least intrusive response is made, balanced with the level of risk.

Protection:
Adults are offered ways to protect themselves, and there is a coordinated response to adult safeguarding.

Partnerships:
Local solutions through services working together within their communities.

Accountability:
Accountability and transparency in delivering a safeguarding response.

The policy and procedures aim to make sure that:

- The needs, interests and human rights of adults at risk are always respected and upheld

- A proportionate, timely, professional and ethical response is made to any adult at risk that may be experiencing abuse

- All decisions and actions are taken in line with the Mental Capacity Act 2005 and other relevant legislation.

What are the types of abuse?

The Care Act 2014 has introduced an additional four safeguarding domains to create the following types (*2015/16 % Data for England*):

- Neglect and acts of omission – *34%*

- Physical – *26%*

- Financial and material – *16%*

- Emotional/psychological – *15%*

- Sexual

- Institutional (i.e. where the abuse is systemic, not just due to a few workers)

- Discriminatory (e.g. abuse which also involves racism or homophobia).

New domains:

- Domestic violence

- Modern Day Slavery

- Sexual Exploitation
- Self Neglect.

What should happen if you believe someone is being abused?

Do:

- Make sure that the adult at risk is safe
- Let the adult at risk know that you may have to tell other people what has happened
- If you are a Community staff member, tell your manager
- Make sure the police are contacted if a crime may have been committed
- Make sure the allegation is passed on to the Safeguarding Adults Team.

Don't:

- Confront the person you suspect of causing harm
- Promise the adult at risk that everything will be kept secret
- Start investigating yourself.

How are safeguarding concerns responded to?

The Safeguarding Adults Team should be informed of all concerns about possible abuse. The team will then find out whether the adult at risk is known to social services or health services and ask the appropriate department to commence enquiries. If the person is not known then Hackney's Information & Access Team (or a local equivalent) will take the lead.

Each enquiry is led by a trained Safeguarding Adults Manager or SAM. The SAM identifies all those who can help to protect the adult at risk or help with the enquiry. These may be family members, service providers, health professionals, the police, or the Local Authority Affairs team.

An initial risk assessment is completed to determine what response is needed. If further action is required then a strategy meeting will take place chaired by the SAM. This will confirm the protection plan for the adult at risk and identify who will carry out any further enquiries.

Further meetings will be arranged to confirm the outcome of the enquiries and to review the protection plan. The person and their carer /family will be supported to be as involved as much as possible, or an advocate will be offered to provide support where there is no family or friends.

Sometimes the person causing harm is also an adult at risk of abuse. In these cases the Safeguarding process will consider whether they need their own protection plan to help them avoid facing any accusations in future.

What are the outcomes?

The Care Act has introduced more person centred outcomes, moving away from the previous substantiated / partly substantiated / unsubstantiated and inconclusive outcomes. The outcomes are now linked to the risk that the person believes that they are now exposed to (*2015/16 % Data for England*):

- Action taken and risk reduced – *47%*
- No Action taken – *25%*
- Action taken and risk removed – *20%*
- Action taken and risk remains – *8%*.

There will be occasions where the risk will remain, although the person will be provided with support to manage the risk more confidently. In cases where a crime has been committed or the person causing the harm is employed to undertake care, the action may lead to the person being referred to the Disclosure & Barring Service which may result in that person no longer being able to work with other adults at risk.

The outcomes for these situations use the principle of "balance of probabilities" – in other words, is it possible to say that the abuse is more likely to have happened than not?

The desired outcome is for the adult at risk to feel safer and have a better quality of life, even if the allegations have not been substantiated. If the person cannot make their own decisions about their care then they may need to be protected in their best interests.

Types of protection include:

- Increased monitoring – e.g. more frequent reviews, more contacts with staff
- Enabling the adult at risk to stay away from people causing harm
- Better management of the finances of the adult at risk
- Application to the Court of Protection.

Whenever possible the person causing harm should be held to account. This can be done by the criminal and/or civil law, or by their employer.

Further reading

http://www.hackney.gov.uk/safeguarding-vulnerable-adults.htm#who

http://londonadass.org.uk/wp-content/uploads/2015/02/Pan-London-Updated-August-2016.pdf

Contact your Local Authority Safeguarding Adults Team

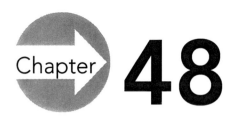

Chapter 48

Domestic Abuse

Safeguarding adults has always been a priority for the Police and Local Authorities, but the Care Act 2014 (implemented in April 2015) increased the awareness of the problem, introducing new statutory requirements, equating to those already in place for children's safeguarding. Of particular note in the new legislation was the requirement for each Local Authority to establish an Adult Safeguarding Committee with representatives from all Bodies involved in adult care.

The Act gave emphasis to Domestic Violence, where 30% of women and 16% of men had experienced some form of abuse during their lifetime. The violence is predominantly male on female; the offender is usually the current or ex-partner: abuse is no respecter of culture, age, sexuality or disability.

The Home Office definition of domestic violence and abuse is:

> 'Any incident or pattern of incidents of controlling, coercive or threatening behaviour, violence or abuse between those aged 16 or over who are or have been intimate partners or family members regardless of gender or sexuality. This can encompass, but is not limited to, the following types of abuse:
>
> psychological; physical; sexual; financial ; emotional.

Other behaviours such as Honour-based Violence and Forced Marriage also fall under the category of domestic abuse due to it happening within the family.

Psychological abuse encompasses a wide spectrum of emotional effects many merging with other forms of abuse: the 2014 Act greatly strengthened legal control in these areas. Perpetrators aim to dominate their victims, gaining power and control, with total dependency, subordination and subservience. Actions may be through threats and coercion, emotional dehumanisation and deprivation.

Threats are real, often based on the previous practice of the perpetrator. They may be threats of violence to the victim, children or family members, or of damage to property or treasured belongings. They can be of disclosure of previous crimes, such as illegal immigration, to friends, employers or the police. At the other extreme they may be the threat of leaving or of committing suicide, all of which amount to coercion and blackmail, aimed at forcing the victim to undertake some unwanted activity, such as sex, drug dealing and crime.

Means of **emotional** destruction of a victim include sarcasm, derogatory remarks and casting blame: belittling them, often in front of others. Such remarks may be directed at their dress, parenting, cooking, sexual or financial skills, and their intelligence.

Deprivation can start with laying down rules, limiting choices and demanding a detailed breakdown of all financial transactions. Limiting financial control may be of clothing, footwear and personal items, and outside activities. Deprivation may extend to medication, care and education, and in the extreme, involve physical restraint and confinement. Neglect leads to isolation and loneliness.

All forms of psychological abuse can lead to depression and potential suicide.

Physical abuse is the most obvious – although frequently covered up and denied by the victim, rather than risk an investigation that in their opinion could be more damageing than the injury. Chargeable grievous bodily harm extends from pushing, slapping, punching, biting and kicking, through strangulation and suffocation, to burns, knife wounds and murder, each carrying appropriate sentencing. [Self harm, including euthanasia, are chargeable in the UK.]

Financial abuse can be used as a psychological weapon, as considered above, such as denying work, withholding access to money and excluding from all financial decisions. More overt use of family funds includes stealing, gambling and running up debt.

Stalking is not usually a domestic problem, but the Care Act made specific reference to stalking and harassment. Abuse includes stalking through texts, telephones, telephone tracking and through social media, at home, during employment and places beyond. It is well established that stalking can escalate to threats and violence.

Sexual abuse presents as a wide spectrum of unwanted and illegal activities. Nonconsensual sex is classified as rape and any forced sexual participation is illegal. Abuse includes criticism and accusation of sexual activity, as well as denial of intimacy and forced pregnancy. Threats made to obtain sex may be to disclose criminal activity or an illegal immigration status.

The **Modern Slavery Act** was introduced in 2015; it includes sexual exploitation, such as forced prostitution and pornographic pursuits, and also labour exploitation, domestic servitude, trafficking to commit crime and organ harvesting.

Honour-based crime does not usually relate to the elderly, but they may become involved through their family connections. Even when these activities incorporate cultural traditions, individuals are subject to the laws of their country of residence, and may be undertaking criminal actions. The latter include female genital mutilation and forced marriage, itself involving deceptive overseas travel with intent.

Acts of exclusion, limitation and punishment are criminal acts, even if linked to cultural and religious traditions, or in response to straying beyond family expectations and values. More obvious criminal intent occurs in dowry theft, child kidnapping and bounty hunting.

Victims

As discussed above, some victims accept abuse to avoid threats of violence or disclosure, as they consider the alternatives would be worse than the state they are already in. Another group of victims that require identification and support are the vulnerable. These include those with mental health problems and the physically disabled – it is reported that the incidence of abuse in the latter is double that of the rest of the population. Other vulnerable groups are those with learning disabilities, drug addicts, alcoholics, and the frail, elderly and demented.

Many victims are in a state of denial that abuse exists, or blame themselves for the situation they are in. However, any abuse is a crime and needs to be identified so support can be offered and discussed with the victim, who can then make a choice on the way forward.

Perpetrators may be identifiable criminals, running prostitution and other forms of modern slavery, and are problems for the police to address. However, perpetrators are not confined to any particular class, ethnicity or other specific group, and their apparent 'normality' can mask detection or the attention given to a victim's plea for help.

In a domestic setting it is sometimes only after abuse has been identified that longstanding signs become apparent. These include a volatile personality, uncontrolled temper tantrums and problems with previous partner-relationships: a history of violence towards animals is another marker for abuse.

There may be a history of mental health problems, including anxiety and depression, it is important to note that escalation towards murderous intent is also linked to an increase of suicide of the perpetrator as well as the victim. Bad signs are the threat to kill and the use of weapons: drugs and alcohol aggravate the situation.

In some domestic violence with domination and intimidation, there are no mitigating features other than being in a position to exert power and control. These situations are no less devastating or less of a risk to the victim, and all those linked to the situation must bring the abuse to the notice of local authorities.

Reporting

It is the responsibility of everyone noting abuse or neglect to report it to the Local Authority: a dedicated confidential helpline is always available. The perpetrators are often known to social services due to repeat episodes, and these are likely to escalate.

If in doubt share information – it may be easier to discuss it with a charity, a family doctor or a religious leader. This information is passed onto skilled professionals and timely intervention can be initiated, ensuring the immediate safety of the victim and the introduction of long term care.

Management process – the first contact with the local authority is an informal discussion with the reporter, addressing concerns, advising and deciding whether formal documentation of the event is appropriate. The immediate concern is the safety of the victim, and if there is a risk of harm to the victim or children, the police may need to be involved. If the victim is not the reporter, steps must be taken to interview them individually in a nonthreatening environment.

The documentation of this interview uses a standardised, nationally applied questionnaire that helps determine the severity of the abuse and the level of support needed. Sharing of information with other departments requires consent from the victim, except where children are involved, and in these matters confidentiality is essential.

Each authority has its own system, usually incorporated into the safeguarding adults team (SAT). In the case of repeat offenders and escalation of the number or severity of the incidents, the report goes to a multiagency risk assessment conference (MRAC), a body of professionals, including the police, where the victim is represented by a fully informed moderator. Mental health problems are directed to a separate board. It is essential that communication and feedback from all these agencies is rapid and programmed into appropriate support.

Action must provide support at all levels, and this must be appropriate and proportional to the level of abuse. Once action is initiated, the perpetrator becomes aware and must be fully appraised of all responses. Immediate removal of the victim and all those at risk to a safe house is the extreme case, and most incidents are of a lesser level. Nevertheless they present some of the most complex problems in social care, frequently needing multiagency involvement.

The victim must be reassured that they are not to blame, and priority given to their safety. The cause of the abuse must be identified, and the perpetrator must be made to realise that they have it in their power to stop the abuse, and must not blame the victim, alcohol, drugs or an uncontrolled temper.

Separation is not necessarily the best solution: it may isolate the victim from a home, children, friends and financial support, and be detrimental to their mental and physical health. It must also be considered that three-quarters of domestic violence related murders follow separation.

The victim has probably already developed a survival policy to address violent episodes, and this is an appropriate place to start a response. The response must be tailored to the victim's needs and wishes, and within a legal framework. Such responses must be fully coordinated, may well be negotiable and conditional on all parties, and fully monitored and followed up by social services. The indisputable message to both victim and perpetrator is that domestic abuse is illegal, unacceptable and inexcusable, and does not have to be put up with.

49

Homelessness

This chapter highlights the diversity of the UK population from which the aged are drawn, particularly within Inner City Environments. Although this only represents a small percentage, and aged rough sleepers even fewer, they are some of the most disadvantaged, vulnerable and socially isolated of our population.

Accessing the homeless is a considerable challenge. They are often with cultural and language differences from the majority of a local community, and others have mental health problems. It emphasises how the aged have to be considered as individuals, requiring specific and unique support. Whereas initial approaches are through carers with knowledge and understanding of the background of individuals, the ultimate aim must be integration within a local community and society as a whole.

This area of activity could be both challenging and rewarding for those readers looking for voluntary work in their retirement – why not approach your Local Council and discuss the opportunities for befriending and building bridges into the minority groups that make up and contribute to our diverse and multicultural society.

Homelessness in The City of London

Davina Lilly

The City of London is a unique local authority. Just one square mile in size it is both the historic and geographic heart of the capital bordered by seven central London boroughs. It is the world's leading international financial centre with more than 6,000 businesses, and is also an important visitor destination and transport hub.

The number of people usually resident in the City is small at around 7,400, with an additional 1400 people who have a second home in the City but live elsewhere. Over the last decade population growth has been slow, but they are projected to accelerate to reach 9,190 by 2021.

The City has 4,390 households and large numbers of people of working age. Compared to Greater London there is a greater proportion of people aged between 25 and 69 and fewer young people. Only 10 per cent of households have children compared to around 30 per cent for London and the rest of the country. Average household size is small and many people (56 per cent) live alone.

The City's population is predominantly white (79 per cent) with the second largest ethnic group being Asian (13 per cent). This group, which includes Indian, Bangladeshi and Chinese populations, has grown over the past decade. The City has a relatively small Black population compared to the London wide population and England and Wales.

This resident population is dwarfed by the City's daytime working population, which at more than 383,000 is some fifty times larger than the resident one. This is projected to grow to 428,000 by 2026.

Its location, size, population and boundaries inform the nature of the City's homelessness challenge. Homelessness and housing needs arise among the City's resident population and its working population. Many who are already homeless, particularly those who sleep rough, come to the City's streets drawn by the busy transport hubs or quieter night time environment of the nonresidential areas.

The most harmful and most obvious manifestation of homelessness is rough sleeping. However, local authorities also assist households who are homeless (but not street homeless) or who are threatened with homelessness. Some may apply for assistance and in certain circumstances a local authority has a legal duty to secure accommodation for them. Others at risk of homelessness, or dealing with issues that can easily lead to homelessness, often seek housing advice from independent agencies as well as the City's services.

Rough sleeping

The rough sleeping population is often very transient, and therefore levels of rough sleeping in the City cannot be separated from trends and issues experienced in London as a whole.

In the last four years the number of rough sleepers seen in the capital has increased dramatically from 3,472 in 2008-2009 to 6,473 in 2012–2013. During this period both the number and proportion rough sleepers from Central and Eastern European nationals has increased dramatically, and they now account for more than a quarter of those seen on the streets.

Over the course of 2012/13 outreach teams recorded a total of 284 people sleeping rough in the City – the sixth highest total in the capital. Of these people, 112 (39 per cent) were new to the streets of London; another 112 (39 per cent) were longer term rough sleepers who had been seen both in the reported year and in the year before, while 60 (21 per cent) were those who had returned to the streets after a period away. Of those who were new to the streets, 50 per cent were seen just once. The vast majority of those met where male (94 per cent) and 85 per cent were aged between 25 and 55 years. In line with the regional trend, the City has experienced a growth in rough sleepers from European countries (other than the UK) with CEE nationals accounting for 28 per cent of those seen on the streets.

In the last 10 years there has been a predominance of long term rough sleepers on the City street whose rough sleeping pattern has been over 10 years and the maximum 45 years. This group tends to be white, older men. They have been helped with the introduction of personalised budgets and The City developing innovative options to accommodation like The Lodge. If you see a rough sleepers in the City, please contact the outreach team on 020 7426 9610 or report to Street Link 0300 500 0914.

Chapter 50

Choosing a Care Home

Pam Hibbs

Deciding to move into a Care Home or looking for one for another person is a big decision and needs careful planning for the transition to be successful. Unfortunately a crisis often makes careful planning and collecting information impossible, and you may find that things that are important to you are not available in these circumstances.

Planning ahead and talking to your relatives about your wishes, as well as finding out about the Care Homes available in your area, enable you to think about the Care Home you would be most happy to live in. **Advance Planning** means that your wishes are known and will be considered if the time comes when you are unable to make the move yourself.

Independent Age, a charity that offers Advice and Support for older people, has produced two very helpful documents to give you the tools that enable you to make a good choice. They are available from their website and called:

- How to find the right care home, and

- Their own Care Home Quality Indicators.

Your local **Health Watch** organisation may well have information from the Enter and View visits.

The Independent Regulator of Care Homes is called the **Care Quality Commission** (also known as the CQC): it is the independent regulator of care homes in England. The Commission regularly inspects them to check that they meet government standards: they do planned and unannounced inspections. You can check on their website for all local care homes to see how they have been rated. Ratings range from outstanding to inadequate, and you can see previous reports to see what progress they are making.

All the above information will give you some idea of the organisations near you and also give you the preparation required before you consider going on any visits.

After gathering information your next step is to contact the Social Services of your Local Council to arrange a **Care Needs Assessment** – if you happen to be in hospital the social worker will do this for you. During this needs assessment make sure that your wishes and your views are heard, if you disagree with the assessment ask for further advice.

Financial Assessments

Even if you feel you have the funds to pay for your care do not miss out on having a care needs assessment, as care is very expensive and you will need some guidance on the selection of the correct home. As care needs escalate, so the cost rises, and you may well qualify for some financial support from the Council. At present if you have capital and savings above £23,250 you will be expected to fund all your care. The new cap of £72,000 does not come into effect until April 2020, and then only includes nursing costs, not room or board. SAGA has worked out that you need £380,000 for ten years of care, and even good pensions do not cover this amount.

Paying for care is complex and very expensive and if the council is paying you may only have the right to choose a care home from the selection of homes they work with. You may be able to choose a more expensive home if you, a friend or a relative can pay the difference.

If you have complex and enduring health and care needs, you may be eligible for NHS continuing care. You will need a separate assessment to work out whether you qualify for this, but if you do qualify, the NHS will pay for all your care needs, including the care home fees: only a few homes provide this level of care so there will be less choice. If you are unable to qualify for continuing care you may still qualify for a nursing care payment of £156.25 per month, but these allowances are only awarded in a Registered Nursing Home.

Residential Care Homes offer twenty-four hour help with personal care, this includes washing, dressing and going to the toilet: although nursing care is not included, they will help with taking medication.

If you have a medical condition that is likely to deteriorate, and require twenty four hour nursing care, in order to avoid an additional move, you may be better in a Care Home that offers some nursing care places or a registered nursing home that has a registered nurse on duty day and night.

There are available Specialist Care Homes that offer support and care for people with Dementia.

Moving to be near relatives requires a search for available local homes. The Elderly Accommodation Counsel has a list, and so does the Local Council, and this will enable a check on the Care Quality Commission Web site to assess standards.

Every Care Home has a registered Manager, who will send a brochure and give details of fees, but this is not enough, and a visit will be required. Before a visit it is important to know what you expect to find, so go with a checklist and all the questions you would like them to answer. During the visit it may be possible to ask for a trial stay if the home looks possible.

Although moving into a care home is a major life style change, for some elderly people it improves their lives considerably, with good food, new friends, interesting activities and no more worries about maintaining a house – they see their health and wellbeing improve considerably and take on a new lease of life.

First impressions are important: does the home look bright, clean and welcoming, are the residents happy and well looked after, do they look clean and well dressed and engage with staff? Are they happy to talk to you about their life in the home and the activities they enjoy; also consider whether you would enjoy living with them?

The rooms may vary and not all will have their own toilet and washing facilities, but you may be able to bring your own furniture.

Health Care within the care home is important to establish. They may have a relationship with a local General Practice, so find out if it is easy to see a General Practitioner whenever you want to, and will you be looked after, as you would be if living at home. You have the same rights to see all other Health Professionals as the general public, these include: dentist, chiropodist, community nursing and physiotherapist.

Good Care Homes try and involve the residents in the smooth running of the home, so ask if you can see these minutes, also a look at the recent complaints gives a good idea of how the home runs.

Your friends and family should be able to visit freely, and homes that are not isolated from their community, bring in welcome new faces and activities.

If you like the home and the Manager, and the staff are welcoming and caring, ask if you can pop in unannounced one day or even come to stay for the night.

Pets are welcome in some homes where they can give a lot of pleasure to residents, but if this is not so, the Cinnamon Trust will always help with the welfare and care of the pets so loved by old people.

Further reading

Independent Age: a charity that provides advice information and support for older people; also provides a comprehensive document on how to choose a care home and standards required; and provides expert advice with any difficulties during the care needs assessment or the access of care.

Care Quality Commission: the Independent Regulator of Care Homes – their web site provides information relating to quality of care

Elderly Accommodation Counsel: provides an up-to-date list of all accommodation for older people

Cinnamon Trust: finds solutions to help older people care for their pets.

Chapter 51

Planning for Your End of Life

Usha Grieve, Jennifer Noel & OPG

Planning for the end of life is something that few of us want to do when we are healthy. Many people do not start to think about the end of life seriously until the first symptoms of an illness or the death of a loved one. Research tells us that the majority of us would not want our lives artificially prolonged if we were dying with little or no prospect of recovery. However, most of us are unaware of **what** our end-of-life rights are. In this section we aim to set out exactly what **your rights** are and how you can ensure that **your wishes for treatment** and care are recorded so that your family and friends know about them and, crucially, so that healthcare professionals can act on them should you lose the ability to communicate.

Did you know? 71% of us report feeling comfortable talking about dying and 60% of us would feel comfortable discussing end-of-life care wishes with your GP.

Your rights

Modern medical treatments such as mechanical ventilation, and artificial nutrition and hydration offer considerable benefits to vast numbers of seriously ill patients. However, many people are concerned that these treatments should not be used to prolong the dying process if their disease or condition cannot be reversed, or their quality of life improved.

You have the right to refuse these and any other types of treatment as long as you have capacity to make and communicate your decisions (i.e. you are of sound mind). You can also refuse any treatment in advance, in case you lose capacity and can no longer make or communicate your decision in the future, for example, if you developed severe dementia, had a stroke or were in a coma. These treatments can be withheld even if they may shorten your life. It is important to remember that regardless of what treatment you may refuse, the healthcare professionals looking after you are duty-bound to keep you comfortable and as pain free as possible. Your wishes can be recorded in advance by completing a legally-binding form called an **Advance Decision** (previously known as Living Wills) or by making a Lasting Power of Attorney for Health and Welfare (**LPA**). We will discuss these in the section 'What if you can't communicate your wishes?'

Did you know? The majority of the general public do not discuss their end-of-life wishes with friends and family, however the majority of the general public say they feel comfortable discussing dying.

Compassion in Dying

Compassion in Dying is a national charity working to inform and empower people to exercise their rights and choices around end-of-life care. We provide information and support to the general public, and health and care professionals, on the legal rights and choices that enable people to plan for their end of life. We have a free Information Line (0800 999 2434) which receives around 350 enquires per month from people requesting Advance Decisions and information on end-of-life issues. Compassion in Dying is funded by donations. We also campaign to get end-of-life rights more widely promoted within the healthcare system.

Did you know? Almost half of us wrongly believe that we have the right to make healthcare decisions on behalf of a dying loved one if they cannot make decisions for themselves.

The Mental Capacity Act and decision-making

Capacity is the ability to make a decision for yourself. It is time and decision-specific. This means that whether or not you have capacity depends on when the decision needs to be made and what the decision is. Having 'capacity' means being able to understand and retain information relating to the decision, understanding the consequences of the decision, and taking that information into account when making your decision. The Mental Capacity Act is designed to protect people who can't make decisions for themselves, and sets out who can and cannot make decisions on that person's behalf. The Mental Capacity Act only applies in England and Wales, although there is a similar Act in Scotland called The Adults with Incapacity Act.

If you have capacity and can communicate your thoughts then you can make decisions about what treatment you want from the options offered by the doctor. The doctor should explain your options in clear language and it is entirely up to you which treatment you choose. You can refuse treatments even if this results in a hastening of your death. The Mental Capacity Act also ensures that you can record your wishes to refuse treatment in advance in a legally binding way in the event that you lose capacity. In other words, you can set out what life-prolonging treatments you would not want in the event that you could no longer speak for yourself.

Did you know? Whilst 70% of us state that we would want comfort care only or limited intervention to prolong our life, only 4% of us have an Advance Decision or a Lasting Power of Attorney for Health and Welfare.

What if you can't communicate your wishes?

There are two ways you can refuse treatment in advance in accordance with the Mental Capacity Act:

i)   You can make a written Advance Decision

ii) You can make a Lasting Power of Attorney for Health and Welfare (LPA) to give someone else the power to make decisions for you.

The key difference between them is that an Advance Decision is a document that sets out your treatment preferences in the event that you lose capacity and an LPA is a document that allows you to appoint people to make these types of decisions for you when you lose capacity. You can of course do both but there are issues to consider if doing so. The section 'things to consider when deciding between an Advance Decision or Lasting Power of Attorney' covers this in more detail.

Advance Decision

Advance Decisions are a direct communication between you and the doctors treating you.. Advance Decisions are a good option if you have strong ideas about the kind of treatment you would want to refuse or accept in *specific* circumstances. An Advance Decision is valid as soon as it has been signed and witnessed correctly, and **it can only be used once you have lost capacity**.

You can contact Compassion in Dying if you would like a free Advance Decision. You can also contact us if you have any questions about making sure that your Advance Decision is completed in a legally binding way.

MyDecisions

www.MyDecisions.org.uk is the UK's first website that allows you to draft an Advance Decision or Advance Statement online for free.

MyDecisions was developed following consultation with over 300 people, which helped to make the process straightforward whilst at the same time encourageing people to consider what is important to them in relation to their future treatment and care.

The site guides you through different scenarios in which you might be unable to make your own decisions and prompts you to consider what you would want in these situations. These scenarios include dementia, brain injury and terminal illness. Comprehensive guidance is offered at each step. You can save your progress and return to it later, allowing you time to consider and talk to others about you wishes. At the end you get a personalised Advance Decision or Advance Statement to print, sign, witness and then share.

Recording your wishes in your Advance Decision

Think about what end-of-life preferences you want to record in your Advance Decision. It might be helpful to speak to your doctor when you are deciding what treatments you would or would not want. They will be able to tell you about the treatment that you are likely to be given in particular circumstances, what sort of quality of life you might expect if you consent to life-prolonging treatments. This could help you decide which treatments you would want to refuse or allow.

- Should your life be prolonged artificially what would be an acceptable quality of life following any recovery? Are there basic things that you feel you must be able to do in order to feel that life is worth living – for example recognising loved ones, eating and drinking or speaking?

- How long would you want to be kept alive artificially if there was little or no prospect of recovery?
  - would you want to be resuscitated if your heart stopped beating?
  - would you want to receive artificial feeding, for example through a tube?
  - would you want to be helped to breathe by a breathing machine?
  - would you want to receive antibiotics or other medication if you became ill?

- Do you have a serious illness or are you relatively healthy? If you were to be diagnosed with an illness or your preferences change **you can change your Advance Decision**.

Medical treatments you can refuse

1 Cardiopulmonary resuscitation (CPR) is used if the patient is not breathing properly or if their heart has stopped

2 Mechanical /artificial ventilation is used when the patient cannot breathe on their own

3 Artificial nutrition or hydration is used when a patient can no longer eat or drink by themselves. A tube is fed through the nose or stomach

4 Antibiotics might be used to clear up a localised infection (e.g. caused by an intravenous drip) or for something more serious like pneumonia. You can set out what is an acceptable level of antibiotic use.

Comfort care

Care professionals have a duty to give you adequate pain relief and to make sure you are comfortable. Even if you have refused life-sustaining treatment, medical staff will still do everything they can to keep you comfortable and free from pain.

Requesting treatment

You do not have the legal right to request a treatment – your doctor will always make the decision about whether a treatment is appropriate for you. However, it is a good idea to include information about the treatments you would want in your Advance Decision, or tell your appointed Attorney (if you have one) about them. This will be used to guide doctors when they are deciding how to treat you. You cannot use an Advance Decision or LPA to ask for medication to end your life.

Ensuring your Advance Decision wishes are known

It is important that your loved ones and the healthcare professionals treating you know about your Advance Decision. There are a few things you can do to make sure the people looking after you are aware that you have one:

- Ask your GP to keep a copy of your Advance Decision with your medical records. It is advisable that your GP signs your Advance Decision. This demonstrates that you have capacity at the time of writing it and that you have had a discussion about the content

- Give a copy of your Advance Decision to those who would be contacted in an emergency

- Keep a copy of your Advance Decision yourself and make sure other people know where it is

- If you are receiving specialist care, give a copy of your Advance Decision to everyone who is regularly involved in your care. For example, a consultant, health visitor or local hospital

- You could also speak to your GP about the possibility of recording your Advance Decision with your local ambulance service or about noting that you have an Advance Decision on your Summary Care Record (an electronic record of information about your medical needs).

Legally binding – witness and GP signature

As long as an Advance Decision is valid and applicable then any refusal of treatment within it is legally binding within England and Wales. This means that if a doctor was to knowingly ignore an Advance Decision they could face criminal prosecution or civil liability.

For your Advance Decision to be valid you must:

- be 18 or over, and have capacity to make your Advance Decision

- not have been forced by others to make your Decision

- say what treatment you give or refuse consent for (this can be in everyday nonmedical language)

- say the circumstances in which you want to refuse treatment

- if you want to refuse life-saving treatment, clearly state that your Advance Decision applies if your life is at risk or shortened as a result of refusing treatment (Compassion in Dying's Advance Decision form includes this wording)

- have signed and dated your Advance Decision in the presence of at least one witness, who must also have signed and dated the Advance Decision in your presence.

Your Advance Decision is applicable if:

- you lose capacity

- and it covers the circumstances you are in and the treatments available to you

- and there are no grounds to believe that changes in circumstances since you made your Advance Decision would have changed the decisions you made in it.

Updating your Advance Decision

You can review and update your Advance Decision at any point, for example if your health changes, or if you are going into hospital for serious treatment or surgery. You can also update your Advance Decision regularly, even if your health is stable. If you lose capacity and your Advance Decision was updated in the last two years, the doctor treating you can be confident that what you have said in your Advance Decision is still what you want.

Read through the document and think about if it still reflects your wishes. If you are happy with it and *don't* want to make any changes:

1 Sign and date your Advance Decision next to the phrase 'I have reviewed my Advance Decision and reaffirm that the wishes stated in this document are my own.' Compassion in Dying's Advance Decision form has space on the front page to do this

2 Give updated versions to everyone who has a copy of your original Advance Decision, and ask them to discard the old copies.

If you *do* make changes you need to sign and date them and make sure that you photocopy the page(s) that have been changed and give copies to your GP and anyone else who has a copy of the Advance Decision. **You do not need to get changes witnessed.**

Making a Lasting Power of Attorney for Health and Welfare

There are two types of Lasting Power of Attorney (LPA); Property and Financial Affairs LPA, which covers areas of your life where money and property are involved, and one which deals with your Health & Welfare, which relates to decisions about your health, personal care and welfare. This chapter firstly considers a Health and Welfare LPA; this is followed by information on the Property and Finance LPA.

A Lasting Power of Attorney (LPA) allows you to give someone you trust the legal power to make decisions on your behalf in case you later become unable to make decisions for yourself. In an LPA for Health and Welfare, your attorney can make decisions about anything to do with your health and personal welfare. This includes decisions about medical treatment, where you are cared for and the type of care you receive, as well as day-to-day things like your diet, how you dress and your daily routine.

You can list any instructions that your attorney must follow, or any preferences that you would like them to take into account when making decisions on your behalf. Your appointed attorney or attorneys only begin to act for you if you lack capacity, for example if you had severe dementia or were in a coma. Your attorney could not make decisions for you if you were able to do so yourself.

When making an LPA you must choose whether or not you want your attorney to be able to make decisions about life-sustaining treatment. If you don't want them to make decisions about life-sustaining treatment they can still make decisions about all other aspects of your health and welfare.

Who should I appoint as an attorney?

It is important to appoint someone you trust, who understands your wishes and will respect them. To help you decide who to appoint, ask yourself these questions:

- Do they understand my end-of-life treatment wishes?
- Will they respect my values?
- Could they stand up for what I want, even if the doctor disagrees?
- Do they live near me?
- Can they be contacted in an emergency?

How do I make an Lasting Power of Attorney for Health and Welfare?

There are 3 key steps to the process:

1 Choose your attorney(s) and all the other people you need to be involved in your LPA

2 Complete the form (available from the Office of the Public Guardian – https://www.gov.uk/power-of-attorney or 0300 456 0300)

3 Register your LPA with the Office of the Public Guardian.

Who is the Office of the Public Guardian?

The Office of the Public Guardian (OPG) is part of the Ministry of Justice. They manage the LPA registration process and maintain a register of all LPAs. They also deal with any complaints if, for example, someone feels that an attorney is acting wrongly.

Who is involved in appointing a Lasting Power of Attorney?

There are a number of people involved in making an LPA. They include:

a) Your attorney(s)

Your attorney(s) can be any person over the age of 18 who has mental capacity. It is important to appoint someone you trust, and who understands your wishes. You can also appoint a replacement attorney to take over if your original attorney cannot continue to act.

You can appoint more than one person if you wish. If you choose to do so, you can appoint your attorneys to act in one of three ways:

• **Jointly:** this means that your attorneys will have to make decisions together and agree on all decisions made. It also means that if one attorney dies or is untraceable, your LPA will become invalid and ineffective

• **Jointly and Severally:** this means your attorneys can make decisions together but they can also act alone. If one of your attorneys dies or is untraceable, the LPA will remain in place and can be used by your remaining Attorney

• **Jointly for some decisions, and jointly and severally for other decisions:** this means the donor can specify the decisions that should be made together and the decisions where the attorneys can act alone.

Your attorney will have a lot of responsibility for your health & welfare so there are a number of safeguards in place to ensure they use their power safely and make decisions in your best interests. As well as the possibility of appointing joint attorneys, the requirements listed below reduce the chance of any abuse or misuse.

b) Certificate provider

A valid LPA must be signed by an independent person who has known you well for at least two years, or who has the relevant professional skills to enable them to confirm that, in their opinion:

- you understand the purpose of the LPA and the scope of the authority conferred under it

- no fraudulent activity or undue pressure is being used to make you to create the LPA

- there is nothing else that should prevent the LPA being created.

c) Person(s) to be told

On your LPA, you can list up to 5 people (not the attorney or certificate provider) who know you well. Before registration of an LPA, these 'person(s) to be told' are notified of the LPA and given an opportunity to raise concerns or objections. This acts as a further safeguard against fraud or undue pressure. If you decide not to have any 'person(s) to be told', you must have two 'certificate providers'.

d) Witness

The witness is the person who witnesses your signature on the LPA form. They are not the same as the attorney(s). There are various restrictions as to who can act as a witness, in particular:

- you and your attorney must not witness each other's signature

- it is not advisable for your spouse or civil partner to witness your signature.

If you are unable to sign for yourself, you can make your mark or direct someone to sign for you in the presence of a witness.

The Form

You can either:

a) ask the Office of the Public Guardian to send the form to you

b) download it from their website

c) complete it online using their digital tool. The digital tool offers step-by-step guidance as you fill it in, relevant guidance at the point you need it and it automatically chooses and fills in the parts of the form you need using the information you provide. You still need to print out the form once completed for people to sign but the tool is designed to make the process quicker and easier. The form is in three parts and must be signed in the correct order. Please refer to Office of Public Guardian guidance for further information.

How much does it cost?

It costs £110 to register a Lasting Power of Attorney (please note that if you are also completing a Property and Financial Affairs LPA the fee is applicable to each form separately). You may be eligible for a reduction in the fees. For example some people on low incomes or certain benefits can apply for a reduction. More information on this can be obtained from the Office of the Public Guardian.

Advance Decision or Lasting Power of Attorney? Issues to consider when deciding which you'd prefer

1. Timescale: An Advance Decision comes into effect as soon as it has been signed and witnessed correctly, whereas the LPA can take up to 12 weeks to register and is only valid once it has been registered with the Office of the Public Guardian

2. Flexibility: An Advance Decision is in your own words and represents your decisions so you do not need to rely on another person to make choices for you. However, Advance Decisions are only applicable to the specific treatments and circumstances you choose to detail within it. It is therefore a good idea to try to complete it in as much detail as you can, while bearing in mind different medical situations that might arise and are important to you.

In an Advance Decision only the refusal of treatment is legally binding. An LPA, on the other hand, can apply to a wider range of healthcare situations. Your Attorney will be able to make any health & welfare decision on your behalf, this could mean deciding where you live and how you are cared for, your diet and what you wear, as well as making decisions about life-sustaining treatment if you give them that power. You therefore need to trust your attorney to understand your wishes, respect your values and make the best decision for you. Your attorney must also feel confident and comfortable making potentially life-changing decisions on your behalf

4. People involved: In order to complete your Advance Decision you only need one person to witness it (although we recommend having two witnesses, and also getting your GP to sign to say you have capacity).

To appoint a Lasting Power of Attorney you need one or more people to act as your attorney, as well as a witness, application certificate provider, and up to five persons to be notified of the application

3. Cost: An Advance Decision is a cheaper and less complicated option as there are no registration fees and you only need your witnesses and GP to sign it. An LPA currently costs £110 to register, although you may be eligible for reduced fees

5. Accessibility: Both an Advance Decision and an LPA are legally binding. In practical terms, however, you need healthcare professionals involved in your care to know that you have made an Advance Decision or an LPA. This happens in different ways.

An LPA is approved for registration by the Office of the Public Guardian and then entered on a register, which is searchable by healthcare professionals caring for you. It would also be advisable to let your GP know that you have an LPA.

Advance Decisions are not centrally registered but you can give a copy to your GP or local hospital; some Ambulance trusts are happy to record that you have one, or you can carry a Notice of Advance Decision card or wear a Medic Alert bracelet.

Should I have both an Advance Decision and a Health & Welfare LPA?

You can have both an Advance Decision and an LPA. If you do, the one that you made more recently will take priority when a decision needs to be made about your treatment and care. For example:

If you make an LPA after making an Advance Decision – your attorney will be able to override what is written in your Advance Decision as long as, when you made the LPA, you gave them the power to make the decision in question (for example, by choosing that they can make decisions about life-sustaining treatment).

If you make an Advance Decision after making an LPA – your attorney will not be able to override what is written in your Advance Decision. In this situation, if a decision needs to be made about something that you haven't detailed in your Advance Decision, then your attorney will still be able to act on your behalf.

If you have both an Advance Decision and an LPA you should make sure that you tell your attorney about your Advance Decision and give them a copy.

Making a Lasting Power of Attorney for Property and Finance

The Lasting Power of Attorney for Property and Finance (allowing an attorney to make decisions about paying bills, dealing with the bank, collecting benefits, selling your house, etc.) takes the same format as the Lasting Power of Attorney for Health and Welfare with all of the same safeguards.

The LPA for Health and Welfare can only be used at a time when the donor lacks capacity to make a decision, whereas the property and finance can be used at any time to support the donor with their permission.

The gov.uk website at www.gov.uk/power-of-attorney gives further information about applying for a lasting power of attorney and http://www.justice.gov.uk/about/opg provides further information about the Public Guardians' other roles including safeguarding vulnerable adults. You can also phone the Office of the Public Guardian on 0300 456 0300 for further information.

DNAR forms

DNAR stands for Do Not Attempt Resuscitation. The DNAR form is also called a DNAR order, or DNACPR order. A DNAR form is a document issued and signed by a doctor, which tells your medical team not to attempt cardiopulmonary resuscitation (CPR). The form is designed to be easily recognised and verifiable, allowing healthcare professionals to make decisions quickly about how to treat you. It is not a legally binding document. Instead, it acts as a tool to communicate to the healthcare professionals involved in your care that CPR should not be attempted. The reason that a DNAR form exists is because without one your healthcare team will always attempt CPR.

The form only covers CPR, so if you have a DNAR form you will still be given all other types of treatment for your condition as well as treatment to ensure you are comfortable and pain-free.

If a person is dying, has a terminal or chronic condition or perhaps is very old and frail they may have a DNAR order. If the person has capacity the doctor should discuss the option of resuscitation with them – e.g. exploring why they might want a DNAR order and what their chances of a good recovery after resuscitation would be. If the person does not have capacity and has made an LPA or written an Advance Decision – these should be used to inform whether a DNAR order is issued. If the person does not have their wishes recorded and does not have capacity, their relatives or friends must be consulted to help the care team make a DNAR decision, however the care team are under no legal obligation to consult with others. The decision making process should be recorded.

Conclusion

We hope this summary of your end-of-life rights is helpful. We have touched on the basic principles of recording your wishes within an Advance Decision or appointing an LPA and given some practical tips and questions to consider when you are thinking about your medical care if the time comes when you do not have capacity to make decisions. For further information you can call Compassion in Dying's Information Line on 0800 9999 2453 (free from landline) or visit our website at www.compassionindying.org.uk. The Office of Public Guardian can be contacted on 0300 456 0300.

Chapter 52

Probate

When you die all your assets (bank accounts, belongings, property) are frozen until an authorised person sorts out your **estate** (affairs/possessions). This person (**personal representative**) can be chosen by you in your will (an **Executor**) or, in the absence of a will, and/or an executor, an **Administrator**, is appointed by the Probate Office – a Government body that has to be informed of your death. The probate office validates any will and must issue the **grant of presentation** (a **probate** – also referred to as a grant of probate; letters of administration; or letters of administration with a will), required before your estate can be distributed.

The probate office documents up to four executors, but more can be appointed, perhaps dealing with different parts of an estate. An executor can refuse the position (renouncing probate), or be considered unsuitable by the courts, such as having a criminal record. The administrator is drawn from your family, in a legally prescribed order (see below); if none is available or willing to commit to the task, a nonfamily official is appointed.

If you want to have a say in the distribution of your possessions, you should write a **will**. You have to be of sound mind (know what you are doing), and have **two witnesses**, who are not receiving anything from your estate. These must **add their signatures to your own** and the **date** at the end of the will – the witnesses do not read or need to know the content of the will. Anything written below your signature is ignored. A new will replaces all old ones, but you can add and amend bits (**codicils**) provided they are signed, dated, and witnessed, and signed by two similarly uninvolved individuals.

If your requests are not very specific you should take legal help on the wording to ensure your wishes are followed – they may still be challenged, and your executor should be fully engaged in your (the testator's) wishes. In most cases, with some forethought, it is possible for your descendants to sort out your affairs without involving a solicitor.

In general a spouse or civil partner, and charities, can inherit an estate free of inheritance tax, and capital gains are not required on property that is not to be sold. **Inheritance tax** to HM

Revenue and Customs (HMRC) on property, monies, possessions, and gifts above a certain threshold is currently 40%: on gifts this reduces in increments to zero over seven years during your lifetime. However, inheritance laws are complex and subject to change by Parliament, legal advice may be needed in this area.

Executors

If you are an executor/administrator you can be a beneficiary from the estate, but other than incurred expenses, you cannot be remunerated for your duties, unless you are also an expert in the field, and being employed as such. A number of tasks are involved, taking many hours of work. These can be daunting when first encountered, particularly as you can be held personally responsible if you get some of the financial bits wrong. Fortunately a great deal of information is available from banks, government departments and legal sources. The fees of the latter can be substantial; they may include a percentage fee linked to the size of the estate, and if you are paying by the hour, these soon mount up. If you intend to use a solicitor or other legal help (such as a company specialising, and usually advertising, in this area) – obtain an all-inclusive estimate at the outset.

The following notes consider some of these tasks and the sources of information. Government web sites are numerous, but require a lot of searching to find specific answers. Talk to all departments when a telephone service is offered, as well as reading their documents. Banks and other agencies require proof of death. In general: obtain at least three copies of all documents – purchase these or make copies yourself if they do not require an official stamp – the probate office retains the original will.

Carry personal identification (e.g. passport, driving license) to present on all matters related to your executor duties. Take a witness with you when you are sifting through any belongings related to the estate. Make a working list of the things you have to do (you still have to provide all the details, even when you are paying for legal support!)

The following notes refer to the practice in England and Wales, elsewhere in the UK and further afield, obtain advice from local experts, these may be found through the Law Society or the Foreign Embassy concerned.

- **Will**: if not easily found, search all potential hiding places in all properties; if intestate (no will) you are more likely to face debate and possible conflicts of interests. The probate office will advise on searches for a will through official registers (the office also provides extensive advice on all the following areas, but cannot give legal help) [www.gov.uk/search-will-probate; www.gov.uk/wills-probate-inheritance/overview; probate helpline 0300 123 1072]
- **Death certificates**: obtain this from the local Register Office; take the medical certificate showing the cause of death; as many documents relating to the deceased as possible

(passport; birth/marriage certificates; proof of address; your own credentials); obtain the death certificate and pay for at least three extra copies from the Registrar

- The executor is in charge of the body and funeral arrangement, although the immediate family usually arranges the latter. Make sure funds are available (a bank is permitted to release these funds ahead of other legally permitted financial transactions). Ask help from doctors, hospital administration departments, funeral directors and religious ministers re a funeral service, burial and cremation

- If a death is unexpected, violent or in any way unnatural it is reported to the **Coroner** who is then in charge of the body. A postmortem and an inquest may follow and, when all legal issues are completed, the coroner issues the certificate of death and gives permission for the release of the body back to the executor and family, and their chosen funeral director

- **Inform everyone** of the death: this is potentially a long list. As well as the family, it may include: employers; services (banks, credit and debit cards, gas, electricity, water, television, telephones, hire purchases, landlords); mortgage companies; building societies, clubs, shares, bonds, savings; government offices (rates, council tax, pensions, GP, hospitals); return passport, medical appliances, national insurance card, disabled parking certificate, driving license to the DVLA; pension books; library books; and redirect mail – the *Tell us once* government line is a helpful link [www.gov.uk/tell-us-once; phone 0345 606 0265]

- **HMRC**: this department requires a detailed evaluation of the estate; property requires a current valuation (obtain a free estimate from a local estate agent, who would be interested in a sale, rather than an expensive in depth valuation); details of bank accounts; stocks, shares; savings bonds; cash; estimate the value of household goods, with a note of specific valuable items; creditors and debtors. For a full evaluation below £5,000.00 or when no inheritance tax is payable, use form IHT205, if above, use form HIT 400, but discuss this with the department: helpline 0300 123 1072 [www.gov.uk/inheritance-tax]

- **Grant of Probate**: notify the death as considered above. Pass over the original will, which is retained [remember to keep at least three copies]; show the original death certificate; the HMRC document (the estate will be issued a number by the HMRC); submit a completed request form for a grant of probate; helpline 0300 123 1072. Once the probate registry has validated any will, approved you as an acceptable executor/administrator and received the inheritance reference number from the HMRC, you will be asked to attend a probate office or the office of a commissioner of oaths to **swear on oath** that, to the best of your knowledge and belief, the information in the presented documents is correct and complete

- Following this you will receive the **Grant of Probate** that gives you the right to sort out all matters related to the estate – accessing bank accounts and other assets; paying debts and liabilities, and addressing the distribution of the estate as directed in the will, or a legally directed intestacy format

- An individual with an interest in the estate can **challenge** a will (e.g. not the last will and testament; a forgery; made under duress; the testator of unsound mind) or its management (e.g. executor of biased disposition). The applicant submits a written notice to the probate registry that issues a **caveat**, delaying the issue of a grant. The caveat remains in force for six months, or until it is withdrawn by the applicant or cancelled by a court order

- **Distributing the Estate**: if there is any doubt about the inheritance, place a statutory advertisement for creditors and claimants in the London Gazette and a local newspaper: do not commence payments for at least three months, and six if there are any unanswered issues. HMRC expects early payments, including inheritance tax and charges interest for any delays – discuss with them terms, such as incremental payments, to allow time for the sale of property or other valuables, without disadvantageing the estate. Laws of intestacy, concerning the payment to beneficiaries in the absence of a will, may require legal help in their application

In the absence of a will, other than a spouse or civil partner, only blood relatives are legally recognised beneficiaries: these include illegitimate children, and children legally adopted by the deceased, but not stepchildren. Inheritance for entitled individuals under 18 is held in trust for them until their eighteenth birthday

- **Final Accounts**: ensure that you retain all the documents and accounts you have accumulated in winding up the estate.

Check List

1 Register death at Register Office within five days – pay for extra copies of death certificate

2 Inform Probate Office of death (copy will as they keep original)

3 Inform 'everyone' of death

4 Arrange funeral (or appropriate service)

5 Value estate and submit this to HMRC

6 Apply for grant of Probate/ swear oath on honesty of submissions

7 Distribute residuary estate, after sorting creditors, debts and legacies.

Legal order of surviving descendants, for appointing an administrator or the distribution of an estate in the absence of a will:

1 Spouse/civil partner

2 Children or descendants

3 Parents

4 Brothers/sisters or descendants

5 Grandparents

6 Paternal/maternal uncles and aunts

7 The Crown.

[Interpretation of whole and half blood relatives, and claims by other potential beneficiaries requires legal help]

Glossary

Administrator – a person appointed to handle an estate in the absence of a valid executor

Assets – all the possessions of a diseased person

Beneficiary – an individual who benefits from a will or intestacy

Caveat – a document delaying a grant of probate when a will is challenged

Codicil – an amendment to a will

Coroner – an official who investigates unexpected deaths

Death Certificate – official document confirming death and its cause

Estate – the total possessions and liabilities of a deceased person

Executor – a person named in a will to carry out its wishes

Funeral director – a professional manager of all matters relating to a dead body

Grant of probate/grant of representation – authority to sort out an estate

HM Revenue & Customs – body dealing with all taxes related to an estate

Inheritance tax – tax paid from the estate of a deceased person linked to its assets

Intestate/intestacy – dying without a will

Legacy – gift written into a will

Letters of administration (+/- with will annexed) – see Grant of probate

Personal representative – an executor or administrator sorting out an estate

Postmortem – examining a dead body to identify the cause of death

Probate – see Grant of probate

Probate registry/office – body responsible for issuing a grant of probate

Register office – body responsible for issuing a death certificate

Registrar – official responsible for issuing a death certificate

Renouncing probate – refusing the position of executor or administrator

Residuary estate – what is left when all debts, taxes and legacies have been paid

Testator – the person producing and signing a will

Will – legal document stating a person's wishes for the distribution of their estate when they die

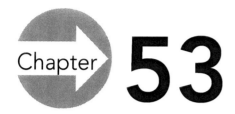

Chapter 53

Spirituality, Health and Wellbeing

Arthur Hawes

In this chapter I will look first at the origins of spirituality and then at the links between spirituality and faith communities, and what they offer. Finally I will outline the practical benefits of spirituality, which encourage health and wellbeing.

Spirituality is a buzzword today and it came to prominence in the 1990s. It is taught in Universities, provides rich material for research and is intrinsic to the work of many of the caring agencies. There is a charity called 'The British Association for the study of Spirituality' which publishes a journal twice a year with articles on research. One of these in the last edition was entitled *'I feel more spiritual. Increased spirituality after a near-death experience'.*

Spirituality has existed in human experience for 70,000 years – far longer than any world religion or faith community. Cave drawings indicate the importance of spirituality for early human beings and witness to the primordial urge to search out the meaning of what it is to be human, and to reflect upon human origins and destiny.

A working definition of spirituality is:

"Spirituality can be understood as that aspect of human existence which relates to structures of significance to give meaning to a person's life and helps them deal with the vicissitudes of existence. It is associated with the human quest for meaning, purpose, self transcending knowledge, meaningful relationships, love and a sense of the Holy" (Swinton J. and Pattison, 2001)

There are very many more definitions and one from a service user is *'One's beliefs about the world and one's place in it, how one lives out these beliefs through reflection and conscious action.'*

Another succinct definition is *'Something that arises within us. A personal quest for understanding and meaning around the big questions of life and death.'* I have also coined my own definition, which is similar to the previous one – *'The awakening in each person of the other side of themselves'.* We are likely to come back to this definition because it speaks of an inner life as well as an outer life.

As a straightforward guide, spirituality is generally considered to involve one or more of the following key aspects:

- Expresses the deepest part of our inner self

- Gives our lives meaning purpose and grounding

- Highly subjective and personal (but can be shared in a religious/faith community)

- The source and focus of a person's hopes, values and worth

- Anything or anyone from whom a person derives purpose, hope and self acceptance

- Connecting with ourselves, other people and a sense of the other.

Not everyone understands their place in the world in relation to 'the other' or a 'higher being' and so some may identify themselves as 'spiritual' but not 'religious'.

This moves us to our second consideration that is the link between spirituality and faith. (See 'Spirituality and Mental Health – A hand book for users, carers and staff wishing to bring a spiritual dimension to mental health services', chapter 8, edited by Peter Gilbert and Published by Pavilion – 2011). The faith communities, and there are nine recognised in the U.K. are:

- Baha'i

- Buddist

- Christian

- Hindu

- Jain

- Jewish

- Muslim

- Sikh

- Zoroastrian.

promote spirituality and the spiritual life. At the same time each is encompassed by spirituality which, as we have already seen, predates them. The Humanists wish to be added to this list as the tenth faith community, which makes the point that **spirituality** encompasses all faiths and none. It was Friedman who said of our postmodern world: '*We can choose our own supernatural*' and so this broadens what might count as 'spiritual' ….

- World Health

- The Environment – there are those, especially young people, who gain deep spiritual benefit from the environment.

- Famine
- Poverty and the meaning of being human (*3 billionaires own the same as 600 million of the world's poorest*)
- Art
- Music
- Poetry.

On the one hand there is traditional religion and on the other modern secularism where often there is no room for a higher being or God. What then can link the two? From what has already been said, spirituality is something that can speak to both, and perhaps faith is the spiritual glue to do this. It has been described as a bridge between faith communities and postmodern people and, writes Gary Hartz, '*In the midst of disillusionment and alienation, many find themselves thirsting for spiritual experience and religious community*'.

The value and place of spirituality in services for older people, assessments, community care, and palliative care, is extensively recorded. A further requirement is a summary of the contribution by the faith communities and the role of spirituality in diagnostics and recovery. There are eight main areas where faith communities contribute:

- Faith Communities
- Social Networks
- Pastoral Support
- Healing
- The Paranormal
- Ecclesiogenics
- Vocation
- The Sacred.

1. Each faith community welcomes the enquirer, the visitor, the foreigner, the immigrant, the alienated, and the marginalised and each person is afforded a dignity befitting their humanity

Local faith communities are part of a worldwide network, a universal family with outlets on every continent and in every country. A faith community is committed not only to welcoming people and respecting each person's individuality but also to accepting them holistically. To be human, comprises body, mind, spirit, personality, origins, ethnicity, social milieu and uniqueness. All of this and more contribute to being human. Being human involves not only living a life, but also undertaking a journey, searching the universe for meaning, recognising the possibility of the supernatural and aspiring to values which enhance and enrich human living.

In a faith community a person is offered privacy and, if appropriate, anonymity. Each person is named and sometimes chooses a new name. Naming is reinforced, because it is so often part of the belief system that every person is known by name to God/A higher being, and is cherished and precious. A theological framework offers an understanding of God, an appreciation of what it is to be human, insights into living a holy life in community, and a context for understanding need, sickness or any other adversity. For example, there is an understandable and growing concern for those who suffer from the organic mental illness dementia and the demands and pressures experienced by carers. This extract from a recent paper seeks to reassure not only the sufferer but also the carer from a theological perspective:

'Finally the context of the Christian faith is eternal. Here is real transformation as we are changed 'from glory to glory' – as it says in one Christian hymn. All that assailed us in our human experience is left behind. Here there is no place for mental illness, for dementia, for learning disabilities, and a whole range of other conditions. Here there is wholeness, mystery, glory, wrapped for eternity in the divine embrace of God's love.'

2.   Well resourced and integrated social networks are essential if community and home care are to prosper. Where and how do the housebound meet other people? What opportunity do they have to do what other people do naturally – chat, discuss and pass the time of day? People with mental health problems and learning disabilities are often confronted with a double measure of isolation because their very condition can have a separating effect. Many caught in this trap describe their house as a prison where they fear for their own safety, feel abandoned and lonely. Nor is this restricted to people living at home. There are those in Residential Care who talk of loneliness and isolation. The greatest care must be exercised to ensure that we do not develop a society in which everyone is an island. Faith communities are well placed to offer social networks across a rich variety of different socio/ethnic groups

Moreover all the faith communities have their own buildings. These are rapidly being adapted for increased community use. They can provide "drop-in" centres, café facilities, meeting rooms for a variety of group work and therapeutic/pastoral support (cf. St Marylebone Healing and Counseling Centre, near Baker Street Station)

3.   In addition to social networks, there is the ever present need of support especially in the early stages of recovery. A faith community not only provides the support of the local church/ chapel/mosque/synagogue/ temple/gudwara but also a commitment to holism. This is translated practically in the life of the faith community by the provision of interpreters, advocates and pastoral teams. A pastoral team has trained people available to visit in hospital, nursing homes and a person's own home

4.   As well as care and support, there is also spiritual healing. Germane to most faith communities is a ministry of healing which takes different forms, depending on the particular faith. Prayer and meditation are cross cutting themes in all the major faiths. Meditation is a spiritual exercise, which evokes in the believer an inner peace and tranquility. Research indicates

that 83% of patients view their spiritual beliefs as having a positive effect on their illness. To be remembered in the prayers of a community not only offers the sufferer the efficacy of prayer but also reinforces a feeling of safety and security. Faith communities help people belong. Safety and belonging are prerequisites in any recovery process most especially for a person with a mental health problem

5.   Faith Communities are often called upon to help with the paranormal. The presenting problem is usually disturbances especially in peoples' homes. Sometimes people themselves feel 'possessed' and seek help and guidance to overcome what they describe as 'evil'

6.   There are some conditions which are generated by faith communities themselves (ecclesiogenics) and they usually focus on existing problems. For example, instead of encourageing confidence and hope, a person is left feeling isolated and more guilty than they were previously

7.   A core element in faith communities is the concept of a "calling". People feel called to a particular role, profession or ministry. Some feel called to the religious life, some to working with people on the fringes of society and others to devote their lives and skills to care for people with profound and enduring disabilities

Today's postmodern world mitigates against the idea of vocation with its emphasis on regulations like the European Working Time Directive.

The question is how, in future, are people who want to serve their neighbour, to be committed to caring for others and seek to value the individual, to identify and express their vocation? These are people who want to be 'on-call', comfort the dying and befriend the lonely. For the person who genuinely wants to care for their neighbour, it is becoming increasingly difficult to offer the milk of human kindness. Welcome to the postvocational age where the calling is taken out of caring.

8.   There are places set aside as sacred and here the worshipper, the visitor, the enquirer can experience wonder, mystery, otherness, the numinous, transcendence, and for some the very presence of God. Here is a place to be uplifted; to be taken beyond the physical and immediate to the spiritual and eternal. Here is a place to reflect, meditate, dream, and pray. Here is the possibility, as I have already said, of *the awakening in each person of the other side of themselves*.

Benefits

We turn now to the final section of the chapter to look at the practical benefits of spirituality. Spirituality encourages a positive approach to human growth and development and seeks to provide resources for the sufferer.

Cognitive Behavioural Therapy focuses on our thinking. The principle underlying it is that changing our thinking will change our behaviour and the way we feel about ourselves. So think positively and you will have positive feelings. This naturally informs wellbeing or 'being well'. The opposite of wellbeing is bleakness, which feels cold and uninviting. Rather, a basic human need is to feel safe and secure in order to enjoy being well. This is true both of the environment around us and within ourselves – our outer and inner lives. We need only to think of the most awful explosion in Manchester to realise how positive expectations can so easily be destroyed. Hundreds of young people felt safe going to the concert. By the end safety and security had, in a flash, turned to insecurity and disaster.

We have on the statute book the Disability Discrimination Act, the Children Act, and designated places of safety all of which help us feel safe. We provide asylum for refugees, always have done and hopefully always will. The old asylums were envisaged as places of safety, though the meaning has changed over the years. Religious buildings traditionally have been places of safety where asylum has been available. They also offer a quiet place and space for reflection, meditation and somewhere to find inner peace, integration and wholeness rather than fragmentation, all of which contribute to our wellbeing.

Spirituality seeks to give meaning to human life and implies that human living and experience extend beyond the womb and the tomb. Many people coping with grief find this a great comfort. Because spirituality values individuals, it naturally emphasises the importance of human dignity and privacy. It is clear in this chapter that one of the main components of spirituality is meaning; privacy provides people with a chance to reflect on what it means to be a human being, especially in a rapidly changing world. This is, of course, offered through the professional therapies from Cognitive Behavioural Therapy to Psychoanalysis. However, faith communities, which provide community resources like drop-in centres, also have trained counselors and listeners. In addition, the wider faith community offers companionship. The word derives from two words, *cum panis*, which means to eat bread with. Central to the idea of companionship is sharing food, something which is happening less and less in modern society. In fact dining rooms are rapidly becoming a thing of the past!

The opposite of companionship and friendship is loneliness. This is a scourge of our age. One million older people speak to another person only once a month. One vicar reported that he asked a parishioner why she came to church regularly but never made her communion. She replied that he blessed those who came to the rail but did not receive communion and she preferred this. She said it was the only human contact she had from one week to the next. Such loneliness can be helped considerably by promoting community living, where neighbours look out for one another. Faith communities are a good example of this, especially as they welcome all comers. Community living has the advantage too of being a vehicle to encourage people to live together in peace, something we need more than ever before.

Safety, peace and community are three of the greatest needs of our age and spirituality has an important part to play in helping to meet those needs.

There are a range of challenges confronting people, as they grow older:

- Immediately, there is the change from going to work to retirement. Preretirement courses are very helpful but many who have recently retired take a long time to readjust to their new role. For some it is the first time in years that they have had to buy stationery! The pressure is greater, if retirement has happened because a person has been made redundant. It is very different from taking early retirement and the two must not be confused

- Faith communities can never have enough volunteers and many churches and other communities are staffed by bands of retired volunteers

- Pensions often mean fixed incomes and there can be worries about having enough money for oneself and, at the same time, wanting to help children and grandchildren financially. An added worry is the fear of becoming a financial burden on family and friends. Having somewhere to go and someone to talk to can be of great benefit

- It is part of the human condition that, as we age, long term and life limiting conditions develop which can be painful, restricting, and worrying to the point of leading to depression. More and more parishes are being encouraged to provide visitors for residential and nursing homes in the local vicinity. Visiting is an activity that is greatly appreciated by people who have restricted mobility and no visitors, but visiting is often forgotten and many are left feeling lonely and isolated

- The passing years can lead to restricted activity and a loss of independence. For many this provokes anxiety and they feel embarrassed talking about it for fear of being thought foolish. My own pet worry is when I will no longer to able to shave every morning with piping hot water. It would definitely be my luxury on **the** desert island. For me shaving is the best start to the day

- Finally in this list is the whole question of loss. I have referred to many areas of loss. The most difficult, of course, is the death of a loved one whether expected or unexpected. There is a well documented grief process that follows a death and, in order to readjust, it has to be completed. Wise advice is not to make any major decision within 12 months of the death and to expect to be grieving for a minimum of two years.

Each person's spirituality, I hope, will provide them with inner resources to cope with the daunting list of vicissitudes outlined above. Spirituality includes values and most of the following list are values. However, we begin with the core principle, which is acceptance. This is vital because it is the foundation underpinning the other values. It is about being realistic and accepting the changes taking place. There is a well known prayer which sums up acceptance:

God grant me the serenity to accept the things I cannot change, the courage to change the things I can, and the wisdom to know the difference

There is a need to develop an inner strength, which has probably been developing within each person over the years. It is a valuable resource because it gives hope and confidence to deal with what confronts us. Hope has to be realistic and, at the same time, move us forwards. It is not realistic to hope that a terminal illness will vanish, but it is realistic to hope that pain can be controlled. There are miracles and the spiritual value of faith opens the possibility of miracle. However, even though medical science has expanded extraordinarily rapidly, there are still swathes of untapped knowledge about the human condition and there is an understandable mystery about it. The last 'M' after miracle and mystery is magnificence. This describes the person who, against all odds, shows courage and fortitude in dealing with a host of problems, like the person who is partially sighted, has mental health problems and is diabetic.

It helps to embrace the value of grace and to live according to the maxim 'Do as you would be done by'. So, if you smile at people, most will return your smile.

Finally the spiritual values of meaning and purpose provide a framework that helps us cope now and also to plan for the future. As all these come into play, then an inner peace and tranquility will blossom and it is infectious.

Chapter

54

Palliative Care

Yvonne Pettingell

Palliative care, unlike most branches of medicine, does not have the cure of disorders as its principle aim. Instead it focusses on the **quality of life** of the individual where cure is no longer possible. The emphasis is on a whole person approach which is aimed at controlling a person's pain and other physical symptoms while meeting their emotional, social and spiritual needs.

We know that "Every minute somebody dies somewhere in the UK" (1) and a recent report looking at the future needs for hospice services, (2), has highlighted the escalating demand for palliative care that an ageing population creates. More people are now living into their ninth and tenth decades, often with complex health conditions. Providing high quality palliative care for these people as they approach the end of life is a huge challenge for the health service. Pressures on the system are already increasing as the number of people dying each year rises. As services become more stretched individuals need to increase their awareness and understanding of the dying process in order to access appropriate help.

Palliative Care

End of life care may last for a few days, or for months, or even years for some patients with incurable, chronic diseases. The General Medical Council considers patients are approaching the end of life when they are assessed as likely to die within the next 12 months. This group of patients would include those with:

- General frailty and coexisting conditions that mean they are likely to die within 12 months

- Existing conditions if they are at risk of dying from a sudden crisis in their condition

- Life threatening acute conditions caused by sudden catastrophic events such as accident or stroke

For many dying patients, either at home or in care homes, who are not burdened by unpleasant physical or psychological symptoms, care can and should be provided by the patient's GP and the local community services, i.e. district nurses, social service carer workers or care home staff. However, if a patient's symptoms are difficult to control for whatever reason, referral to a palliative care service may be sought.

Palliative care is based on the principles expounded by Dame Cicely Saunders, the founder of the modern hospice movement:

"You matter because you are you. You matter to the last moment of your life, and we will do all we can not only to help you die peacefully, but to live until you die."

It is a proactive approach to caring for the whole person with advanced, progressive disease, aiming to manage any **pain** and **physical symptoms** while also providing **emotional**, **social** and **spiritual support**. Palliative care therefore:

- Affirms life and regards dying as a normal process

- Provides relief from pain and other distressing symptoms

- Integrates the psychological and spiritual aspects of patient care

- Offers a support system to help patients live as actively as possible until death

- Offers a support system to help the family to cope during the patient's illness and in their own bereavement. (1)

Palliative care is provided by **multiprofessional teams**, usually made up of doctors and nurses, and often including social workers, chaplains, physiotherapists, occupational therapists and complementary therapists. The size of the team depends on local resources and needs, however, the range of skills available enable the team to provide holistic (i.e. **whole person**) care for the patient and their family.

Palliative care teams can be based at a local hospice, which may be an independent charity; within the NHS as part of the community primary care team; or in a hospital. In some areas several different teams provide services, depending on the location of the patient; in other areas all palliative care is managed by one provider. The different teams enable patients to receive palliative care in their own home or care home, in a hospice or in hospital.

Accessing Palliative Care

Referral to a specialist palliative care service is usually made by the healthcare team caring for the patient, either in the hospital or the community. Most palliative care services accept referrals from any healthcare professional involved with the patient, e.g. hospital doctors, clinical nurse specialists, GPs and district nurses. It is also possible for patients, or their families, to self refer, however where that happens the palliative care team will need the permission of the patient's GP and/or hospital team before they can accept the referral. The **GP** and/or **hospital team remain responsible for the care** of the patient and therefore the palliative care team need to work alongside them in supporting the patient.

Palliative Care at Home

For many people being able to stay at home for their end of life care is their preferred option, but they are often concerned about the burden this might place on their families. With appropriate help and support, for both the patient and their family, **dying at home** should be possible in most instances, but current figures on place of death, indicate that the majority of people die in hospital. For this trend to be reversed there needs to be access to adequate palliative care support for all dying patients.

In the community setting, the patient's GP is the key healthcare professional responsible for the patient's care. They can arrange for district nurses to provide nursing care and either the GP or district nurse can help families to access practical support and equipment from the local social care services. Some patients may need to pay for some of these social care services if they have a high level of income or savings, but this will be assessed by the local authority. To help with these costs most people in receipt of palliative care are entitled to either Personal Independence Payment (PIP), if under the age of 65, or Attendance Allowance, if over the age of 65. These benefits are not means tested. Those patients considered to be in the last six months of life can apply for PIP or AA under special rules. The patient's doctor completes a form ensuring the claim is given priority and enabling payment of the benefit at the highest rate.

The GP can also refer to the local community palliative care services for additional support for patients at home. For most patients a referral results in a home visit by a clinical nurse specialist in palliative care, (many, but not all, of these nurses are titled MacMillan Nurses if their post has been funded by the charity: **MacMillan Cancer Support**). These nurses are able to offer the patient and their family advice on how to manage the symptoms of their illness together with practical, psychological and emotional support. They also have access to the wider palliative care multiprofessional team if the patients' needs are more complex.

The number and frequency of visits to a patient by the clinical nurse specialist depends on the patient's level of need and complexity of symptoms, together with the resources the palliative care team has available. As patient numbers are increasing more community palliative care services are offering support to patients through outpatient clinics, resulting in fewer home visits. This pattern is likely to become more widespread as services struggle to provide support for a greater number of patients within limited resources.

As the patient's condition deteriorates they may require increasing levels of support and care. This is particularly pertinent if the patient is having **disturbed nights**, as the main carer is likely to become exhausted and very quickly unable to cope in these circumstances. Many localities are able to access, usually through the district nurses, additional support and night sits from Marie Curie nurses, or from local hospices where they provide Hospice at Home services. Receiving this support when the patient reaches the terminal stages of their illness can make the difference as to whether the patient is able to stay at home or needs to be admitted to the local hospice or hospital for the final stage of their illness.

Palliative Care in Care Homes

For patients who are already residents in a care home, palliative care can be accessed, by the GP or the nursing staff at the care home, in the same way as it is accessed in a patient's home. Some care homes are registered to provide palliative care and have their own trained staff able to care for most patients who are dying. They are also able to request more specialist help from the local palliative care services for patients with more complex needs or uncontrolled symptoms. Some palliative care services provide regular support for staff in care homes in their area, while others visit individual patients in care homes who are referred to them. With appropriate advice and planning for the final stages of their illness, most patients should be able to stay in their care home when they are dying, unless there is an unexpected acute deterioration resulting in the need for a transfer to hospital.

People requiring more complex care, that cannot easily be met in their own home, may need to move into a care home during their final illness. There are various options regarding the funding of a placement in a care home. It can be:

- Self funded – where the individual pays all the costs of the care home

- Local authority funded – where the local authority pays all, or part of, the costs of the care home. In this option the choice of care homes may be limited by the amount the local authority is prepared to pay, unless the patient, or their family, are prepared to make up the difference.

- NHS Continuing Health Care funded – where it can be identified that the patients' needs are health related, the NHS funds the care home fees, including the cost of accommodation, personal and other needs. An assessment is carried out to decide whether someone is eligible for this funding.

The healthcare professionals involved in supporting the patient at the time when a decision to move to a care home is being made, are usually the people best placed to advise the patient regarding their funding choices depending on their individual circumstances. For some independent, more general advice, organisations like Age UK (www.ageuk.org.uk) may also be able to help.

Hospice Care

Hospices are specialist units providing palliative care. They are not just buildings, but a way of caring for people and have been leading providers of palliative care for many years. Most hospices are **charitably funded**, though some are funded by the NHS. The hospice teams work closely with colleagues in other settings in the local community, care homes and hospitals, to identify people who may benefit from their care and provide it appropriately.

Hospices employ a multiprofessional team in order to offer a range of services, these may include:

- Pain and symptom control

- Psychological and social support

- Rehabilitation, where appropriate, to enable patients to stay independent for as long as possible

- Complementary therapies such as massage and aromatherapy

- Spiritual care

- Family care, looking at all the family members' needs

- Practical and financial advice

- Bereavement care

Hospices are now caring for people with a **range of different diseases** including cancer, heart failure and lung disease. There are hospices for adults, and for children and young people.

Many hospices provide a community palliative care team, as described previously, to support patients in their own homes. Hospices may also provide a Hospice at Home service, allowing people to receive hospice care in their own homes. Some of these teams are able to offer nursing care 24 hours a day to care for patients approaching the end of their life, or to give the patient's family/carers a break or to provide care during a difficult time, e.g. if symptoms are suddenly worse or a family member/carer is ill and unable to support the patient.

Day care at a hospice enables many patients to stay at home but visit the local hospice during the day at least once a week. The care and support offered may include:

- Medical and nursing care and review

- Rehabilitation to encourage independence for as long as possible

- Creative therapies such as art therapy and music therapy

- Complementary therapies

Attending day care at a hospice allows patients to meet other people in similar circumstances in an environment where they can share their experiences and support each other. It also provides the patients' carers with some regular respite and time away from the caring role.

Hospices also provide some inpatient care although the number of beds available is usually small. The main reasons for admission to a hospice are for:

- Symptom control, where symptoms are complex and/or difficult to control
- Respite to enable carers to have a break
- Terminal care, where the prognosis is felt to be very short

Most admissions to a hospice are for a short period of 10 to 14 days only. They do not provide long term care and patients are either discharged home to be supported by their GP and community services, or to another care setting such as a care home.

There is no charge for hospice care, but patients need to be referred by the healthcare professionals responsible for their care, i.e. their GP or hospital doctor, or their district nurse or clinical nurse specialist.

Hospital Palliative Care

A specialist palliative care service is available in most general hospitals working alongside the hospital doctors, nurses and other health and social care professionals. The service can be made up of a multiprofessional team of doctors and nurses, plus a social worker and chaplain, or it may be a nurse led service. Referral to the palliative care service is through the hospital team caring for the patient.

The role of hospital palliative care teams is to provide education, training and advice on pain and symptom management to the hospital medical and nursing staff. They also provide emotional support to patients referred to them and their families during their hospital stay. While they are not responsible for arranging a patient's discharge from hospital, they are often asked to advise on planning care for when a patient goes home, or transferring to another setting, e.g. a care home or hospice.

Advance Care Planning

Every individual has different ideas about what a "good death" may look like, and what they may prefer when they are dying themselves. For most people it is important to be treated as an **individual with dignity and respect; to be free from pain and other symptoms; to be able to**

stay in familiar surroundings; and to have the company of family and close friends. The End of Life Care Strategy (2008) (3) identified that "people approaching the end of life need to have their needs assessed, and their wishes and preferences discussed".

Advance Care Planning (ACP) is a process to make clear a person's wishes in anticipation of their condition deteriorating in the future. In normal circumstances all decisions regarding a person's care and treatment are discussed with them at the point decisions need to be made. An advance care plan is only used if a person loses their mental capacity and/or ability to tell people their wishes regarding treatment choices. ACP is a voluntary process between an individual and those who provide them with care, e.g. a doctor, a nurse, or a care home manager. Usually one of the healthcare professionals involved with the patient supports them in drawing up an advance care plan, and communicates any wishes and decisions that impact upon the patient's care, e.g. that the patient wishes to die at home, to all relevant members of the caring team.

By the time they reach the end of their lives people may have multiple conditions and complex needs. Not everyone wants, or is able, to participate in ACP, however they may have strong views about what they would, or would not, like to happen at this time and, unless there is a record of their views, they will be unable to influence decisions being made on their behalf.

Drawing up an advance care plan facilitates a **period of dialogue**, with discussions about the likely changes in a person's condition as their disease progresses. A record of a person's preferences and goals of care, both now and in the future, can then be made. This record can be adjusted and **amended at any time** if the patient's views change. The process of dying affects individuals in many different ways, and these cannot always be predicted. Their stated goals and preferences may change, so it is important to keep any advance care plan current and updated. These recorded choices and preferences will be referred to by those responsible for an individual's care, (whether healthcare professional or family carers), to assist with decision making should the individual lose their capacity to make decisions themselves as the illness progresses.

ACP can cover a whole range of decision making from the very simple to the quite complex. Each decision is important for individuals for different reasons, but some of the things people may want to consider are:

- Where they wish to be cared for, e.g. at home or in a care home

- Whether they would want to be resuscitated

- Where they would like to die, e.g. home, hospice, care home or hospital

- What is important about their care that they wish people to know, e.g. food likes and dislikes, what they like to wear, whether they prefer baths or showers.

- Whether there are any important religious or cultural activities that they would want observed

- Whether there are any treatments they want to refuse

- If they would like to donate their organs if it is possible

- Funeral plans

- Future care plans for any dependants

Some of the above issues may need to be addressed through legal documents such as wills, lasting power of attorney and advance decisions to refuse treatment, while for others it is sufficient to record the individuals preferences and make sure people are aware that this record is available to refer to when needed.

In summary ACP can take the form of:

1. An advance statement to inform subsequent best interest decisions. This provides a record of the individual's preferences and wishes, beliefs and values about future care. It is not legally binding, but should be taken into account by all those involved in the patient's care if they are unable to participate in making decisions

2. Advance decisions to refuse treatment (ADRT) covers refusal of specified treatment in the event that an individual has lost the mental capacity to make these decisions. It must be written, signed and witnessed by an individual when they have mental capacity to make these decisions and contain a statement that it will apply even if the person's life is at risk. It is **legally binding** if the ADRT is assessed as complying with the Mental Capacity Act, and is both valid and applicable to the particular circumstances at the time

3. Do not attempt cardiopulmonary resuscitation (DNACPR) only covers the decision about withholding cardiopulmonary resuscitation (CPR). It is completed by a clinician with responsibility for the patient. It documents either that CPR cannot be successful and therefore should not be attempted and/or an individual's decision to refuse CPR. It is legally binding if it is included in a patient's ADRT, otherwise it is advisory only. Patient consent is only sought if cardiac arrest is anticipated and CPR might be successful

4. Appointment of a Lasting Power of Attorney (health and welfare and/or property and affairs) (page 345).

Planning for the Future

Most people, even if they have thought about death and dying, have not made any arrangements to ensure that their wishes, and those for their next of kin after their death, are known. People are reluctant to start "putting their house in order" when they are fit and healthy, but there are some key things that people can organise at any point, rather than waiting until they are ill and dying, and therefore less able to organise their affairs.

Writing a will is one of the tasks that people always intend to do at some point, but many never get around to doing. Drawing up a will does not mean that the person is likely to die in the near future, but is a means of ensuring that what a person wants to happen to their money and possessions after they die happens. If someone dies without having made a will, their money and possessions (known as their estate) are allocated to their nearest relatives, according to set rules, and these are not necessarily the same people a person would wish to be their next of kin. It is possible to write a will oneself using the will-writing packs available for purchase in some high street shops, or online, but it is usually advisable to employ a solicitor to check that everything is in order. Once written a will can, and should, be revised and updated at any point when a person's circumstances and or wishes change. Again, it is always advisable to do this with the help of a solicitor to avoid any possibility of a dispute over the contents of the will after death.

Thinking about and **planning one's own funeral** is another task that most people are reluctant to consider until they know they are dying. At this point they may lack the time or energy to put any arrangements in place, and it can be difficult for next of kin to make arrangements for the funeral, when struggling with their own grief and loss. Knowing an individual's preferences with regard to their funeral can make the task of organising it very much easier. A plan, or record of what someone would like, does not need to be complicated, but there are a number of options to consider, e.g. burial or cremation, religious service or humanist ceremony, any preferred music, hymns, prayers or readings, as well as the cost of the funeral. Funerals are expensive, but it is possible to set up a prepaid funeral plan with a funeral director, where the costs are spread over time and paid in advance. This can be done at any time, not just when someone knows they are dying in the near future.

Practicalities after somebody dies

Registering the Death

All deaths in England, Wales and Northern Ireland must be registered with the Registrar of Births, Deaths and Marriages **within five days** of the death, (eight days in Scotland),unless the death has been referred to the coroner. Deaths are registered at the local registry office in the district **where the person died** (not where they lived).

If the cause of death is uncertain, or possibly from an industrial disease, or was unexpected or unnatural, there may be a need for a post mortem before a death certificate giving the cause of death can be issued. A post mortem can be requested by the medical team caring for the person, or by the coroner. Permission is not required if the coroner requests a post mortem, however the deceased person's next of kin needs to give their consent for one requested by the person's medical team. Once a medical certificate is issued, either immediately following the death or after the post mortem, the death can be registered.

Anyone can register a death provided they have the correct documentation and information. The person registering the death needs to give to the Registrar the medical certificate giving the cause of death. They also require the following information:

- The date and place the deceased was born (the person's birth certificate provides this information) and the place they died

- The deceased's full name (including any maiden name) and address

- The deceased's occupation

- The name, date of birth and occupation of their spouse and civil partner

- Whether the deceased was in receipt of a pension or any state benefits

If they are available it is helpful for the Registrar to see the deceased person's:

- Medical card and NHS number

- Birth and marriage, or civil partnership, certificates

Once the death has been formally registered the Registrar issues:

- The death certificate

- The certificate for burial or cremation giving permission for the body to be buried, or for an application for cremation to be made. This certificate needs to be given to the funeral director.

- A certificate of registration of the death, (form BD8 in England and Wales, form 14 in Scotland, or form GR021 in Northern Ireland), to be competed and returned to the local social security office if the deceased was in receipt of any benefits.

It is advisable to **purchase a few copies** of the death certificate at the time of registering the death. The deceased's executor needs some original copies for dealing with the person's will, bank accounts and other organisations that may request an original copy, (i.e. not a photocopy), of the death certificate. It is always possible to obtain further copies from the Registrar at a later date, but most people find it easier, and less time consuming, to request additional copies at the time of registering the death.

The Registrar will also usually give the person registering the death the Department for Work and Pensions (DWP) **booklet DWP1027** entitled "What to do after a death", this contains clear advice on probate and other administrative issues that need to be resolved following a person's death.

Arranging the funeral

A funeral can usually only take place after the death has been registered. The deceased person may have left instructions about their funeral either as part of their will, or separately. If there are no clear wishes the person's executor and/or nearest relative needs to decide what type of funeral will take place, including whether the person is buried or cremated, and whether it will be a religious or nonreligious service.

Most people use a funeral director to help them arrange a funeral. The person organising the funeral with the funeral director is responsible for paying the bill so it is important to check what money is available from the person's estate, or prepaid funeral plan, or insurance policies before making any arrangements. It may be possible to obtain some help with funeral costs by applying for a grant from the Social Fund, but there are strict rules regarding eligibility for assistance and to qualify the person responsible for the funeral must be in receipt of benefits.

If using a funeral director they should be a member of either the National Association of Funeral Directors or the Society of Allied and Independent Funeral Directors (see glossary). Both organisations have codes of practice and members must provide a price list on request, enabling a comparison of costs.

It is possible to organise a funeral without a funeral director by contacting the cemeteries and cremation department of the local council. Some local councils also run their own funeral services and the British Humanist Association (see glossary) will also assist in arranging non-religious funerals.

Organisations to be contacted after a death

As previously identified, the Registrar will give the person registering the death a certificate to be completed and returned to the deceased's local Social Security or Jobs & Benefits office. Most local councils now run a service called **Tell Us Once** and this enables the reporting of a death to most government organisations in one go. The registrar will explain how to use the Tell Us Once service and provide a unique reference number to access the service. Tell Us Once will notify:

- HM Revenue and Customs (HMRC) – to deal with tax and cancel benefits
- Department for Work and Pensions (DWP) – to cancel benefits, e.g. income support
- Driver and Vehicle Licensing Agency – to cancel a driving licence
- Passport Office – to cancel a passport
- The Local Council to cancel housing benefit, a Blue Badge, inform council housing services and remove the person from the electoral register.

Following notification by Tell Us Once, and within 30 days of the death, HMRC send form **R27 to the deceased's executor**. The information on the completed and returned form is used to calculate any tax due. If the deceased was self employed, or paid voluntary National Insurance, the National Insurance Contributions Office needs to be notified within one month of the death. In addition all the deceased's bank, mortgage, pension and insurance providers need to be notified of the death in order to close, or change the details of their accounts.

Dealing with the estate of the deceased

The legal process of distributing the estate of a deceased person is known as probate (or Confirmation in Scotland). If there is a will, the executor identified in the will (which may be the person's next of kin, a nominated person, or a solicitor) needs to apply to the Probate Registry (the local Sheriff Court in Scotland or the Probate Office in Northern Ireland), for a grant of representation.

If there is no will the person is said to have **died intestate**. In these cases the law sets out who should deal with the deceased's affairs and who should inherit their estate (property, personal possessions and money). Anyone administrating the estate needs to understand these rules, or take legal advice, before undertaking this role. Usually a close relative like a spouse, child or parent has the legal right to sort out the estate of the deceased person, but they need to apply to the Probate Registry for a grant of letters of administration. On receipt of the grant the person becomes the "administrator" of the estate. However, if Inheritance Tax is due on the estate some, or all, of this must be paid before a grant of administration is issued.

The grant of representation or administration provide proof to banks, building societies, insurance companies and other organisations that the person has the legal authority to access and distribute funds that are held in the deceased's name.

The **Principal Probate Registry** gives information and advice to anyone dealing with an estate in England and Wales, whether they left a will or died intestate. Alternatively organisations like Age UK may be able to help.

Further reading

National Council for Palliative Care, Dying Matters (2011)

The Commission on the Future of Hospice Care. (Help the Hospices 2013)

The National End of Life Care Programme. (Department of Health 2009)

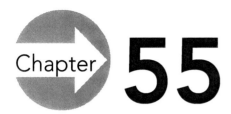

Chapter 55

Bereavement

The older you get the more likely you are of experiencing the death of friends and acquaintances. However, in no way do these events prepare you for the pain that occurs when the death is of someone close to you, such as a parent, child or a partner.

You are not alone in this grief, as evidenced by the large number of authors describing their own traumatic experiences. In many cases writing their book is probably part of their own grieving process.

Bereavement is the period of grief and mourning that you go through when someone close to you dies. **The time taken to accept and adjust to this loss is unpredictable, as are the effects that they will have on you**. There is a great variation in people's response, and whatever time it takes, this is the normal for you. For a small number of people grief may last a very long time and be very intense, stopping you from doing the normal things you need to do. In these circumstances, sometimes referred to as a prolonged grief reaction, it may be helpful to talk to your GP or a bereavement counsellor.

Bereavement and grief is accompanied by a wide range of emotional responses that cannot be predicted. It is important that you do not try to interpret these emotions as reflecting hidden attitudes towards your lost love one. They may well include anger and bitterness, as well as the sadness that you are anticipating. Anger may relate to your being left alone, a sudden death leaving unsaid goodbyes or unfinished business that has been lost to the world. Equally, the experience may leave you numb, withdrawn and depressed, and a worry to those around you.

Studies of bereavement have identified four stages that people go through, although you may not conform to this pattern.

1 **Denial** – it is at first difficult to appreciate and accept the death of someone so close to you – perhaps a loved partner for many decades. You still think it is all a mistake, and that they will just turn up. The shock is likely to leave you emotionally drained and too overwhelmed to contemplate the effect on your future existence. It may take a two or

three months before you can accept that the death has occurred. On occasion you may even think that you can hear or see the person you have lost. This is a normal part of the response to loss and does not mean that you are developing an illness

2 **Intense concern** – the realisation that the death has actually happened brings with it the intense pain of grief. The death and associated pain are constantly on your mind and in your conversation. Although the funeral, wake and other rituals were evidence of your loss, it is only now that you are able to say farewell to your loved one. This mourning is an important part of bereavement and usually lasts for more than six months

3 **Despair and depression** – the gradual realisation and acceptance of a new order brings with it new problems and responsibilities. The emotional turmoil of the previous months, that may have included, pain, sadness and possibly anger or guilt, now give way to a wide range of feelings including loneliness, isolation, anxiety and depression. You are still susceptible to bouts of intense grief, feelings of despair and being unable to cope. Unexpected and unwanted tasks appear, such as sorting out life insurance policies, bank accounts and household tasks. To these may be added the requirements made by different cultures, concerning traditional dress and expected rituals. This stage lasts for at least a year

4 **Recovery** – grief does not go away. However, over time, you gradually find ways to cope, redirecting your energy and emotions into new activities that fill the gap that has been left in your life. The memories that usually persist are the happy ones.

Various attempts have been made to classify the outcome of bereavement; one such classification separates individuals into five groups:

1 **Normalisers** – individuals who return to their previously active state (at least as seen by the outside world)

2 **Memorialists** – who extend their mourning by preserving some form of memorabilia, be this an action, deed or a physical object, that becomes part of their every day life

3 **Nomads** – who lead a secluded existence, never fully resolve, understand or come to terms with what has happened

4 **Activists** – individuals who throw themselves into alternative exploits, often helping others suffering from the disease that the loved one died of

5 **Seekers** – where the alternative activity involves a religious or spiritual pursuit.

Other workers have suggested that individuals fall into one of four types of grief:

1 **Resilience** – those who, at least outwardly, are able to suppress emotional involvement in bereavement, retaining an unaltered stable existence in their lifestyle

2 **Recovery** – those who gradually are able to return to normal activity

3 **Chronic dysfunction** – one who never returns to their previous state of existence, and exhibit prolonged suffering

4 **Delayed grief** – one who initially shows signs of normal recovery, but later is prone to bouts of severe delayed grief.

Knowing that you fall into a specific category may be helpful and reassuring, but most people require time, solace and reassurance that grief gradually fades, and that they can expect, albeit in a number of years, to return to a peaceful existence, and happy memories.

One of the problems for a clinical specialist looking after you during bereavement is differentiating grief from psychological depression. Both conditions lead to personal neglect, malnutrition, insomnia, and loss of the desire to get out of bed in the morning, to go to work or to carry on living. Generally grief comes in bouts and can be temporarily relieved by outside distractions, such as participating in group activities with friends. Depression, however, is a constant state and may have additional symptoms, such as confusion, incoherence of speech, and difficulty in completing mental or physical tasks.

There are no right and wrong ways of expressing grief, but it helps to be able to talk through your emotions. If you do not have a close acquaintance to talk to you should discuss this with your GP. They will be able to advise and, if necessary, put you in contact with a bereavement counsellor. Your loved one may have died in a care home or hospital, and these can also direct you, possibly through their chaplain, to a counsellor: the glossary also has suggestions in this area.

Counsellors are trained to listen, and have the experience to clarify and resolve areas of conflict; they are able to reassure and encourage you through difficult times. It is usually you, rather than the counsellor, that decides your sessions are no longer required. Seeking help from a counsellor is not a personal failure. **It is important to remember that it is normal to go through a period of turmoil following the death of someone close to you**. You are not alone in this experience: the time it takes to overcome these problems varies and whatever this is, it is the normal for you.

 # Glossary of Medical Terms

The descriptions are of commonly encountered terms and conditions.

Abscess – localised collection of pus. The site is added (sometimes with a prefix): subphrenic, subungual, subcutaneous (under the diaphragm, nail, skin); intrahepatic (in the liver), para/perinephric (around the kidney); retrocaecal, retroperitoneal (behind the caecum, peritoneum)

Accommodation – the process of focusing an image onto the retina, through ciliary muscle contraction

Accommodation reflex – changes in the pupil size that occur on changing between distant to near vision

Acquired immunodeficiency disease (AIDS) – viral infection producing a defect in cell-mediated immunity

Acromegaly – clinical syndrome due to increased growth hormone

Acute – sudden onset; also used to define severe and to differentiate an acute inflammatory response to certain bacteria from the chronic inflammatory granuloma produced by others

Adhesions – sticking together of two normally separate parts, e.g. loops of gut, visceral and parietal, pleura and pericardium

Agnosia – inability to interpret a sensation, e.g. visual

Akinesia – paucity of movement

Allergy – body's reaction to foreign material (the substance may not be identified)

Alveoli – terminal air sac in the lungs

Anaemia – reduction of circulating red cells, haemoglobin or packed red cell volume

Anaesthesia – loss of sensation, local or general

Anaphylaxis – acute hypersensitivity to a foreign substance, such as a protein, drug or mismatched transfusion, giving rise to a state of shock

Anatomy – study of body form

Aneurysm – localised dilatation of a blood vessel, usually an artery

Angina – chest pain from myocardial ischaemia

Antibiotics – drugs that kill bacteria

Antibody – a substance produced by the body to neutralise foreign material: as part of the immune response

Antigen – a foreign protein the body attacks by producing antibodies

Aphasia – inability to speak; may be partial, as in nominal (loss of names), jargon (senseless speech)

Apnoea – cessation of breathing

Arrythmia – abnormal heart contraction

Arthritis – inflammation of a joint, usually qualified by the type, e.g. **osteoarthritis** – wear and tear of cartilage covering the articular surface; **rheumatoid arthritis** – a chronic inflammation involving cartilage and soft tissues

Ascites – collection of intra-peritoneal serous fluid

Asthma – respiratory disease, with spasm and infection of the bronchi; usually starting in childhood

Ataxia – loss of control of voluntary movement

Atheroma/atheromatous/arteriosclerosis – arterial occlusive disease

Atrophy – wasting of a tissue, as in malnutrition or muscle denervation

Audiometry – test of hearing

Bacteriology – study of bacteria

Benign – nonmalignant tumour; a disease with mild characteristics or a good prognosis

BMI – body mass index: a measure of body fat, calculated from height and weight

Bronchiectasis – bronchial dilatation with infection

Bronchitis – inflammation of bronchial mucosa

Bruising – bleeding into tissues

Cachexia – extreme general state of ill-health, with malnutrition, wasting, anaemia and muscle weakness

Calculus – an abnormal concretion, usually of inorganic matter; occurring in reservoir organs and ducts

Carbohydrate – a generic name for sugar containing foodstuff, also used as **carbs** to define the amount of energy provided by a food

Carcinoma – malignant epithelial tumour, characterised by invasion and metastasis

Caries – tooth decay

Catalyst – a substance that promotes a chemical reaction without itself being changed

Cataract – opacity of the lens and/or its capsule

Cholecystitis – inflammation of the gall bladder

Cholesterol – one of the varieties of fat

Chronic – persistent, e.g. pain, discharge or infection. In the latter, the term has a specific pathological meaning, with production of a granuloma

Cirrhosis – chronic perilobular fibrosis of the connective tissue of the liver

Clubbing – digital disorder, usually of the fingers, characterised by longitudinal and lateral curving of the nails, and bulbous endings: occurring in a number of conditions, including congenital cardiac, chronic pulmonary and inflammatory bowel disease

Colic – painful powerful contractions of a muscular tube, usually due to obstruction of the intestine, ureter or biliary tree

Coma – unrousable state of consciousness

Conjunctivitis – inflammation of the conjunctiva

COPD – chronic obstructive pulmonary disease, incorporating both bronchitis and emphysema

Coronary – pertaining to the heart, e.g. coronary artery; also used to denote a heart attack

Crepitus – abnormal noise or palpable feeling on moving abnormal tissues, as with a fractured bone, osteoarthritic joints, inflamed tendons or gas in tissues

CT – computed tomography: X ray technique for demonstrating body parts

Cushing's disease – clinical syndrome due to hypersecretion of adrenal cortical hormones, in response to a local abnormality, an extrinsic stimulus, or from an ectopic site

Cyanosis – blue discolouration of the skin and mucous membranes due to an abnormal amount of reduced haemoglobin, usually due to pulmonary or cardiac disease

Cyst – retained collection of fluid, from a variety of sources, e.g. exocrine and endocrine glands, congenital rests (dermoid, hypoglossal), degenerative, e.g. pancreatitis and parasitic (hydatid)

Dehydration – reduced body fluid due to low intake or loss

Diabetes mellitus – clinical syndrome due to the lack of, or of an abnormal response to, insulin

Diarrhoea – increased frequency and/or quantity, and looseness of stool

Diplopia – double vision

Discharge – leaking of fluid from the body through a normal (e.g. nose or anus) or an abnormal opening (e.g. an ulcer or fistula)

Dislocation – loss of the normal proximity of structures, usually the bones of a joint

Diverticulum – pouch or cul-de-sac on a hollow organ or duct

DNA – a molecule that carries the body's genetic instructions for development and function

Dossett box – container for dispensing pills in an organised way

DVT – deep vein thrombosis

Dysfunction – general term for impaired activity of an organ or part

Dyspepsia – general term covering symptoms from the upper alimentary tract

Dysphagia – difficulty or pain on swallowing

Dysphasia – difficulty in speaking

Dyspnoea – difficulty or discomfort in breathing when lying flat, as in bed, usually secondary to left heart failure

Dysuria – pain or difficulty in passing urine

ECG – a machine that records the electrical activity of the heart

Effusion – fluid collection, such as in a joint or pleural cavity

Electrocardiogram (ECG) – a record of the electrical activity of heart muscle

Embolism – sudden blocking of a blood vessel, usually an artery, by thrombosis, clumps of bacteria or other foreign marerial transported in the circulation

Emphysema – dilatation of pulmonary alveoli

Empyema – pus in the pleural cavity

Encephalitis – inflammation of the brain

Endocrine gland – one of a system of glands that regulate body function

Enzyme – a biological catalyst

Epilepsy – cerebral disorder producing excessive and disordered discharge of cerebral neurons, resulting in paroxysmal recurrent movements, often with tongue biting and urinary incontinence, and usually accompanied by unconsciousness – the **epileptic fit**

Exophthalmos – prominence or protrusion of the eyeball

Failure – end stage loss of function of an organ, e.g. cardiac, pulmonary, hepatic or renal failure

Fibrillation – spontaneous independent contraction of the auricular or ventricular muscle; spontaneous contraction of recently denervated skeletal muscle

Fibroid – resembling fibrous tissue; smooth muscle tumour (fibroma) commonly of the uterus

Fissure – deep groove, may be normal, e.g. in the brain, but may be a breach of a normal lining, e.g. the longitudinal ulcer of an **anal fissure**

Fistula – an abnormal connection between epithelial/endothelial surfaces, e.g. anal (from anal canal to external skin), between two loops of gut or arteriovenous

Fit – see epilepsy

Fracture – discontinuity of a structure usually a broken bone

Fructose – a simple sugar

Gallstone – concretion within the biliary tree

Gangrene – death and anaerobic putrefaction of ischaemic tissue

Gastroenteritis – inflammation of the stomach and intestine

Glasgow coma scale (GCS) – system of assessing cerebral damage

Glaucoma – increased intraocular pressure

Glucose – the simplest form of sugar (carbohydrate)

Glycogen – a form of sugar stored in the liver and muscle as an energy source

Goitre – enlargement of the thyroid gland

GP – general practitioner

Haemarthrosis – bloody joint effusion

Haematoma – discreet collection of blood in the body following a bleed

Haematuria – blood in the urine

Haemoglobin – a protein in the red blood cell that transports oxygen

Haemoglobinopathy – abnormal haemoglobin

Haemolysis – release of haemoglobin from damaged red cells

Haemoptysis – coughing of bright red blood from the lungs, bronchi and trachea

Haemorrhage – bleeding; the escape of blood from any part of the vascular system

Haemorrhoid (pile) – swelling at the anal margin

Haemothorax – collection of blood in the pleural cavity

Hemiplegia – paralysis of one side of the body

Hepatitis – inflammation of the liver

Hernia – protrusion of the contents of a cavity through its wall

Hormone – substance secreted by an endocrine gland

Hydrocele – circumscribed collection of fluid around the testis

Hyper/hypo – abnormal increase/low level (e.g. measures of cholesterol, sodium, calcium, glucose)

Hypertension – high arterial blood pressure usually in the systemic circulation. It may also be in the pulmonary arteries, secondary to lung disease, and in the portal venous system, due to liver disease

Hypertrophy – an increase in the size of the cells of a tissue; **ventricular hypertrophy** – enlargement of heart muscle

Hypoglycaemia – low blood sugar concentration

Hypokalaemia – low body potassium

Hypothyroidism – clinical syndrome, due to thyroid hormone insufficiency

Iatrogenic – disorder produced by therapy

Idiopathic – disease of unknown cause

Immune response – the body's reaction against harmful foreign material and organisms, such as bacteria

Impaction – forceful driving of one structure into another, such as broken bones, a maldirected tooth or faeces into a poorly evacuating rectum

Impotence – inability to perform the sexual act

Infarct – area of dead tissue, with or without haemorrhage, produced by obstruction of an end-artery

Infection – invasion of the body by pathogenic organisms, and their subsequent multiplication

Inflammation – body's response to cellular damage, whether this be physical or chemical injury, bacterial invasion or other disease

Intermittent claudication – skeletal muscle pain on exercise, due to inadequate blood supply

Intracranial pressure – pressure within the skull

Ipsilateral – occurring on the same side of the body

Ischaemia – insufficient blood supply to a part to sustain its normal function

Jaundice – clinical syndrome of excessive circulating bile pigments, giving rise to yellow discolouration of the sclera, skin and mucous membranes

Ketosis – excessive ketones within the body

Kyphosis – spinal curvature in which the concavity of the curve is in a forward direction, generally seen in the thoracic region

Lesion – nonspecific term for a pathological abnormality

Leukaemia – disease of the white blood cells

Lordosis – spinal curvature in which the convexity of the curve is in a forward direction, generally found in the lumbar region

Lymph – tissue fluid that is collected in a fine network of lymph vessels and returned to the blood stream

Lymphoedema – excess tissue fluid, due to failure of lymphatic drainage

Malignant – life threatening pathological process, usually characterised by invasion and metastases

Mammography – soft tissue radiographic technique for examining the breasts

Menarche – onset of the menses

Menopause – cessation of the menses

Metastasis – spread of malignant disease from its primary site to distant parts of the body, by way of natural passages, blood vessels, lymphatics or by direct continuity.

MI (myocardial infarction) – death of a segment of heart muscle due to ischaemia

Motor neurone disease – progressive degeneration of motor neurons

MRI – magnetic resonance imageing: medical imageing technique for demonstrating parts of the body

Multiple sclerosis – demyelinating disease of the brain and spinal cord

Myocardial infarct (MI) – death of a segment of heart muscle due to ischaemia

Myxoedema – a clinical syndrome, due to reduced thyroid hormone production

Nausea – feeling of sickness with the desire to vomit

Neoplasia – generic term for a new growth, whether benign or malignant

Neuropathy – altered neuronal function

Nocturia – getting up at night to pass urine

NSAID – nonsteroidal anti-inflammatory drugs

Oedema – excess of tissue fluid

Organ – a functioning body unit made up of cells and tissues

Orthopnoea – breathlessness on lying flat

Orthosis – mechanical aid

Osteomalacia – decalcification of the bones

Osteoarthritis – degenerative joint disease associated with wear, tear and ageing

Osteoporosis – rarefaction of bone

Palpitations – awareness of the heartbeat, often because of increased force, rate or irregularity

Pancreatitis – inflammation of the pancreas

Paralysis – weakness of neural or neuromuscular origin

Parkinson's disease – chronic neurological disease producing muscle weakness, rigidity and tremor (**parkinsonism**)

Pathology – study of disease

Photophobia – aversion to light

Pile – see haemorrhoid

Plasma proteins – the proteins in the fluid part of the blood

Pleura – membrane covering the lung and the inside of the chest wall

Pleural effusion – fluid collection in the chest cavity

Pleurisy – inflammation of the pleura

Pneumonia – inflammation of the lung

Pneumothorax – gas within the pleural cavity

Presbycusis – age related deafness

Prolapse – bulging of a lax wall, e.g. vagina into the rectum, or of cardiac valves, e.g. mitral valve

Proteins – a food product; also a body constituent

Pulmonary – pertaining to the lungs

Pulmonary effusion – fluid in the pleural cavity

Pulmonary embolus – thrombus carried by the blood stream into the lungs, usually from the legs

Pulmonary oedema – fluid in the alveoli

Pulsatile – beating with the pulse (see also expansile)

Pyrexia – raised temperature

Ramsay Hunt syndrome – herpes zoster infection of the geniculate ganglion of the seventh cranial nerve

Rash – cutaneous eruption

Reflux – back flow, e.g. through an incompetent gastro-oesophageal junction, or through valve-less lower limb veins

Regurgitation – reversal of flow, as with swallowed food into the mouth

Respiration – the process of breathing in oxygen and blowing off carbon dioxide; also the process by which oxygen is converted into energy at a cellular level

Resuscitation – restoration of life or consciousness, in the apparently dead or collapsed patient

Retention – retaining substances in the body that are normally excreted

Rheumatism – nonspecific term applied to pain of musculoskeletal origin

RNA – a cellar molecule replicated from DNA that carries out body functions

Sciatica – leg pain due to pressure on a spinal nerve

Scoliosis – lateral curvature of the spine

Secondary – see matastasis

Sickle cell – hereditary abnormality of haemoglobin

Spasm – sudden, powerful, involuntary contraction of muscle

Spasticity – persistent muscle contraction, producing stiffness and rigidity, or loss of controlled movement, usually following an upper motor neuron lesion

Splenomegaly – enlarged spleen

Sputum – material expelled from the respiratory passages by coughing or clearing the throat

Starch – a complex sugar (carbohydrate) obtained from plants, where it is used to store glucose

Stoma – opening, such as a colostomy on the abdominal wall

Strangulated hernia – gut ischaemia due to constriction of the lumen and blood vessels at the neck of a hernial sac

Stroke – sudden paralsis, due to cerebral damage; **stroke volume** – blood ejected by a contraction of the left ventricle

Sucrose – a simple sugar

Tachycardia – rapid beating of the heart

Thalassemia – hereditary anaemia, due to a haemoglobin abnormality

Thrombosis – intravascular coagulation

Thrombus – blood clot in a vessel

Thyrotoxicosis – clinical syndrome, due to an overactive thyroid gland

Tinnitus – subjective noise in the ear

Tone – tension in normal muscle; altered by neuromuscular disorders

Trachea – the windpipe

Tracheostomy – opening in the trachea, usually to relieve an obstructed airway

Tremor – rhythmic, involuntary, purposeless, oscillating movement, resulting from the alternate contraction and relaxation of opposing muscle groups

Tumour – swelling

Ulcer/ulceration – discontinuity of epithelium

Varicose veins – dilated thin tortuous superficial veins, usually of the lower limbs

Vasodilatation – widening of a blood vessel

Vasoconstriction – narrowing of a blood vessel

Vertigo – giddiness, a sense of instability, often with a sense of rotation

Virology – study of viruses

Vomiting – oral evacuation of gastric contents

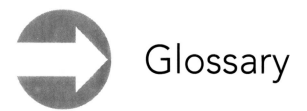# Glossary

This glossary directs you to valuable websites, supplementing (and where appropriate duplicating) those already included in the relevant chapters

www.abilitynet.org.uk - help for disabled people using the Internet

www.affordablewarmthgrants.co.uk - government scheme for people in need: supporting energy saving initiatives

www.ageuk.org.uk - the major UK charity for the aged

www.ageofcreativity.co.uk - inspiring art for the older age

www.alcoholics-anonymous.org.uk - fellowship of men and women who share their experience to help individuals stop drinking

www.alzheimers.org.uk - Alzheimer Society: leading the fight against dementia

www.bbc.co.uk/webwise - BBCguide to the web

www.bhf.org.uk - British Heart Foundation

www.campaignetoendloneliness.org - addressing loneliness in older age thoughout the UK

www.cancerresearchuk.org - cancer research

www.carers.org - carers trust: making carers count

www.carersuk.org - helping carers and their family

www.cccs.co.uk - free expert advice on problems of debt and their solution

www.citizensadvice.org.uk - provides free, independent and confidential help on legal, money and related problems

www.communitydance.org.uk - creating oportunity for people to experience and participate in dance www.communityhowto.com - suggestions for community web tools

www.crusebereavementcare.org.uk - provides support, advice and information to anyone affected by bereavement

www.csv.org.uk - UK voluntary and learning charity: activities include befriending and other help for the elderly

www.diabetes.co.uk - education and research into diabetes

www.digitalunite.com - helping the online digital community

www.dyingmatters.org - raisng awareness of dying, death and bereavement

www.facbook.com - social media site

www.facetime.org.uk - online free video communication link for apple-mac users

www.go-on.co.uk - promoting digital skills

www.gov.uk - UK Government site

www.gov.uk/browse/benefits - UK government site

www.gov.uk/carers-allowance - UK Government site

www.gov.uk/place-retirement-income - UK Government site

www.gov.uk/power-of-attorney - UK Government site

www.helpthehospices.org.uk - hospice consortium for education and training

www.homesandcommunities.co.uk/housing-ageing-population... Cached - panel recommendation on housing needs for older people

www.hpc-uk.org - Health and Care Professions Council: regulating health care workers

www.humanism.org.uk - British Humanist Association

www.independentage.org - online and telephone advice and fact sheets on many questions on ageing

www.justice.gov.uk/about/opg - Office of the Public Guardian: Ministry of Justice

www.linkedin.com - social media site

www.macmillan.org.uk - cancer support, including resourcing health and social care workers

www.mariecurie.org.uk - provides cancer care through nurses and hospices

www.myageingparent.com - providing elderly care advice

www.nafd.org.uk- National Association of Funeral Directors

www.naturaldeath.org.uk- independent funeral advice

www.ncpc.org.ukNational Council for Palliative Care

www.nhs.uk/carersdirect - NHS support, and advice on social care

www.patient.co.uk - patient information site

www.publicguardian.gov.uk - Office of the Public Guardian

www.pensionsadvisoryservice.org.uk- independent advisory service on pensions

www.ramblers.org.uk- advising on walking for health and with disability

www.saif.org.uk - National Society of Alied and Independent Funeral Directors

www.scpod.org - Society of Chiropodists and Podiatrists

www.skype.com - online free video communication link

www.ukonlinecentres.com - supporting communities through digital technology and training

www.unbiased.co.uk - independent financial advice

www.u3a.org.uk - University of the Third Age: etensive network of activity for the elderly

 www.walkingforhealth.org.uk - supporting activity and listing walks in your locality

www.webopedia.com - concise definition of Internet terms

Index